ATLAS OF OTOLOGIC SURGERY AND MAGIC OTOLOGY

Volume 1

System requirement:
- **Windows XP or above**
- **Power DVD player (Software)**
- **Windows media player 11.0 version or above (Software)**

Accompanying DVD ROM is playable only in Computer and not in DVD player.

Kindly wait for few seconds for DVD ROM to autorun. If it does not autorun then please do the following:
- Click on my computer
- Click the **CD/DVD drive** and after opening the drive, kindly double click the file **Jaypee**

DVD Contents

ATLAS OF OTOLOGIC SURGERY AND MAGIC OTOLOGY

The International Team Approach Based on Pathogenesis

Volume 1

Editor

MARCOS V GOYCOOLEA MD, MS, PhD

and Friends.

Series Editor

CHRIS DE SOUZA MS, DORL, DNB, FACS

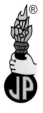

JAYPEE BROTHERS MEDICAL PUBLISHERS (P) LTD

New Delhi • Panama City • London

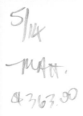

 :: **Jaypee Brothers Medical Publishers (P) Ltd.**

Headquarter
Jaypee Brothers Medical Publishers (P) Ltd
4838/24, Ansari Road, Daryaganj
New Delhi 110 002, India
Phone: +91-11-43574357
Fax: +91-11-43574314
Email: jaypee@jaypeebrothers.com

Overseas Offices
J.P. Medical Ltd.
83 Victoria Street, London
SW1H 0HW (UK)
Phone: +44-2031708910
Fax: +02-03-0086180
Email: info@jpmedpub.com

Jaypee-Highlights Medical Publishers Inc.
City of Knowledge, Bld. 237, Clayton
Panama City, Panama
Phone: 507-317-0160
Fax: +50-73-010499
Email: cservice@jphmedical.com

Website: www.jaypeebrothers.com
Website: www.jaypeedigital.com

© 2012, Jaypee Brothers Medical Publishers

Atlas of Otologic Surgery and Magic Otology (Volume 1)

First Edition: **2012**

ISBN 978-93-5025-519-3

Printed at: Ajanta Offset & Packagings Ltd., New Delhi

Dedicated to...

This book is dedicated to those who believe in friendship, magic and harmony.

There are moments in the lives of people and teams in which magic happens. When this occurs, the groups emerge way above average and all the members become one and one becomes all. These are moments in which friendship, honor, loyalty and happiness prevail, and there are ideals and purposes. These group feelings of invincibility and eternity necessarily result in great success.

Through generations people dream of having these moments, which have been exemplified by Camelot and the Knights of the Round Table; by The Three Musketeers, and in our days by the Jedis who fought and defeated the Evil Empire.

These moments may last for a period of time, but in the hearts and spirit of the participants they last forever, and while those privileged individuals who have lived them may at some time part, wherever they might be, a bond remains, that will last a lifetime.

I have been privileged to have lived these moments at Home, at School, and then at the Department of Otolaryngology in Minneapolis Minnesota, where I did my ENT training. We were and we are a group that can make magic happen and I want to believe that I have also done my part and that part of the shining glare provides from my own magic wand.

I want to dedicate this book to our group and to add a special thanks to three master jedis, who in their own character and style have contributed to strengthen my "otologic force within"—

Anna-Mary Carpenter; Steven K Juhn and Michael M Paparella.

ANNA-MARY CARPENTER MS, PhD, MD

January 14, 1916–February 4, 2003

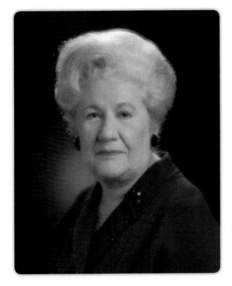

Professor Carpenter ("Anna-Mary") was born in Ambridge, Pennsylvania. She received her BA from Geneva College in Beaver Falls, Pa, in 1936; an MS in 1937 and PhD in 1940 from the University of Pittsburgh. She received her MD from the University of Minnesota in 1958 and joined the Anatomy Department at the University of Minnesota, where she became Full Professor in 1963 and remained in that position until 1982, becoming then Professor Emeritus.

In spite of all her degrees, scientific deeds and international recognition (innovations in diabetes, quantitative morphology, and being first to "section" a pancreas using computer stimulation), her greatest achievements came from her teachings of her discipline. She trained several generations of graduate students (including myself), postdoctoral fellows, and over 5,000 medical students. Her extraordinary teaching ability and capacity were the result of her profound knowledge and understanding of morphology. Her personal interest and dedication to all of her students gained her the legendary nickname "Ma Carpenter." Anna-Mary represented an exceptional breed of true scholar and scientist. As one of her students and with the conviction of representing all of them, I want to assure that those scientific and university values taught for over 50 years are alive and very strong in all of us, that her teachings will persist for generations, and that she will live forever in our hearts.

STEVEN K JUHN MD, MS, Dr Med

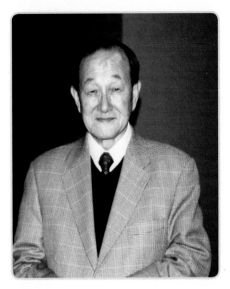

Professor, Director of Biochemistry Laboratory, Department of Otolaryngology, Adjunct Professor, Department of Neuroscience, University of Minnesota.

Dr Juhn ("Steve") was born in Daegu in the south-eastern part of Korea. His father was an otolaryngologist. He received his MD degree at Kyung-Pook University (KPU) School of Medicine, Daegu, in 1957, and an MS (Biochemistry) at Seoul National University (SNU) College of Medicine in 1961. In 1963, while working as a research assistant and instructor of biochemistry at SNU and KPU, he won an International Atomic Energy Agency fellowship and went as a postdoctoral fellow to the University of Bologna.

The following year, he was appointed as a research fellow at the University of Hamburg. In 1966, he started working as a research associate in the Inner Ear Research Laboratory under Professor S Rauch at the University of Düsseldorf, where he completed his doctoral thesis in biochemistry of the inner ear.

In 1967, Michael M Paparella became Professor and Chairman of the Department of Otolaryngology at the University of Minnesota and was looking for the right person to establish an auditory biochemistry laboratory and develop the graduate program for residents in otolaryngology. His longtime friend, Dr David Lim did one more of the many good things he has done for Otolaryngology when he recommended that Michael should incorporate Steve Juhn to the Minnesota team. Steve accepted and since that time, he has devoted himself to research and teaching at the University of Minnesota.

It is not easy to summarize Steve´s vast contributions in both middle and inner ear research. He has authored more than 230 publications and 10 book chapters. He has been a pioneer in the study of biochemical events taking place in the pathogenesis of otitis media, in middle and inner ear interaction as well as in inner ear physiology and physiopathology.

While his scientific merits are vast and internationally known and recognized, Steve´s additional activities have resulted in great achievements in other aspects that are as much if not more transcendent than the above mentioned. In 1988, he helped establish the faculty and student exchange program between the University of Minnesota and the Karolinska Institute in Sweden. The idea for this program stemmed from a conversation between Dr Juhn and former Minnesota Governor, Wendell Anderson in the streets of Stockholm during a casual encounter, while both were just walking around in the evening (both were in Stockholm for totally different activities) and Steve recognized the Governor and started talking to him. In addition to the scientific exchange, this resulted in close ties and friendships with the Swedish otolaryngologists that persist until today. Moreover, in 1993, Steve also participated in the development of the Biomedical Research Center at the Korea Institute of Science and Technology (KIST) in Seoul, Korea, where he served as the first director.

He has published two nonscience books in Korean entitled, "Dreaming Traveler" in 1996 and "Mississippi Minnesota-Dream and Hope of a Sojourner" in 2007. These books contain essays and poems crystallizing his thoughts and wisdom from daily life, and are not only entertaining with quiet humors, but also full of educational and heartwarming true stories. Behind his many accomplishments is the unfailing, dedicated support of his wife, Jane. They have three sons, Peter, Martin and Paul and four grandchildren.

Steve has made an outstanding impact as a teacher in the full sense of the word. In addition of orienting and helping through the years, all the residents of the Department in their laboratory rotations; under his direct supervision, 28 otolaryngology residents finished research projects, some with masters, others with doctoral degrees. He also supervised and helped 25 international research fellows and had many students doing research in his laboratory. Many of his former fellows became professors, chairs and leaders in their fields.

Above all, his sincere Christian concern for other people, his optimistic attitude towards life and his wisdom made a positive influence to many students and colleagues alike and contributed to change their lives for the better. Without Steve, the Department would have never reached the levels of excellence that it achieved since pure science is not enough. Wisdom, love, sense of humor and friendship are essential ingredients for success and Steve was one of the main sources of these magic ingredients for our Department.

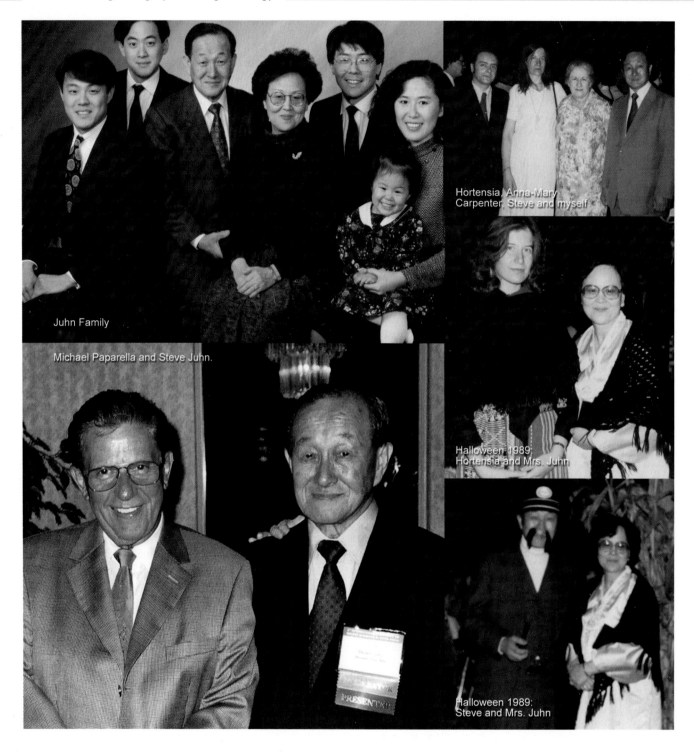

Juhn Family

Michael Paparella and Steve Juhn.

Hortensia, Anna-Mary Carpenter, Steve and myself

Halloween 1989: Hortensia and Mrs. Juhn

Halloween 1989: Steve and Mrs. Juhn

MICHAEL M PAPARELLA MD

Michael was born in Detroit, Michigan on February 13, 1933

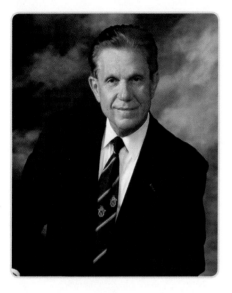

He received his MD degree at the University of Michigan (Ann Arbor) in 1957, and completed his residency in Otolaryngology at Henry Ford Hospital, Detroit, Michigan, United States in 1961. During his residency he started doing animal experiments in a small house that was adjacent to the Hospital (I visited it) and started developing his passion for understanding the mechanisms of disease. Once he finished his residency, he was sent (Military Service) as Chief of Ear, Nose and Throat to the US Army Hospital at Nuremberg, Germany.

In 1963, he came back as a staff member at the Massachusetts Eye and Ear Infirmary and Harvard Medical School. In 1964, he was offered the position as Director of the Otological Research Laboratory, Ohio State University College of Medicine in Columbus Ohio and Staff Member of the Department of Otolaryngology. He remained in this position until January 1967 when—being 33 years old—he became Professor and Chairman of the Department of Otolaryngology, University of Minnesota Medical School, Minneapolis, Minnesota. He held this position until retirement as Emeritus Professor, and founded the Minnesota Ear, Head and Neck Clinic (today the Paparella Ear Clinic after being pressured to change the name by his former students and colleagues) and the Hearing Research Foundation, remaining as Director of the Otopathology laboratory which he founded and is world renowned.

Describing his sites of training and positions has been easy, however, summarizing Michael´s scientific and academic achievements would be quite complex and would require a book. To put it in brief, Michael is a world legend in Otolaryngology and it would be simpler to summarize Michael Jackson´s musical achievements. Michael has been awarded practically all the honors that can be awarded to a specialist, has won all the Grants that somebody would like to have and belongs and has belonged to all the Otolaryngology Societies, Specialty Committees, Boards, Editorial Boards, etc. that are worth belonging to. His papers are in hundreds and so are his chapters and books, including the classic textbook of our specialty—"Otolaryngology" with its three editions. His contributions to the field include major concepts in otitis media pathogenesis and treatment, including silent otitis media, sensorineural hearing loss and otitis media, labyrinthitis ossificans pathogenesis, the concepts of POM, SOM, COM, ROM, design of PE tubes (Paparella PE tubes), surgical procedures such as flexible approach, IBM, sac surgery, and many others that are known by everybody in our field.

However, while his scientific achievements are self evident and respected all over the world, there are important aspects about him that have to be mentioned because they are not that known, since, believe it or not, Michael is a shy man when it comes to describing his deeds.

Michael has two sons from his first marriage (his wife died), Mark and Steve, and one adopted daughter (Lisa). Michael is above all a great father, friend and leader and a wonderful human being. From the very beginning he organized a Department oriented to research and to the study of pathology and pathogenesis. In the process he brought together people from all areas and created an environment of creativity and friendship that gradually developed into a group full of spirit and mystique on its way to glory. In addition, he opened his Department and lab to the world and his Department became a United Nations, not of pompous Professors with impressive language, but instead of natural and spontaneous friendly people. In this environment we all learned from each other and received inputs from people of different cultures and backgrounds, at the same time that we were enjoying life and having fun. Naturally, from this group and this environment came the largest numbers of papers and emerged

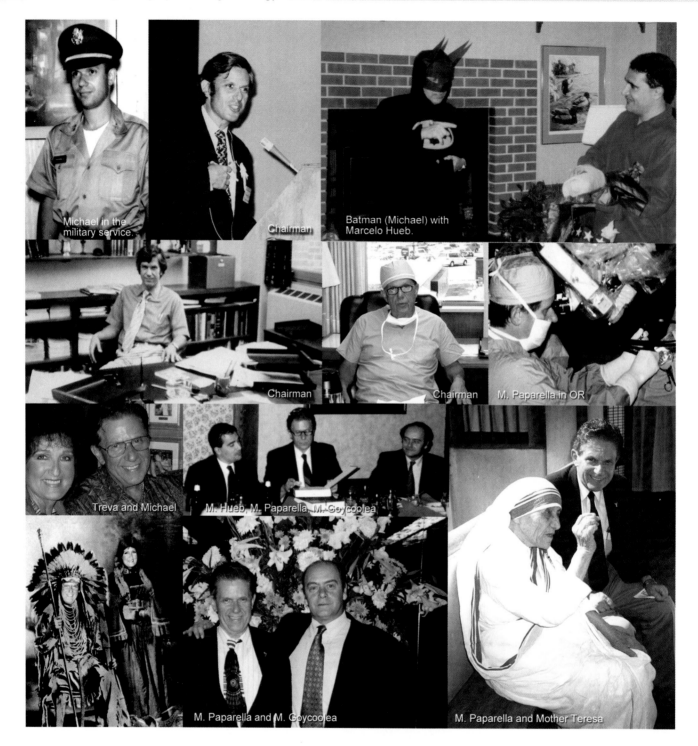

Michael in the military service.

Chairman

Batman (Michael) with Marcelo Hueb.

Chairman

Chairman

M. Paparella in OR

Treva and Michael

M. Hueb, M. Paparella, M. Goycoolea

M. Paparella and M. Goycoolea

M. Paparella and Mother Teresa

the largest amount of Chairmen than in any Department of the world at the time, and the largest number of members from a single Department at the Collegium which is in my opinion one of the... if not the... most prestigious otolaryngology society in the world. More important than this were the human bonds that developed that linked all of us forever, bonds that will be described in the last chapter of the book. I mentioned earlier that Steve Juhn was one of the most important sources of magic ingredients for the formula of success of the Department. Well... the other source has been and is Treva Paparella, his wonderful companion through the years and the heart and soul of the group. Without Treva nothing of this would have happened either.

Michael, Treva, Steve and Anna-Mary

It has been an honor and a privilege to have met you. You have been and are an important part of our lives and in some way, you have become part of us. Many of the authors are former residents and fellows, and many others are also your friends and we are sure that they share our feelings and our sincere appreciation for you.

Marcos V Goycoolea

Motto

"Learn to learn from everything you do and everybody around you."
Marcos Goycoolea, 1989

"Research is at the same time an art, a feeling, a vision, a dream and a passion."
Marcos Goycoolea, 2007

"Plain beauty might be in the mind of the beholder; however, the beauty of harmony, function and of proportion is in the neuronal circuits of everybody."
Marcos Goycoolea, 2010

Key Concepts

Anatomy, Function, Pathogenesis, Research,
Open mind, Common sense, Dedication, Integrity, Decency,
Honesty, Loyalty, Purpose

This book is written for otolaryngologists at all levels including residents. It is our aim to make it a dialogue with you beginning with the preface itself. We want to cast a spell with it so that this book means something to you, and hopefully makes a difference in the way you see and practice otology.

The origin of this book goes back to my first year of residency in Otolaryngology. Although many good texts were available, I felt that I needed a book that went back to basics in clear and understandable language, and that would provide me with the essential concepts from which to start. It seemed to me that a complicated organ such as the ear could be made, at least at that stage, a little simpler (not simple). Over time I thought of different aspects that I felt to be important and useful for this purpose, and I asked different contributors to do the same. Accordingly, we have tried to create a book that emphasizes the basics, rather than one that shows our methods. In this same spirit, this book has different authors who have different approaches for the same aims and purposes.

In the same context, this atlas is only intended to complement other texts on the subject. Because this is primarily a conceptual atlas, we have made no attempt to provide detailed discussions of evaluations and indications; such discussions are provided by the works cited in the list of selected references. Because of the extent of these subjects, the works available number in the thousands; we apologize and request the understanding of those authors whose important publications are not cited. This is not because we want to ignore their contributions and pretend to make them our own, but because of lack of space. We are aware that this edition will need improvements. It is our hope that these will come from your criticisms and suggestions.

This book has a number of thoughts and general philosophies that I believe are useful. I do not expect you to agree with them, but to be exposed to them and think. Some of them will make sense, some will not. I hope that some of the latter will make sense to you in time.

Otologic surgery, like medicine and life itself, is a never-ending learning process. Moreover, otology in particular, is a very humbling specialty because unwanted results and recurrences do happen. Those otologists who do not have them, most probably have their patients consulting somebody else. You are never too good to learn from everybody else. Seeking advice is not a sign of weakness but of maturity. Learn to use your senses; observe and listen to other surgeons and specialists, the operating team, your patients, and others. Learn positively from those who want to help you and from those who want to harm or use you. Learn to learn from everything you do and everybody around you.

A few words on the edition of a previous atlas in 1989 by WB Saunders Company in Philadelphia. The medical illustrator was Gwenn Afton. At the time she was finishing an MS program in Medical Illustration at the Medical College of Georgia. She needed a thesis and the Atlas was just what she needed. Fortunately for her and me, she was just what I needed. I had the privilege of writing the temporal bone dissection manual that she illustrated as her master's thesis. In spite of her being by far the youngest member of the team, her professionalism, dedication, interest, and talents were those that I would have expected from an experienced and famed medical illustrator. I worked directly with her on each and every drawing (in all chapters) in the atlas. Her efforts gave fruit, since these drawings gained her the national USA medical illustration award that same year. We have been asked to lend many of the illustrations (only those designed by Gwenn and me) to Michael Paparella for the otology volume of his text and I have used these drawings in different publications. In 1995, I contacted Saunders Company regarding a new edition of the atlas, but at the time they were already involved in other books, and gave me back the original drawings and pictures as well as a release letter. I had told my friend and former fellow Chris de Souza about my intentions of writing a new Atlas and last year he not only came up full of ideas and enthusiasm, as he usually does, but he brought along the interest and expertise of Jaypee Brothers Medical Publishers as well. In addition, they informed me that the publication was going to be in English, Spanish and Chinese. This seemed to me like a good idea and I accepted, with the understanding that the drawings and pictures remain my property and the drawings of the different chapters would remain as property of the authors. At that point I contacted the different contributors and I must say with positive emotion, that they responded positively. Due to the complexity of putting everything together properly, I convinced Celeste Valencia to be our coordinator and general organizer and Dr Gloria Ribalta (with whom I have worked for over 15 years at our ENT Department in Clínica las Condes) to be a co-editor, particularly of the video section. Their work, the contributions of my friends and my modifications to the original book resulted in this new edition of this atlas which I hope you like as much as I do. The opinions in this preface, as well as the selection of the dedication, key concepts, motto and surgical comments in the atlas, are my own, and do not necessarily represent the opinions and choices of the contributors to this atlas.

Marcos V Goycoolea

Contributors

Nicolás Albertz
Surgeon
University of Chile
Master of Public Health
Universidad de Chile, Chile

Matti Anniko MD, PhD
Chief Editor
Acta-Oto-Laryngologica
Professor and Head
Department of Otolaryngology
Head and Neck Surgery
University Hospital
Uppsala, Sweden

Santiago Alberto Arauz MD
Chief Resident
Arauz Foundation
Buenos Aires, Argentina

Santiago Luis Arauz MD
President
Oto-Rhino-Laryngology Institute
Faculty of Medicine Universidad de Buenos
Aires
Professor
Graduate School Medical Association of
Argentina
Co-Director
Otolaryngology Specialty Course
Faculty of Medicine
Universidad de Buenos Aires, Argentina

Miguel Arístegui
Associate Professor of ENT
Department of Otolaryngology
Hospital Universitario Gregorio Marañón
Madrid, Spain

Bernard Ars MD, PhD
Professor of Otolaryngology
Bruxelles, Belgium

Marcus D Atlas MD, MBBS, FRACS
Professor of Otolaryngology
University of Western Australia
Director of Ear Science Institute of Australia
Australia

Manuel Tomás Barberán MD
Professor of Otolaryngology
Hospital Universitario Son Espases
Palma de Mallorca, Spain

Ricardo Bento MD
Professor and Chairman
Department of Otorhinolaryngology
University of Sao Paulo, Brazil

Manuel Bernal-Sprekelsen MD, PhD
Head of ENT Dept
Hospital Clinic, Barcelona, Spain
Tenure Professor for Otorhinolaryngology
University of Barcelona, Spain
Privat-Dozent for Otorhinolaryngology
Ruhr-University, Bochum, Germany

Hormy Biavatti MD, MSc
Master's degree in Otolaryngology from
Universidade Federal do Rio Grande doSul
Porto Alegre, Brazil
Federal University of Rio Grande doSul

Gonzalo Bonilla MD
Department of Otolaryngology
Clinica Alemana
Faculty of Medicine
Universidad del Desarrollo
President
Chilean Society of Otolaryngology
Santiago, Chile

Silvia Breuning
Hospital Pediatric Audiologist
"Prof Dr Juan P Garrahan"
Director of the Center for Audiology
Research
Otoaudiológicas - CIOA
In charge of Audiology "Audiology and
Institute
Language"
Audiology Supervisor "Team Tucumano
Cochlear Implant"
ETTIC

Robert Briggs MD, MBBS, FRACS
Chairman
Department of Otolaryngology

Royal Victorian Eye and Ear Hospital
Clinical School
The University of Melbourne, Australia

Verónica Briones
Scrub nurse
Department of Otolaryngology
Clínicalas Condes
Santiago, Chile

Patricio Burdiles MD
Professor
University of Chile
Department of General Surgery
Academic Director
Clínica las Condes
Santiago, Chile

Miguel Caballero Borrego MD
Department of Otorhinolaryngology
Hospital Clínic of Barcelona, Spain

Luis Cabezas
Department of Otolaryngology
Clínica Las Condes, Santiago, Chile

Jorge Caro Letelier MD
Associate Professor
Department of Otolaryngology
Catholic University of Chile
Chief Editor
Chilean Journal of Otolaryngology and
Head and Neck Surgery
Former President
Chilean Society of Otolaryngology
Member of the Educational Council of the
Chilean Society of Otolaryngology
Santiago, Chile

Miguel Casals MD
Radiology Department
Hospital Padre Hurtado
Director of Radiology
San Vicente de Paul Institute
Santiago, Chile

Jason Chae-Hyun Lee MBBS, BMedSci, MS
Clinical Researcher
Royal Victorian Eye and Ear Hospital
Melbourne, Victoria, Australia

Edgar Chiossone MD
Associate Professor of Otolaryngology
Central University of Venezuela
President of Otological Foundation of
Venezuela

Juan Armando Chiossone MD
Professor and Head of the Department of
Otolaryngology
Central University of Venezuela
Executive Vice-President of the Otological
Foundation of Venezuela

Richard A Chole MD, PhD
Professor and Chairman
Department of Otolaryngology
Washington University School of Medicine
Saint Louis, MO, USA

Axel Christensen MD
Emeritus Chief and Head
Department of Otolaryngology
Clínica las Condes,
Santiago, Chile

Mauricio Cohen MD
Department of Otolaryngology
Cochlear Implant Program
Clínica las Condes
Santiago, Chile

Tim Connolly, Master of Surgery
Graduate Student
Department of Otolaryngology
The University of Melbourne
Australia

José Miguel Contreras MD
Associate Professor
University of Chile
Department of Otorhinolaryngology
Hospital San Juan de Dios de Santiago
Clínica Alemana de Santiago
Chile

Leopoldo Cordero MD
Director
Center for Research Otoaudiológicas
Cochlear Implant Program Consultant
Hospital, De Pediatria Juan P Garrahan
ENT Hospital Service Chief, Cesar Milstein
Argentina

Pedro Cubillos MD
Department of Anesthesiology
Clínica Las Condes, Santiago, Chile

Carlos Curet MD, PhD
Professor of Otorhinolaryngology
National University of Cordoba
Professor of Audiology
Universidad Nacional de San Luis
Professor of postgraduate teaching in
Otorhinolaryngology
Instituto Georges Portmann, France
Director of COAT:
Centro Otoaudiológico-Córdoba-Argentina

Viviana Dalamón PhD
Engineering Research Institute
Genetics and Molecular Biology
National Research Council
Scientific and Technical
Buenos Aires, Argentina

Paul Délano MD, PhD
Assistant Professor
Department of Otorhinolaryngology
Clinical Hospital, University of Chile
Program of Physiology and Biophysics
ICBM, Faculty of Medicine
University of Chile, Chile

Luis Dentone MD
Ass. Professor
Department of Otolaryngology
University of Chile, Clinical Hospital
Santiago, Chile

Romina Di Iorio MD
Second year resident
Arauz Foundation, Argentina

Vicente Diamante MD
Professor
Department of Otolaryngology
Faculty of Medicine Universidad del Salvador
and
Faculty of Medicine Universidad de Buenos
Aires
Emeritus Professor Universidad de Ciencias
Empresariales y Sociales
Director Professor
Diamante Cochlear Implant Center
President of Otorhinolaryngological
Foundation
Buenos Aires, Argentina

Ana Belén Elgoyhen PhD
Principal Investigator
Engineering Research Institute
Genetics and Molecular Biology Council
National Research and
Techniques, Buenos Aires, Argentina

Adjoint Professor
Department of Pharmacology
Facultad de Medicina
Universidad de Buenos Aires, Argentina

Josefina Ernst
Medical Technologist
Department of Otorhinolaryngology
Clínica Las Condes
Santiago, Chile

Patricia Faletty MA
Master in Audiology
Professor of Audiology
Universidad del Museo Social Argentino
Regional Director for South America of
Cochlear Americas, Argentina

Luis Ferrán de la Cierva MD
Hospital Universitario Son Espases, Palma de
Mallorca, Spain

Ugo Fisch MD
Professor of Otolaryngology
Head and Neck and Base of Skull Surgery
Director of Otolaryngology
University of Zurich (1970–99)
Head of Otolaryngology ORL Center Clinic
Hirslanden, Zurich, Switzerland

Rick Fox MD, FRCS(C)
Assistant Professor
Department of Otolaryngology - Head and
Neck Surgery
University of Toronto
Chief
Department of Otolaryngology
St Joseph's Health Centre
Toronto, Ontario, Canada

Richard Gacek MD
Professor of Otolaryngology
University of Massachusetts Medical School
(UMMS)
Worcester, MA, USA

William P R Gibson MD
Tyree Professor of Otolaryngology Surgery
Central Clinical School
University of Sydney
Director
The Sydney Cochlear Implant Centre
Sydney, Australia

Elisa Gil-Carcedo
Associate Professor
Department of Otolaryngology
University of Valladolid, Spain

Luis María Gil-Carcedo
Professor and Chairman
Department of Otolaryngology
University of Valladolid, Spain

Michael B Gluth MD
Assistant Professor
Department of Otolaryngology
University of Melbourne
Melbourne, Australia

Jose Miguel Godoy
Head of Otolaryngology
Clínica Las Condes
Santiago, Chile

Carlos Gómez Velasco MD
Otology Division
Department of Otolaryngology
Complejo EP Hospital Costa del Sol
Málaga, Spain

Donald E Hayes PhD
Director, Audiology
Unitron Hearing Ltd

Sten Hellström MD, PhD
Professor and Head
Dept of Audiology and Neurotology
Karolinska University Hospital
Stockholm, Sweden

Peter Hilger MD, FACS
Professor
Division of Facial Plastic Surgery
Department of Otolaryngology
University of Minnesota
Minneapolis, Minnesota, USA

William House DDS, MD
Otologic Medical Group (now the House
Clinic)
Founder of Hearing for Children
Past President of the American Otological
Society

Marcelo Hueb MD, MS, PhD
Professor and Head
Department of Otolaryngology
Federal University of the Triángulo Mineiro
Uberaba, Brazil
Director of Minas Gerais Otorhinolaryngol-
ogy Foundation
President Elect
Brazilian Association of Otorhinolaryngology
and Cervicofacial Surgery (2012)

Timothy E Hullar MD, FACS
Assistant Professor
Department of Otolaryngology
Washington University School of Medicine
Saint Louis, MO, USA

Hudaifa Ismail MBChB, FRACS (part I), MS
Department of Otolaryngology
University of Melbourne, Australia

Steven Juhn MD, MS, Dr Med
Professor and Director of Biochemistry
Laboratory
Department of Otolaryngology
Adjunct Professor
Department of Neuroscience
University of Minnesota, USA

Timothy T K Jung MD, PhD
Inland Ear Head and Neck Clinic, Riverside
California
Clinical Professor and Director of Research in
Otolaryngology
Loma Linda University School of Medicine
Otologist and Staff Surgeon at
Jerry L Pettis Memorial Veterans Medical
Center
Loma Linda, California, USA

Chong Sun Kim MD,PhD
Clinical Professor
Department of Otorhinolaryngology-Head
and Neck Surgery
Seoul National University
Bundang Hospital
Seongnam-si,Gyeonggi-do, Korea

Ricardo Larrea MD
Associate Professor
Universidad del Valparaíso.
Postgraduate adjunct Professor University
de Chile
Otolaryngologist
Clinica Ciudad del Mar
Valparaíso, Chile

Michelle Lavinsky MD
Professor
Department of Otorhinolaryngology
School of Medicine
Universidade Federal do Rio Grande do Sul
Member of the Otology and Otoneurology
Research Group
Hospital de Clínicas de Porto Alegre/CnPQ
Otorhinolaryngologist, Clínica Lavinsky
MSc in Otorhinolaryngology, Porto Alegre
RS, Brazil

Joel Lavinsky MD
Otorhinolaryngologist at Clínica Lavinsky
Member of the Research Group in Otology
and Otoneurology, Hospital de Clínicas de
Porto Alegre/CNPq, MSc student, Otorhino-
laryngology, Porto Alegre, RS, Brazil

Luiz Lavinsky MD
Professor
Department of Otorhinolaryngology
School of Medicine, Universidade Federal do
Rio Grande do Sul. Coordinator, Otology and
Otoneurology
Research Group, Hospital de Clínicas de
Porto Alegre/CnPQ. MSc, PhD and Post-PhD
in Otorhinolaryngology, Porto Alegre, RS
Brazil

Angel Lede Barreiro MD
Department of Otorhinolaryngology
Hospital da Costa
Burela, Lugo, Spain

Raquel Levy
Medical Technologist ORL
Audiologist
Department of Otolaryngology
Cochlear Implant Program
Clínica Las Condes
Santiago, Chile

Juan Cristobal Maass
Otolaryngology Service
Clínica Alemana of Santiago, Chile
Clinical Hospital, University of Chile
Academic Instructor, University of Chile
Member of the Chilean Society of
Otolaryngology
Chile

Raquel Manrique Huarte MD
Resident
Department of Otorhinolaryngology
Clínic University of Navarra, Spain

Manuel Manrique MD
Consultant
Department of Otorhinolaryngology
Clínic University of Navarra
Professor of Otorhinolaryngology
Faculty of Medicine
University of Navarra, Spain

Chandler Marietta MD
Fellow
Paparella Ear, Head and Neck Institute
Minneapolis, Minnesota, USA

Gumaro Martínez MD
Emeritus Chief and Head
Otolaryngologist
Chilean Military Hospital
Santiago, Chile

Ismael Mena MD
Emeritus Professor Radiological Sciences
UCLA School of Medicine
Doctor Honoris Causa
Universite d' Auvergne, Clermont Ferrand
France
Department of Nuclear Medicine
Clínica Las Condes
Santiago, Chile

Fernando Mendonca MD
Otorhinolaryngologist and Medical Illustrator
Director – Circulo Médico
Lisboa, Portugal

Carmen Gloria Morovic MD
Pediatric Plastic Surgeon
Plastic Surgical Unit
Dr Luis Calvo Mackenna Hospital
and Clínica Las Condes, Santiago, Chile

Luis Henrique Motta MD
Otorhinolaryngologist, Fellow
Department of Otorhinolaryngology
School of Medicine
Universida de Federal do Rio Grande do Sul
MSc degree student, Otorhinolaryngology
Porto Alegre, RS, Brazil

Sonia Neubauer
Head of Department of Nuclear Medicine
Clínica las Condes, Santiago, Chile

Luis Nicenboim MD
Instituto del oido
Rosario, Argentina

Rick Nissen
Otolaryngologist
Facial Plastic Surgery
Bloomington, Minnesota, USA

Mauricio Noschang da Silva, MD
Fellow in Otology and Neurotology
Service of Otolaryngology, Head & Neck
Surgery. Hospital de Clínicas de Porto
Alegre, Brazil
Staff Physician of the Otology and
Neurotology Division. Sistema Hospitalar
Mãe de Deus, Porto Alegre, Brazil

Stephen O'Leary MBBS, BMedSc, PhD, FRACS
William Gibson Chair of Otolaryngology
The University of Melbourne
Prinicipal Otolaryngologist
The Royal Victorian Eye and Ear Hospital
Melbourne, Australia

Sharon Oleskevich PhD
Senior Research Fellow
Group Leader, Hearing Research Program
Garvan Institute of Medical Research
Conjoint Senior Lecturer
Faculty of Medicine
The University of New South Wales, Australia

Viviana Orellana
Medical Technologist, ORL
Head Audiologist
Audia,
Santiago, Chile

Primitivo Ortega
Chairman
Dept of Otolaryngology
Móstoles Hospital, Madrid, Spain

Armando Ortiz
Department of Neurosurgery and
Otolaryngology
Base of Skull Unit
President
Ethics Committee, Clínica Las Condes
Santiago, Chile

Norma Pallares
Speech therapist, Master of Audiology
Prof Holder " Therapeutic Audiology" LIC
Audiology, Faculty of Medicine
Univ of Savior
Prof Head "Music Therapy Clinic" LIC
Music Therapy Medical Fac
Univ of Savior
Co-Director, Cochlear Implant Center
"Prof Diamond" Buenos Aires, Argentina

Michael M Paparella MD
Emeritus Professor
Department of Otolaryngology
University of Minnesota Medical School
Director
Otopathology Laboratory
President
Paparella Ear, Head and Neck Institute
Minneapolis, Minnesota, USA

Marisa Pedemonte MD, DSc
Professor of Physiology
Faculty of Medicine, Instituto Universitario

CLAEH
Punta del Este, Uruguay

Pablo Pérez MD
Otorhinolaryngologist
Córdoba, Argentina

Leticia Petersen Schmidt Rosito MD, MSc
Otologist
Department of Otolaryngology
Head and Neck Surgery
Hospital de Clínicas de Porto Alegre
Staff Physician of the Otology Neurotology
Division
Sistema Hospitalar Mae de Deus, Porto
Alegre, Brazil

Franco Portillo
Director
International Operations
MED-EL North and Middle America
Miami, Florida, USA

Rodrigo Posada-Trujillo MD
Centro Asociado
Fisch International Foundation
Bogotá, Colombia

Carlos Ramírez MS
Clinical Psychologist
Máster in Psychology
Pontificia Universidad Católica de Chile
Clinical Psychologist Department of
Otolaryngology
Clinica Las Condes, Santiago, Chile

Angel Ramos
Head of Department of Otolaryngology
University of Las Palmas
CH Universitario Insular de Gran Canaria, Spain

Gloria Ribalta L MD
Associate Professor
University of Chile
Co-Director
Cochlear Implant Program
Department of Otolaryngology
Clínica Las Condes, Santiago, Chile

Ernesto Ried Goycoolea MD
Otology Division and Cochlear Implant
Program
Department of Otolaryngology
Clínica Las Condes, Santiago, Chile

Ernesto Ried Undurraga MD
Institute of Otology
Santiago, Chile

Luz Adriana Rincón
Esp Audiología

Alejandro Rivas MD
Vanderbilt University Medical Center
Department of Otolaryngology
Head and Neck Surgery
Nashville, USA

José Antonio Rivas MD
Otolaryngologist, Otologist, Neurotólogo
Clinic President, Jose A Rivas
Professor of Otolaryngology and Otology
University of New Granada
Bogotá, Colombia

Adriana Rivas MD, AuD
Audiology Department
Director of Clínica Rivas
Bogotá, DC Colombia

Claudia Romani MD
Specialist in Otolaryngology
Member of the Cochlear Implant Team
Córdoba, Argentina

Héctor Rondón Cardoso MD
Professor of Otolaryngology
Faculty of Medicine
Universidad Nacional de San Agustín
Arequipa, Perú
Head of the Otolaryngology Department
Hospital Regional Honorio Delgado
Arequipa, Perú
President of the Otorhinolaryngological
Foundation of Arequipa
Director and Editor of Revista Anales
Otorrinolaringológicos del Perú
General Secretary of IFOS for Central and
South America

Carlos B Ruah MD, PhD
Clinica ORL Drs Ruah
Lisboa, Portugal

María Inés Salvadores Esp Aud
Phonoaudiologist, Child Audiologist
(Bordeaux)
Cochlear Implant Programming
Cordoba, Argentina

Jorge Salvat
Consultant and Head
Department of Neurosurgery FLENI

Consultant to the Spanish Hospital of
Buenos Aires since 1978, Argentina

Andrea F Santos MD
Otorhinolaryngologist, Otological Group
Hospital das Clinicas
University of Sao Paulo, Brazil

Arturo Samith MD
Emeritus Chief and Head
Otolaryngologist
University of Valparaiso, Chile

Homero Sariego MD
Otolaryngology
Adjoint Professor, Dept of Neurological
Sciences, Campus
Oriente, U de Chile
Neurosurgery Institute Dr Asenjo
Santiago, Chile

Valter Seibel MD, MSc, PhD
Professor of the Department of
Otolaryngology, School of Medicine
Universidade Federal do Rio Grande
Rio Grande, Brazil
Otolaryngologist at
Clínica Lavinsky, Porto Alegre, Brazil

Sady Selaimen da Costa MD, MSc, PhD
Associate Professor
Department of Otolaryngology, Head and
Neck Surgery, School of Medicine
Universidade Federal do Rio Grande do Sul
Brazil
Chief of the Otology and Neurotology
Division, Sistema Hospitalar Mãe de Deus
Porto Alegre, Brazil
Director of the Continuing Medical
Education
Brazilian Association of Otolaryngology
Head and Neck Surgery

Fabio André Selaimen MD
Teaching Assistant
Department of Otolaryngology
Head and Neck Surgery
School of Medicine; Universida de Federal do
Rio Grande do Sul, Brazil

Jose Miguel Selman
Department of Neurosurgery and
Otolaryngology, Base of Skull Unit
Clínica Las Condes, Santiago, Chile

Levent Sennaroglu
Head of Department of Otolaryngology
Hacettepe University Medical Faculty
Ankara, Turkey

Adriana Severina MD
Specialist in Child Otorhinolaryngology
Córdoba, Argentina

Víctor Slavutsky MD
Garraf-Service Medical Group ENT
Barcelona, Spain

Antonio Soda M MD
Professor of Otolaryngology INER-UNAM
Member of the Mexican National Academy
of Medicine and the Mexican National
Academy of Surgery
Former President of the Mexican Society of
Otolaryngology, Head and Neck Surgery
Former President of the Mexican Council of
Otolaryngology, Head and Neck Surgery
Mexico

Francisco Soto Silva MD
Director
Intraoperative Monitorization Program
Clinical Neurophysiology Laboratory
Department of Neurology
Clínica Las Condes
Santiago, Chile

Jorge E Spratley MD, PhD
Professor of Otorhinolaryngology
University of Porto Medical School
Head of Pediatric Otorhinolaryngology
Hospital S João, EPE, Porto, Portugal

Carlos Sttot A
Professor
Clinical Hospital Universidad de Chile, Chile

Alejo Suarez MD, MS, BS
Otologist
Dept of Otolaryngology
British Hospital, Montevideo
Hospital de Niños Pereira Rossell
Montevideo, Uruguay

Hamlet Suárez MD, PhD
Director
Lab of Otoneurology
CLAEH School of Medicine, Uruguay
Chairman
Dept of Otolaryngology, British Hospital
Montevideo, Uruguay

Mariela Torrente
Ass. Professor
Department of Otorhinolaryngology
University of Chile
San Juan de Dios Hospital
Member of the Chilean Society of
Otolaryngology

Mirko Tos MD, Dr Sci
Emeritus Professor from ENT Department
Gentofte Hospital
University of Copenhagen, Denmark
ENT Professor at the University of Maribor
Maribor, Slovenia

Rafael Urquiza de la Rosa MD
Professor and Director
Department of Otolaryngology

Complejo EP Hospital Costa del Sol
Professor of Otolaryngology
University of Málaga
Marbella, Málaga, Spain

Enrique Valenzuela
Head of Otolaryngology
Chilean Military Hospital
Santiago, Chile

Luis Angel Vallejo
Professor and Vice Chairman
University of Valladolid, Spain

Ricardo M Vaz MD
Assistant of Anatomy, University of Porto
Medical School
Chief Resident of Otorhinolaryngology
Hospital S João, EPE, Porto, Portugal

Ricardo A Velluti MD, DSc
Professor of Physiology
Faculty of Medicine
Experimental Neuro-Otology Division, ORL
Hospital de Clínicas, Universidad de la
República, Montevideo, Uruguay

Carlos Young Ordoñez MD
Médico especialista en Otorrinolaringología
Otorrinolaringología Infantil
Honduras

José Francisco Zuma e Maia MD, MSc, PhD
MSc and PhD in Otorhinolaryngology from
Universidade Federal do Rio Grande do Sul
Member of the Otology and Otoneurology
Research Group, Hospital de Clínicas de
Porto Alegre/CnPQ, Porto Alegre, RS, Brazil

General Considerations

The shaking air rattled Lord Edward's membrane tympani, the interlocked malleus, incus and stirrup bones were set in motion so to agitate the membrane of the oval window and raise an infinitesimal storm in the fluid of his labyrinth. The hairy endings of the auditory nerve shuddered like weeds in a rough sea; a vast number of obscure miracles were performed in the brain and Lord Edward ecstatically whispered, *Bach!* (Aldous Huxley, 1928).

The traveler on foot stumbled over a clod. His head was set in motion so to raise an infinitesimal storm in the fluids of his labyrinth. The otoliths shuddered like weeds in a rough sea; a vast number of stimuli traveled to his brain and the adaptation systems were set in action. The traveler became spatially oriented, straightened up and whispered with relief, *I almost fell!* (Author´s adaptation for the sense of balance).

"The cerebral cortex resembles a garden populated by innumerable trees, the pyramidal cells, which thanks to an intelligent culture can multiply their branches and sink their roots much further, and produce flowers and fruits that are each time more varied and exquisite." (Santiago Ramón y Cajal, 1894).

The ear is a part of the body that is oriented toward two fundamental functions: hearing and balance. In order to fulfill these purposes, it is formed by a structural system that is functionally synergic and harmonic; in which every component is oriented toward the overall function of the ear, which in turn is an integral part of the body. Surgeons must become familiar with these concepts. That is to say, with anatomy and function, and their harmonic and precise operations oriented to its purpose.

We must consider that surgery is not performed in an isolated organ, but in one that interrelates anatomically and functionally with other organs and systems, some of which are of the same embryologic origin. Moreover, this occurs in a person who has unique general conditions and lives in an environment which has an important influence in his/her behavior, function and adaptation. When the aggression factors prevail over the defense system of the body, this harmonic function is disturbed.

The aggression factors of disease might be the same, however, they can manifest in different ways. The structures involved might be the same; however, the individuals that are affected are not the same and may react in different manners. A procedure that is good for somebody might be harmful to another. People and environments are unique and have variations.

This Atlas has a special emphasis in structure, function, pathogenesis and research. This is because of my firm conviction that in order to select, modify or develop a rational therapy, it is essential to have an understanding of the anatomy, function and pathology of the organs involved as well as of the mechanisms of disease. This is what leads to progress and innovation, and also allows for the most important concept of timing.

Under this philosophy, the techniques described in this book are more oriented toward a way of thinking than toward a dogma of doing. Moreover, because our knowledge and ability to define particular states and stages of otologic disease are partial, we hardly can be dogmatic in its treatment. Therefore, this Atlas advocates an open-minded approach that tailors the treatment to each patient rather than fitting patients into rigid treatments.

In addition, it is expected that this atlas will provide information that would contribute to a gradual acquisition of a three-dimensional functional image of the ear. This process implies hours of practice and study until this three-dimensional image is internalized and becomes natural. In reality, this learning process is similar to other activities.

Just as a violinist, an athlete, a golfer or a chess player requires a certain number of hours before internalizing their movements toward maximal efficiency; the same occurs with a surgical act in which every movement is regulated by neuronal circuits that provide anticipation. That is why it is essential to have dedication, passion, and hours and hours of hard work. It is not possible to achieve excellence from 8 to 12 and from 2 to 6 based on good public relations.

The ideal approach towards disease for years has been prevention and early detection. With the current scientific advances, particularly in genetics and molecular biology, we are approaching a personalized predictive medicine that will eventually turn into regenerative and not only of tissues but of full organs. Response to medications and potential allergies or toxicities will be predicted, and therapies will be improved. Moreover, this regenerative medicine is starting to include tissues such as the central nervous system, tissues that nobody would have ever dreamed that could be regenerated.

As suggested in the initial paragraphs, as early as 1894, Santiago Ramón y Cajal described the concept of neural plasticity. He suggested that as a difference with telephone cables, with proper stimulation the central nervous system would develop an increase in dendritic and axonal connections in some of the stimulated neuronal circuits. These concepts have re-emerged in otology especially for sensorineural hearing loss, and we find ourselves working hard in early detection and stimulation. Little did Ramón y Cajal and our own selves just a few years ago, imagine that regeneration of the cells themselves could be possible. We are in the doorsteps of a wonderful new approach to otology, and in particular to sensorineural hearing loss, in which cochlear implants, hearing aids and bone anchored hearing devices are only part of it. Hair cells can be regenerated by different means; nervous tissue can be exposed and responds to neurotrophic factors, hearing aids and implants are making gigantic progress and advances in digital systems and chip technology are completely revolutionizing signal processing. This is truly a great moment, and we are facing a new world of different and stimulating approaches. Based on these firm beliefs is that I have asked the different authors to touch upon these subjects along this surgical atlas since in the not too distant future we will be approaching some of these therapies surgically.

Introduction of the Book
From the Desk of the Series Editor

The textbook edited by Dr Marcos Goycoolea and friends is a first of its kind and is totally unique. Its title says it all.

Dr Goycoolea has put together the finest quality of authors and the finest quality studying material. All the well-respected names have agreed to contribute to this book because of their respect and admiration for Dr Goycoolea.

The material presented in this book is not abstract theory but a living text that provides excellent insight into disorders ranging from the simple to the complex.

This text provides excellent material that can be applied directly into clinical practice.

I have trained under Dr Goycoolea at the University of Minnesota where he conducted excellent research on the round window membrane among many things. I still continue to learn from him and my patients are the better for it.

I am proud to be associated with Dr Goycoolea and his magical wonderful text.

I thank the numerous authors of this text for so graciously and unselfishly sharing their knowledge and experience so that all who read this text can benefit from it.

Dr Chris de Souza MS, DORL, DNB, FACS
Honorary ENT and Skull Base Surgeon
Tata Memorial Hospital, Mumbai, India
Consultant Otolaryngologist and Head Neck Surgeon
Lilavati Hospital and Holy Family Hospital, Mumbai, India

Contents

Section I

Structure and Function

Marcos Goycoolea, Arturo Samith,
Ricardo Velluti, Marisa Pedemonte,
Paul Délano, Miguel Casals,
Ismael Mena, Sonia Neubauer,
Gumaro Martínez, Marcelo Galvez Moya

1.1

General Overview

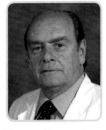

Marcos Goycoolea

The shaking air rattled Lord Edward's membrana tympani, the interlocked malleus, incus and stirrup bones were set in motion so to agitate the membrane of the oval window and raise an infinitesimal storm in the fluid of his labyrinth. The hairy endings of the auditory nerve shuddered like weeds in a rough sea; a vast number of obscure miracles were performed in the brain and Lord Edward ecstatically whispered, *Bach!* (Aldous Huxley, 1928).

This paragraph written in 1928, describes in essence the sense of hearing. Although our understanding of anatomy and function as well as the clarification of some of the obscure miracles has improved, the fundamental concepts described by Huxley have remained unaltered. When an object generates a sound, this sound alters the air that surrounds it. These alterations translate into sound waves—sinusoids of mechanical energy—that travel away from their source of origin at approximately 340 meters per second. This speed is much less than the speed of light. I learned this concept as a child while I watched the bird hunters in a hill nearby. They used gun powder with smoke and when they did the shooting I could see the smoke and only after a while I could hear the noise.

The ear is the organ in charge of transmitting these sound waves to the brain for interpretation. For this to occur, the sound waves must travel through a number of specialized areas of the ear (external, middle and inner ear) prior to reaching the brain.

"The shaking air rattled Lord Edward's membrana tympani…" implies the participation of the external ear and the tympanic membrane in sound transmission.

The external ear includes the pinna and the external auditory canal. The pinna (from the Latin word: feather) allows the sound waves to be funneled to the external auditory canal, at the end of which lies the tympanic membrane. Our pinnas are too small to amplify low frequencies; however, they amplify high frequencies which are important in order to understand a conversation. These components are amplified in the external auditory canal (resonance).

The old "auditory trumpets" were nothing but artificial pinnas of a large size. If a person is near a waterfall, and covers and uncovers the lateral aspect of the pinna with the palm of the hand, that person would notice that the sounds that fluctuate are those of high frequencies. Low frequency sounds manage to reach the inner ear by osseous vibration.

At the end of the external ear canal is an elastic tympanic membrane (from the Greek word tympanon: drum, resonator, diaphragm).

"The interlocked malleus, incus and stirrup bones were set in motion so to agitate the membrane of the oval window and raise an infinitesimal storm in the fluid of his labyrinth…"

The tympanic membrane (ear drum) is connected to the ossicular chain through which these vibrations are transmitted to the inner ear (membranous resonator). In addition to its transmission function, the tympanic membrane seals the entrance from the external ear canal to the middle ear and also avoids that the sound waves reach the round window membrane directly.

The last bone of the ossicular chain is the stapes which is in direct contact with the inner ear fluids as a piston surrounded by an envelope which is the oval window. The middle ear is a cavity that is filled with air and this allows a better transmission of the sound waves. For this transmission to be efficient, the middle ear must function at atmospheric pressure. That role is covered by the Eustachian tube which communicates the middle ear cavity with the posterior pharynx. The Eustachian tube opens when we swallow, allowing pressure equalization in

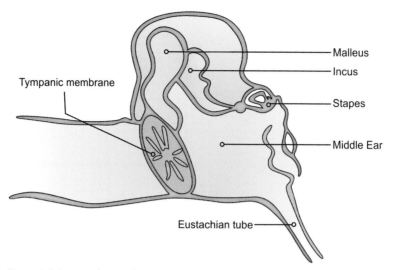

Tympanic membrane

Malleus

Incus

Stapes

Middle Ear

Eustachian tube

Figure 1 Schematic diagram showing anatomy of an ear

the middle ear. It is the Eustachian tube that we open when we climb a hill or are subjected to pressure changes in the ascent or descent of an airplane, in order to equalize pressures (Figure 1).

Fish do not need a middle ear since they live under the water, however, animals that live on the land need middle ears since if sound waves would come directly from air to liquid they would rebound. In addition, sound transmission through liquids is extremely poor. Just imagine what it is to talk to somebody who is under water. That is why not only an air-filled cavity but also an amplification system (e.g. ossicular chain) is needed.

Where does this Amplification Occur?

The first amplification occurs as resonance in the ear canal. Resonance is the "sympathetic" vibration of an object with sound resulting in amplification of the sound or of some of its frequencies. In the external ear canal this occurs at 4,000 cycles per second. The second amplification occurs at the level of the ossicular chain, a system of levers that amplify only 2.5 decibels. That is why an ossicular prostheses, such as a total ossicular replacement prosthesis (TORP) (to be described in ossiculoplasty) is so successful. The third and main amplification is at the level of the oval window (stapes footplate) which is 30 times smaller than the tympanic membrane, yielding an amplification of 25 decibels. This amplification effect is similar to that of the heel of a high heel shoe which concentrates the whole weight in a small surface.

Our amplified wave reaches the liquids of the inner ear located in the vestibule in which our stapes footplate is located. It is at this stage when our amplified waves pass from air to fluid.

"The hairy endings of the auditory nerve shuddered like weeds in a rough sea…"

INNER EAR

The inner ear has receptors for two sensory systems: (1) the auditory system (hearing) and (2) the vestibular system (spatial orientation and equilibrium). The inner ear contains the bony and membranous labyrinths. The bony labyrinth (bone containing a cavity) is filled with perilymph and contains three main cavities: (1) the vestibule (with the utricle and saccule), (2) cochlea and (3) the semicircular canals. These cavities have membranous ducts that are immersed in perilymph and are intercommunicated among them. Internally they contain endolymph (Figures 2 and 3). The semicircular canals (that respond to rotational acceleration), and the saccule and utricle (that respond to linear acceleration) form the membranous labyrinth of the vestibular system. The membranous labyrinth of the auditory system is formed by the cochlear duct which contains the ciliated cells of the organ of Corti (Figures 4 and 5). This duct is located in the cochlea (from the Greek word Cochlos: snail), which bears its name because of its resemblance with a snail.

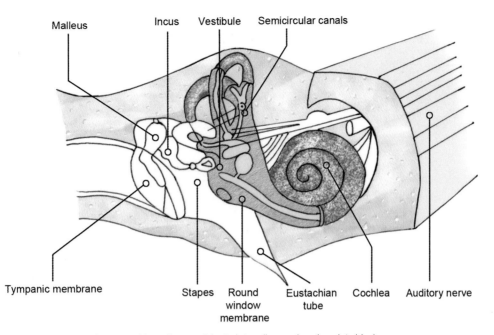

Malleus Incus Vestibule Semicircular canals

Tympanic membrane Stapes Round window membrane Eustachian tube Cochlea Auditory nerve

Figure 2 External auditory canal (membranous labyrinth in yellow and perilymph in blue)

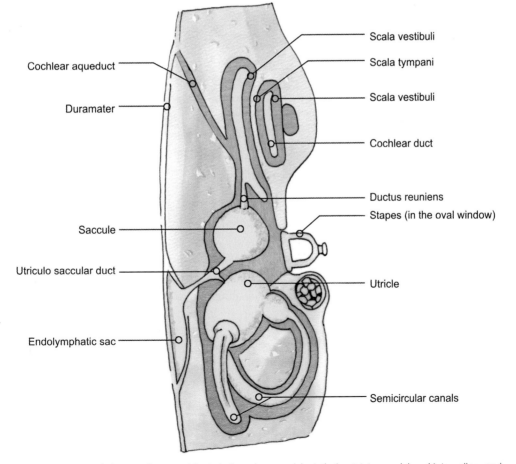

Cochlear aqueduct Scala vestibuli

Duramater Scala tympani

Scala vestibuli

Cochlear duct

Ductus reuniens

Stapes (in the oval window)

Saccule

Utriculo saccular duct

Utricle

Endolymphatic sac

Semicircular canals

Figure 3 Diagram of the membranous labyrinth [membranous labyrinth (containing endolymph) in yellow and perilymph in blue]

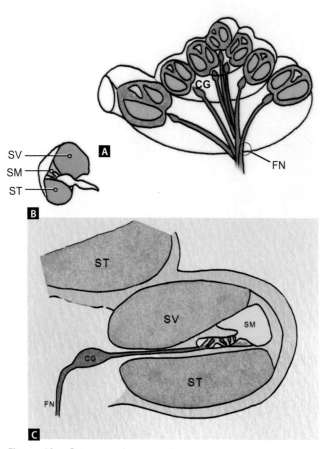

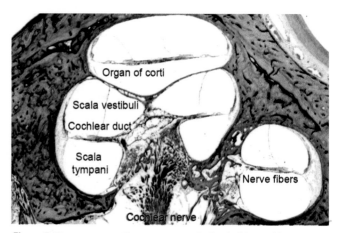

Figure 5 Human temporal bone section at the level of the cochlea

Figures 4A to C Drawing of a section of the cochlea. (Perilymph in blue), ST: scala tympani; SV: scala vestibule. Cochlear duct, also termed as scala media (SM) with endolymph (in yellow). In red: ganglion cells (CG) and nerve fibers (FN) of the auditory nerve

The cochlea is lodged in the petrous portion of the temporal bone, the hardest bone in humans. It contains three ducts filled with fluid that are rolled around the modiolus in an helicoidal fashion (Figure 6). In the superior compartment is the scala vestibuli. The base of this scala is in the vestibule. In the inferior compartment is the scala tympani. The base of this scala is at the round window membrane. Both scala are communicated at the cochlear tip at the helicotrema. Our amplified sound wave reaches the cochlea coming from the vestibuli (stapes footplate) through the scala vestibuli and descends through the scala tympani toward the round window membrane (pressure release valve). During this process the sound wave is transmitted to the basilar membrane that lodges the organ of Corti. It is at the organ of Corti where the mechanical sound waves that reach the endolymph are transformed into electrical impulses.

The organ of Corti (to be described in detail in other sections of the atlas) has the ciliated cells that are in charge of transforming mechanical into electrical impulses. The organ of Corti has two types of ciliated cells; one row of inner hair cells and three rows of outer hair cells (external hair cells) (Figures 6 and 7). Inner hair cells are receptors and transmit signals to the ganglion cells (that originate the auditory nerve fibers).

In addition to their sensory function, the outer hair cells are also motor cells, they contribute to auditory sensibility and selectivity (they contain elastin and have contractile properties), and having a modulator function (fine tuning).

The inner ear will be discussed later; however, for practical purposes the cochlea can be seen from a functional standpoint, as an anatomical area (Figures 6 to 9) consisting of three components:

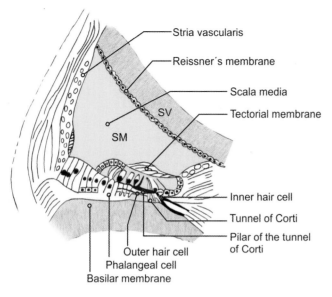

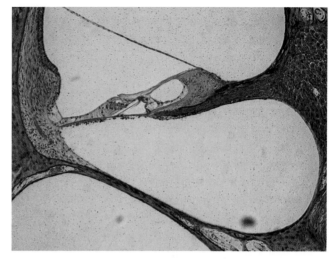

Figure 6 Drawing (radial section) of the organ of Corti (endolymph in yellow and perilymph in blue)
SM: Scala media; ST: Scala tympani; SV: Scala vestibuli

Labels in Figure 6:
Stria vascularis
Reissner's membrane
Scala media
Tectorial membrane
Inner hair cell
Tunnel of Corti
Pilar of the tunnel of Corti
Outer hair cell
Phalangeal cell
Basilar membrane

Figure 8 Scala media with the organ of Corti and stria vascularis

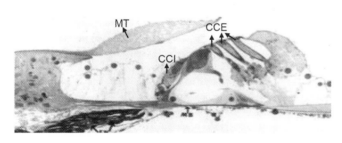

Figure 7 Human temporal bone section at the level of the organ of Corti MT: Tectorial membrane; CCE: Outer hair cell; CCI: inner hair cell; FN: Nerve fibers; MB: Basilar membrane

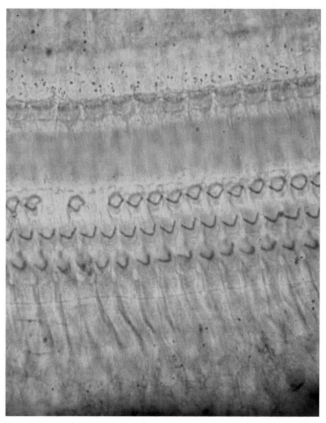

1. The stria vascularis and lateral wall (to be described) that provide the necessary energy.
2. The inner and outer hair cells which act not only as transductors (mechanical to electrical) but also as amplifiers.
3. The supporting cells (to be described) that provide infrastructure. The electromechanical transduction by the hair

Figure 9 View from above: cochlea with cilia in blue, three rows of cilia of outer and one row of cilia of inner cells (stain developed by David Muchow)

cells is caused by the opening of ionic channels of these ciliated cells, opening that occurs following mechanical deflection of their stereocilia.

Finally, the ciliated cells not only transform mechanical sound waves into electrical impulses, but also do this preserving their frequencies. This is in part possible because of their tonotopic organization in the cochlear duct.

The cells in the base of the cochlea are stimulated by high frequencies, while the apical ones are stimulated by low frequencies. This distribution is similar to a piano, except that instead of having 100 keys it has more than 3,500 which is the number of inner hair cells. Each inner hair cell is innervated by approximately 20 nerve fibers, which constitute 90–95% of the cochlear nerve fibers. However, this organization does not fully explain the high degree of resolution of frequency information. This is in part the job of the outer hair cells that are approximately 15,000 to 20,000. In this case each nerve fiber innervates 10 outer hair cells. With this structural organization the inner hair cells seemingly perceive acoustic stimuli, and outer hair cells modulate and perform fine tuning. The nerve endings to which the ciliated cells relate are the dendrites of the ganglion cells that are located in the center of the cochlea (Figures 4 and 5) in the spiral ganglion. Dendrites travel from the spiral ganglion to the organ of Corti by a bony canal termed Rosenthal's canal (Figures 10 to 13). The axons of the ganglion cells form the nerve fibers of the auditory (cochlear) nerve that traverses towards the cochlear nuclei in the brainstem.

It is impressive that hearing—the "youngest" of the senses in the evolutionary process—can function so efficiently with such a small number of receptors in comparison with other senses such as sight and smell. The retina has 100 million receptors that provide around 1,000,000 nerve fibers to the ophthalmic nerve, in contrast to 14,000 hair cells that provide 32,000 nerve fibers to the auditory nerve.

This small number of receptors makes the system more vulnerable and it is here where the highest number of damage occurs, originating a high incidence of sensorineural hearing loss. If in addition we have a sensory organ with a terminal irrigation (similar to the heart) this results in a sensory organ that is highly vulnerable.

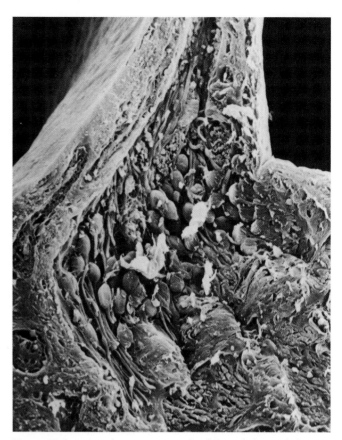

Figure 10 Scanning electron micrograph of Rosenthal's canal showing ganglion cells

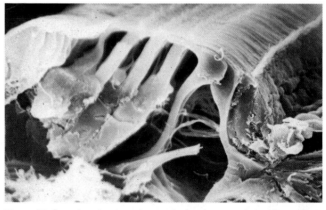

Figure 11 Scanning electron micrograph showing outer hair cells and their stereocilia, within the organ of Corti

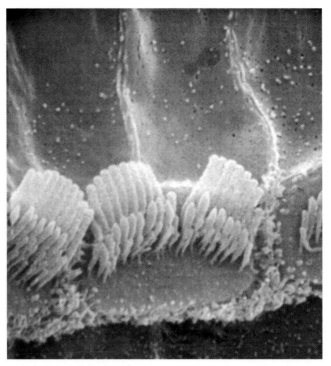

Figure 12 Scanning electron micrograph showing stereocilia of outer hair cells

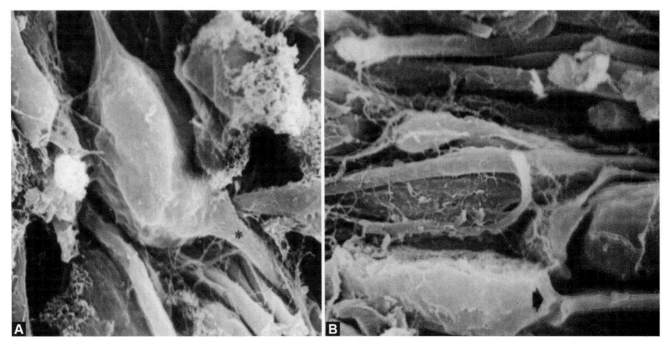

Figures 13A and B Type I ganglion cell with its axon, cell body and dendritic process

CENTRAL TRANSMISSION

Marcos Goycoolea, Ismael Mena, Sonia Neubauer

A vast number of obscure miracles were performed in the brain and Lord Edward ecstatically whispered, *Bach!*

The most established afferent system includes five neurons from the cochlea to the cerebral cortex. The first order neurons originate in the spiral ganglion of the cochlea and end up in the cell body of the second order neurons located in the cochlear nuclei (dorsal and ventral) in the brainstem (central transmission will be described later in detail); from this point on, they follow different routes, being the most established the one that describes the axons of the second order neurons crossing the midline of the brainstem through the trapezoid body to the contralateral superior olivary complex. The third order neurons ascend through the lateral lemniscus to the inferior colliculus, from where the fourth order neurons reach the medial geniculate body of the thalamus. The axons of the fifth order neurons end in the cell bodies of the neurons of the auditory cortex.

Even if this is the most studied pathway, it is not the only pathway. There are many alternative ipsilateral and contralateral pathways—with less and also more synaptic connections—that are well established. The only constant and seemingly obligatory relay station is the geniculate body of the thalamus. Not all the fibers from the thalamus go directly to the cerebral cortex. Some go to the reticular formation. Moreover, there are also interconnecting fibers between both auditory cortical centers (right and left). How much is ipsilateral or contralateral, and under what circumstances, is still to be determined.

Even if it is the most established efferent pathway, this does not mean that it is the only efferent pathway. Its role in the regulation of hair cells is well established, however, there is no sufficient information with respect to other efferent fibers that could also be playing important role in the auditory process. In addition, there are inhibitory and excitatory central nuclei that play a significant role in the process of determining what, how and where the auditory stimuli are heard and processed.

Between the cochlear nuclei and the geniculate body of the thalamus (where all impulses converge) information on localization of sound is processed. This process is essential not

only to determine if a sound comes from left or right but also if it comes from above or below, from front or back and from how far. While for humans this information is extremely important, for some animals it is vital. Such is the case of a predator or for an animal in search of a mate.

Humans go far beyond this stage, by interpreting the meaning of what is heard. This implies a process of interpretation, analysis and selection that is done at the cortical level.

Although functional brain imaging will be described later in this section, the available information in the literature, including our own studies suggest the following:

- The auditory energy that is transmitted by the auditory neuronal system travels through ipsilateral and contralateral pathways. How much is ipsilateral or contralateral, and under what circumstances, is still to be determined.
- The auditory pathway has both excitatory and inhibitory relays.
- Central response is bilateral, regardless of the ear that is stimulated.
- Central response can consist of activation or inhibition. This occurrence should determine not only what reaches the cortex but also where in the cortex a specific stimulus will be processed.
- Although central activation/deactivation is bilateral, this does not mean that it is symmetrical. That is to say, processing of specific information can be done more on one side than on the other, e.g. pure tones can be processed preferentially on the left side, musical perceptions on the right.
- Bilateral central response to acoustic stimuli (auditory energy) involves areas other than auditory centers, such as executive frontal, visual and affective areas among many others; and also involves areas of auditory memory.
- Although central activation/deactivation is bilateral (regardless of which ear is stimulated), central inhibition can be significantly different in the same individual, depending on

which ear (side) is stimulated; suggesting the possibility of the existence of a preferred or leading ear, manifested as functional asymmetries according to which ear is stimulated.

• When an individual receives auditory stimuli, these are not isolated pure tones but a considerable amount of stimuli that become available practically at the same time.

On the other hand, considering all the different pathways (ipsi and contralateral, with more or less synapsis) and stages (excitatory, inhibitory), from a same stimulus, what reaches the cortex is not the single original stimulus but a group of stimuli which are the end result of having traveled through different pathways simultaneously. Therefore the cortex has to analyze, integrate and process this complex information.

Considering the previous observations, one can realize that the process for *"Lord Edward to whisper ecstatically Bach!"* is not just a matter of electrical impulses traveling through ipsilateral and contralateral pathways to the auditory cortex. Hearing and making sense of it requires analysis, integration and processing of complex information (auditory and others, e.g. visual) that is ultimately defined at the cortical level. In addition, the existence of an auditory memory is essential for the hearing sensation to be meaningful (recognizing Bach!) and additional centers are required for this sensation to be "ecstatic".

While this Atlas deals primarily with the surgical aspects of the mechanical aspects of sound transmission, cochlear implants are the beginning of an approach of the central aspects of hearing that we have barely touched upon. The auditory system is not just a receiving and transmitting system but a complete active, and fully integrated circuit where problems occurring in one area can manifest in a different one. Therefore, it is essential for the surgeon who wants to re-establish harmony and function, to understand the auditory system as a whole in order to approach it from a global standpoint.

BIBLIOGRAPHY

1. Binder JR, Rao SM, Hammeke TA, et al. Functional magnetic resonance imaging of human auditory cortex. Ann Neurol. 1994;35:662-72.

2. Gardner EP, Martin JH. Codificacion de la informacion sensorial. In: Kandel ER, Schwartz JH, Jessel TH (Eds). Principios de Neurociencia. Madrid: McGraw-Hill Interamericana; 2000. pp. 411-29.

3. Goycoolea MV, Mena I, Neubauer S (2004). Functional studies of the human auditory cortex, auditory memory and musical hallucinations (Article No. AJ25-2). [online] Alasbimn Journal website. Available from www2.alasbimnjournal.cl/alasbimn/CDA/sec_b/0,1206,SCID%253D11173,00.html. [Accessed May, 2011].

4. Goycoolea M, Mena I, Neubauer S. Spontaneous musical auditory perceptions in patients who develop abrupt bilateral sensorineural hearing loss. An uninhibition syndrome? Acta Oto-Laryngologica. 2006;126:368-74.

5. Goycoolea M, Mena I, Neubauer S, et al. Musical brains: a study of spontaneous and evoked musical sensations without external auditory stimuli. Acta Oto-Laryngologica. 2007;127:711-21.

6. Goycoolea M, Mena I, Neubauer S. Is there a difference in activation or in inhibition of cortical auditory centers depending on the ear that is stimulated? Acta Oto-Laryngologica. 2009;129:348-53.

7. Goycoolea M, Mena I, Neubauer S. Functional studies of the human auditory pathway after monaural stimulation with pure tones. Establishing a normal database. Acta Oto-Laryngologica 2005;125:513-9.

8. Goycoolea M, Mena I, Neubauer S. Functional studies of the human auditory pathway alter stimulating binaurally with pure tones. Presented at the Collegium Meeting in August 2010, Budapest, Hungary. In press Acta Oto-Laryngologica.

9. Griffiths TD, Warren JD, Scott SK, et al. Cortical processing of complex sound: a way forward? Trends in Neuroscience. 2004;27:181-5.

10. Howard D, Patterson K, Wise R, et al. The cortical localization of lexicons. Positron Emission Tomography Evidence. Brain. 1992;115:1769-82.

11. Hudspeth AJ. Audición. In: Kandel ER, Schwartz JH, Jessel TH (Eds). Principios de Neurociencia. Madrid: Mc Graw-Hill-Interamericana; 2000. pp. 590-613.

12. Millen SJ, Haughton VM, Yetkin FZ. Functional magnetic resonance imaging of the central auditory pathway following speech and pure-tone stimuli. Laryngoscope. 1995;105:1305-10.

13. Saunders J, Erulkar S. Neurophysiology of the auditory system. In: Durrant JD, Lovrinic JH (Eds). Bases Hearing Science. Baltimore: Williams and Wilkins Co; 1977. pp. 110-37.

14. Strainer JC, Ulmer JL, Yetkin FZ, et al. Functional MR of the primary auditory cortex. Am J Neuroradiol. 1997;18:601-10.

15. Yetkin FZ, Roland PS, Christensen F, et al. Silent functional magnetic resonance imaging (FMRI) of tonotopicity and stimulus intensity coding in human primary auditory cortex. Laryngoscope. 2004;114:512-8.

1.2
External Ear

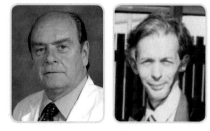

Marcos Goycoolea, Gumaro Martinez

For descriptive purposes the ear is divided into three parts: (1) the external ear consisting of the auricle, the external acoustic meatus and the tympanic membrane; (2) the middle ear (tympanic cavity), associated ossicles and muscles, and (3) the inner ear containing the organs for equilibration and hearing.

AURICLE

The auricular component of the external ear consists of a single cartilaginous plate with a covering skin. This cartilage framework is responsible for the shape of the auricle, and determines all the various prominences and depressions seen on the ear, with the exception of the lobule.

In addition to the features that are superficially discernible, the cartilage plate contains other features that become evident upon removal of overlying skin. These include the following (Figures 1A to C):

- The spine of the helix, projecting anteriorly from the helix near the crus.
- The tail of the helix (cauda helix), the terminal portion of the helix, located at the posteroinferior margin of the auricle.
- The isthmus, the point of continuity between the auricular and meatal cartilages, located immediately posterior to the entrance of the external meatus.
- The terminal incisure, between the isthmus and the tragal lamina of the auricular cartilage. Its inferior extremity is the opening of the external meatus. Superiorly it is marked by the anterior incisure.

The tragus also has a role in the transmission of sound waves toward the ear canal (and this transmission is different if it comes from dorsal, ventral or lateral).

The auricle is attached to the side of the head by the following features:

- Its continuity with the cartilaginous portion of the external acoustic meatus.

- The skin covering the ear and continuing onto the skull. The skin of the auricle is tightly bound to the perichondrium of the lateral aspect of the ear, but is somewhat freer on the medial surface. There is very little fat in the subcutaneous tissue of the ear. Except in the tragal and antitragal regions, the hair of the auricle is rudimentary. Sebaceous glands are present on both the surfaces, and are particularly numerous in the concha and triangular fossa.
- Three extrinsic ligaments. These include:
  1. The anterior ligament, extending from the zygoma to the helix and the tragus.
  2. The superior ligament, extending from the superior margin of the bony meatus to the spine of the helix.
  3. The posterior ligament, extending from the mastoid process to the concha of the auricle.
- Muscles consisting of the following:
  1. An extrinsic group formed of three small muscles (anterior, superior and posterior) belonging to the facial group of muscles and supplied by the facial nerve (Figures 1A to C).
  2. An intrinsic group of six small muscles, which are extremely variable in their development and have no functional significance in humans.

In fact, in humans, these muscles (extrinsic and intrinsic) do not have sound localization purposes as is the case in animals. For example, in deers, their pinnas can move independently of each other, even in opposite directions. In this manner they provide information about the direction of sound. Humans in turn, have to turn their heads.

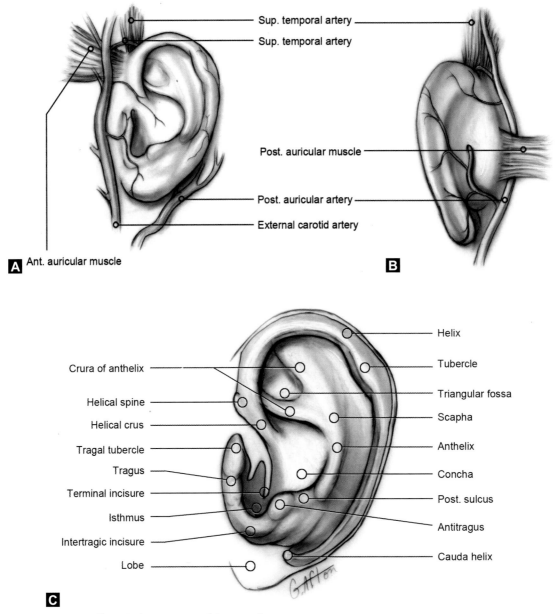

A

Sup. temporal artery

Sup. temporal artery

Post. auricular muscle

Post. auricular artery

External carotid artery

Ant. auricular muscle

B

Crura of anthelix

Helical spine

Helical crus

Tragal tubercle

Tragus

Terminal incisure

Isthmus

Intertragic incisure

Lobe

Helix

Tubercle

Triangular fossa

Scapha

Anthelix

Concha

Post. sulcus

Antitragus

Cauda helix

C

Figures 1A to C The auricular component of the external ear

THE EXTERNAL ACOUSTIC MEATUS (AUDITORY CANAL)

The external acoustic meatus is a bony-cartilaginous canal extending from the concha of the auricle to the tympanic membrane. In its adult configuration, it describes a slight S-shape, with the lateral cartilaginous portion somewhat concave anteriorly and inferiorly, and the medial bony portion slightly concave posteriorly and superiorly. Owing to the obliquity of the tympanic membrane, the posterosuperior wall of the meatus is slightly shorter than the anteroinferior wall (approximately 25 mm and 31 mm respectively). Its internal diameter is 7 mm by 9 mm, and it is elliptical and not circular. In its lateral portion the diameter is larger in a vertical direction, whereas in its medial portion it is in the horizontal direction. The narrowest point is located medial to the osseous-cartilaginous junction (also termed the isthmus). These anatomical relationships explain the usefulness of the oval ear specula. In addition, the cartilaginous portion is slightly concave towards anterior and the osseous portion towards posterior. Therefore, the canal has an italic "S" shape. When placing an ear speculum in an adult, the pinna should be pulled upwards and backwards, and the speculum is "screwed" in. The volume of the ear canal in the adult is approximately 15.4 cm^3. The resonance of the external auditory canal in the adult is approximately 2.5–3 kilohertz (kHz), which are the frequencies in which acoustic trauma occurs.

What is Resonance?

When an object produces a sound, it causes changes in the air that surrounds it. These changes translate into sound waves that travel away from their source. When these sound waves reach an object, this object tends to repel these sounds and to attenuate them. However, certain frequencies are not attenuated and make the object vibrate. These are called the resonant frequencies. All objects have resonant frequencies and this will depend on their size, form, material, etc. Heavy objects resonate with low frequencies; light and small objects with high frequencies and the ear canal with frequencies between 2.5 and 3 kHz.

Osseous Components

Slightly more than half of the external meatus is entirely bony (medially), with the anterior wall, floor and lower posterior wall formed by the tympanic portion of the temporal bone. Its roof and the upper part of the posterior wall are formed by the squamous portion.

The bony components of the external ear (Figure 2) are all part of the temporal bone. They include the following:

The Squamous Portion

The squamous portion, forming a small, superiorly located part of the bony external auditory meatus and the anterolateral portion of the mastoid process. Extending laterally and anteriorly from the inferior part of the squamous portion of the temporal bone is the zygomatic process, which has three roots: (1) the anterior root extends medially to become confluent with the articular tubercle; (2) the medial root forms the posterior wall of the mandibular fossa and (3) the posterior root curves slightly downward onto the mastoid process. This root bears the small suprameatal spine (of Henle) on its dorsal extremity. Hence, the upper portion of the external acoustic meatus is located between the middle and posterior roots. The crest of the posterior root and the posterosuperior portion of the bony meatus are joined by an imaginary line to form the

suprameatal triangle, marking the site of access to the antrum of the middle ear.

The Tympanic Portion

The tympanic portion is forming most of the bony meatus. The greatest part of this component develops after birth and the alteration in form as it develops brings about a shift in the depth of the external meatus as well as in the orientation of the tympanic membrane. In the newborn it is a slight bone ring that is imperfect superiorly. With subsequent growth, small projections of bone arising from its anterior and posterior crura extend into the lumen of the ring, eventually fusing to divide the annulus into the superiorly located acoustic meatus proper and a small, inferiorly situated aperture. Although the latter usually closes with continued development, it may on occasion persist to form what is designated the "foramen of Huschke." The superiorly located discontinuity in the tympanic ring persists into adult life as the tympanic notch (of Rivinus).

Posteriorly the tympanic ring forms, in conjunction with both the squamous and petrous portions of the mastoid process, the tympanomastoid and petrotympanic sutures (frequently designated collectively the tympanomastoid suture). Anteriorly the ring participates in the formation of the squamotympanic and petrotympanic sutures. It is in the latter suture that the foramen transmitting the chorda tympani nerve (the iter chordae anterius) is found. It should be appreciated that the tympanic ring, with its growth, forms a portion of the posterior wall of the mandibular fossa.

The Petrous Portion

The petrous portion, forming the tip and posterior portion of the mastoid process.

Cartilaginous Components

The cartilaginous (lateral) portion of the external meatus forms a trough-shaped structure that is open superiorly and posteriorly. This canal is completed in the latter quadrants by the squamous portion of the temporal bone. In addition to being slightly curved, it is somewhat broader in its lateral aspect, where it makes up approximately two-thirds of the circumference of the meatus. Medially, it makes up roughly one-third of the meatal wall. At its lateral extremity the cartilage of the meatus is con-

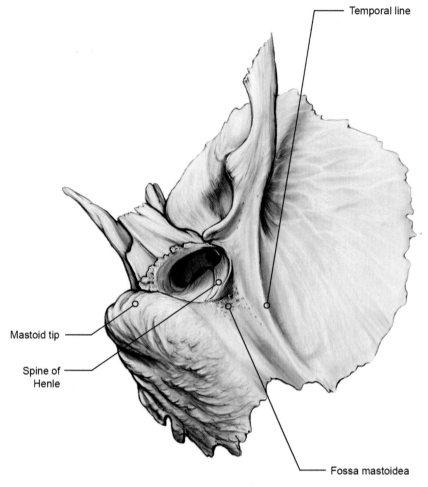

Temporal line

Mastoid tip

Spine of
Henle

Fossa mastoidea

Figure 2 The bony components of external ear

tinuous with that of the auricle through the isthmus; medially, it articulates with the bony portion of the meatus. The anterior wall is characterized by the presence of two fissures (incisures of the cartilaginous meatus or fissures of Santorini), which assist in imparting a limited mobility to the auricle.

The major relationships of the meatus are the following (Figure 3):
- Anteriorly and laterally, the parotid gland. The more medial and anterior relationships include the mandibular fossa and the condyle of the mandible
- Inferiorly, the parotid gland

- Superiorly and medially, the epitympanic recess of the middle ear
- Posteriorly, the mastoid air cells.

The ear canal ends at the tympanic membrane which is inserted in the tympanic annulus, which is incomplete in its posterosuperior portion.

The external auditory canal is covered by skin which is continuous with that of the auricle (that is why the ear canal hurts when the auricle is pulled in cases of external otitis and not in cases of otitis media) and also forms the external layer of the tympanic membrane. Since it is a cavity, it has a pH and

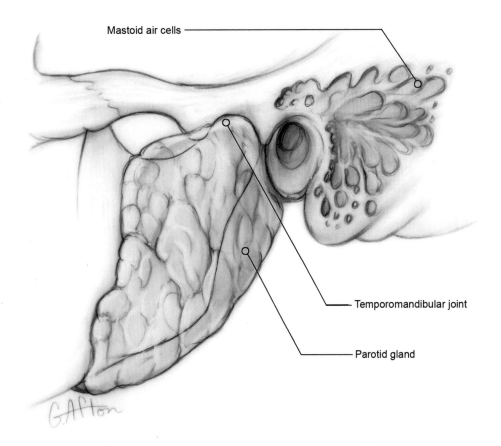

Mastoid air cells

Temporomandibular joint

Parotid gland

Figure 3 The major relationships of the meatus

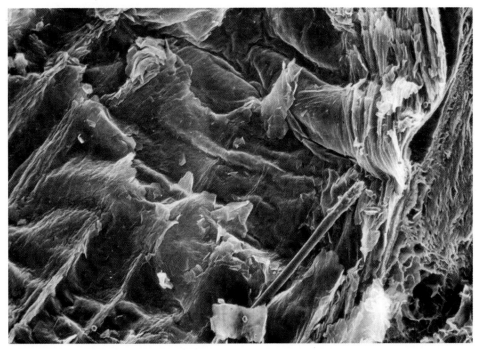

Figure 4 Scanning electron micrograph of skin of the ear canal showing its irregularity and the presence of debris

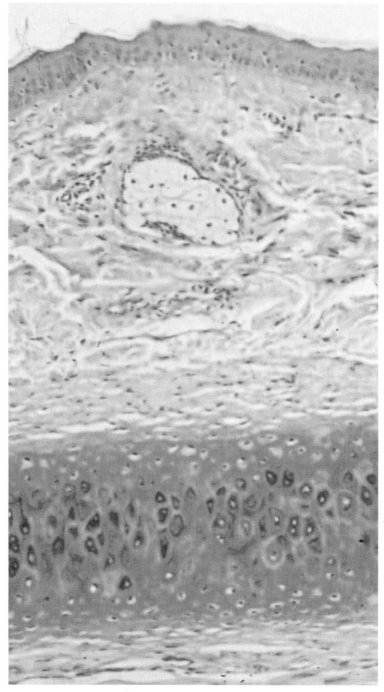

Figure 5 Light microscopy of the skin of the cartilaginous canal

humidity that are quite constant. As all skin does, it has bacteria. Changes in humidity or in pH favor the appearance of infection. As any skin it is also subject to allergic reactions which in turn can alter the local homeostasis and favor infection. When seen with a naked eye or a regular operating microscope the skin seems quite smooth, however, when seen with a scanning electron microscope one can observe that its uniformity and evenness is not so (Figure 4, histology of external ear canal). Therefore, washing and cleansing of the skin of the canal should be done thoroughly.

Skin of the Cartilaginous Canal

The skin of the cartilaginous canal (Figure 5) is tightly bound to the perichondrium (hematomas are common) where it is

relatively thick (0.5–1 mm). Due to its thickness it is preferable to inject local anesthetics at this level in a slow fashion "dissecting medially" ("blanching the ear canal"). The skin has sebaceous and ceruminous glands as well as hair follicles in the superior and posterior portion. Infections and furuncles occur here as well as tumors of the glands and skin (squamous and basocellular) (Figure 6).

Skin of the Osseous Canal

The skin is not firmly bound to the dermis (it can be de-epithelialized completely with surgical instruments) and is continuous with the external (lateral) aspect of the tympanic membrane. It is thin (0.2 mm) and has no glands or sebaceous glands (Figures 7 and 8).

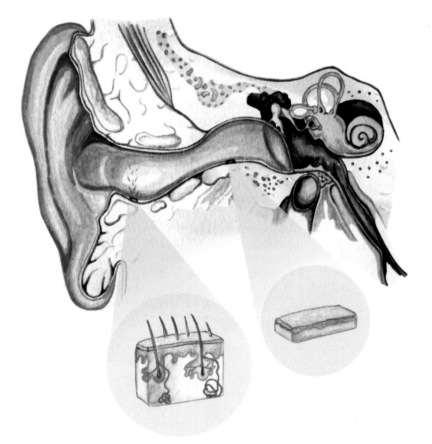

Figure 6 Thickness of the cartilaginous and bony canal skin

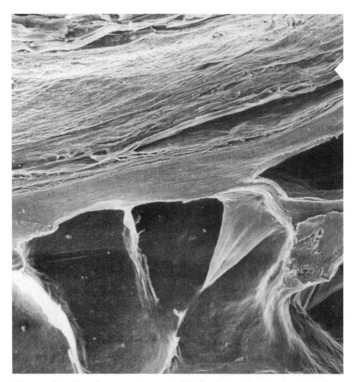

Figure 7 Scanning electron micrograph. Skin firmly bound to the dermis and not so firmly to the underlying bone of the canal located over mastoid air cells

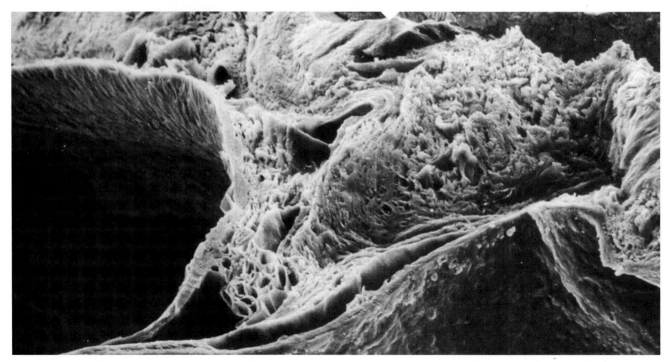

Figure 8 Scanning electron micrograph at the tympanic membrane level showing loose attachment at the level of the annulus and bony canal. This allows the surgical de-epithelialization described in the text

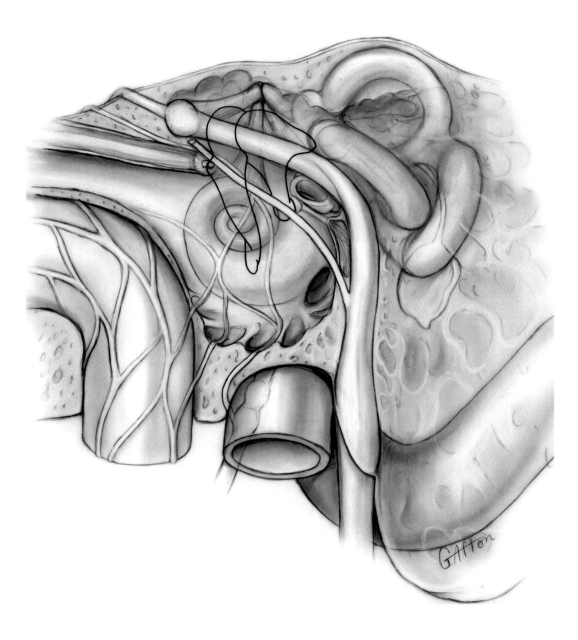

Figure 4 Composite drawing of middle and inner ear contents and major surrounding vessels

tions supplying the margins of the membrane, while the primary nerves descend from the superior aspect of the membrane and parallel the course of the external descending artery, tending to lie slightly posterior to the vessel. The pars tensa of the membrane is not particularly well supplied with sensory nerves; in contrast, the pars flaccida has an extremely rich innervation. Composite drawing of middle and inner ear contents and major surrounding vessels is shown in Figure 4.

1.4
Middle Ear and Mastoid

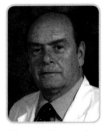

Marcos Goycoolea

THE MIDDLE EAR

The middle ear includes the tympanic cavity, the tympanic antrum (antrum mastoideum) and the Eustachian tube (auditory tube). These constitute a continuous, irregular, pneumatic cavity located within the temporal bone, between the tympanic membrane laterally and the petrous portion of the temporal bone medially. It is an oval-shaped cavity and its greatest dimensions are in the anteroposterior and vertical planes, which measure approximately 15 mm each. The transverse diameter—between the medial and lateral walls (width) varies with location and ranges from 2 mm to 6 mm. It is not a confined space but communicates anteriorly with the nasopharynx through the Eustachian tube, and posteriorly with the mastoid antrum and mastoid air cells.

The middle ear can be divided into the tympanic cavity proper, which is that portion situated medial to the tympanic membrane and the epitympanic recess, which is the upward extension of the tympanic cavity proper above the level of the tympanic membrane.

The parts to be considered are: the walls and contents of the tympanic cavity (excluding the tympanic antrum and mastoid cells), and the Eustachian tube.

The tympanic cavity is bounded by six pairs of walls facing one another that are not clearly demarcated. They are lateral, medial, anterior and posterior walls, the roof or tegmen tympani, and the floor or jugular wall.

For practical purposes the walls will be initially described separately. However, as mentioned earlier, since the middle ear (and the ear as a whole) has to be understood as a three-dimensional unit, the initial descriptions will gradually evolve into such three-dimensional concept.

1. *The lateral wall* (membranous wall) is formed for the most part by the tympanic membrane. Superiorly, within the epi-tympanic recess this wall is formed by a plate of bone (the scutum) derived from the squamous portion of the temporal bone. The head of the malleus and the body, and short process of the incus lie in the epitympanic recess (Figure 1). As will be discussed later, the anterior epitympanic space is a very troublesome area regarding cholesteatoma removal.

2. *The roof* (tegmental wall, tegmen tympani) of the middle ear consists of a thin plate of bone, the tegmen tympani, which separates the epitympanic recess from the cranial cavity (middle cranial fossa) (Figure 2). It is traversed by the petrosquamous suture, which persists into adult life in approximately 50% of the population, and by small foramina that transmit nerves and arteries.

3. *The floor or jugular wall* is a very narrow, irregular surface lying slightly below the level of the meatus and is formed by a plate of bone separating the cavity from the bulb of the internal jugular vein (Figure 3). If the bulb of the vein is small, the floor may be as much as 8–10 mm thick and may contain hypotympanic air cells. This is a point to remember

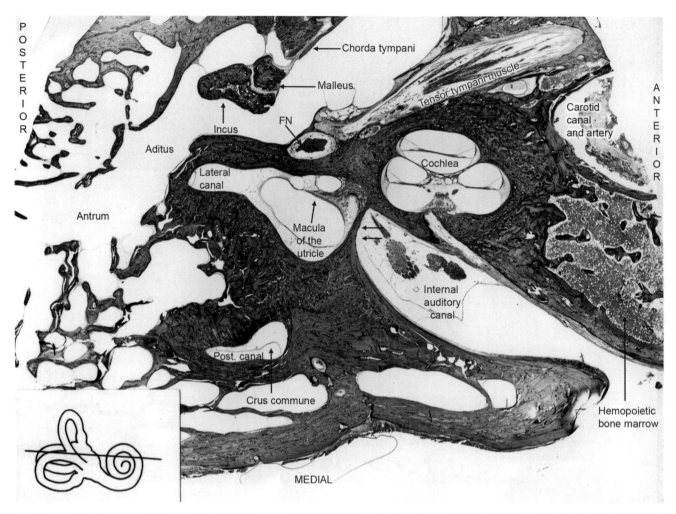

P
O
S
T
E
R
I
O
R

A
N
T
E
R
I
O
R

Chorda tympani

Malleus

Tensor tympani muscle

Carotid
canal
and artery

FN

Incus

Aditus

Cochlea

Lateral
canal

Antrum

Macula
of the
utricle

Internal
auditory
canal

Post. canal

Crus commune

Hemopoietic
bone marrow

MEDIAL

Figure 1 This section is of the area of the epitympanum. It is important to remember that the middle ear cavity extends superiorly above the tympanic membrane. The wide communication between the middle ear and mastoid can be observed as well as the close proximity of the incus and horizontal semicircular canal to the aditus and antrum

when eradicating surgically residual disease. In contrast, a large bulb may cause the floor to bulge upward into the middle ear. In such cases the floor may be imperfect, and the vessel and cavity are separated only by the mucosa of the middle ear.

This anatomical fact has to be always kept in mind when working surgically in this area and even when placing polyethylene (PE) tubes.

4. *The anterior wall or carotid wall* is a very thin bony septum separating the middle ear from the carotid canal (Figures 4 and 5). Perforations in the plate allow the transmission of nerves and vessels from the carotid to the middle ear (caroticotympanic sympathetic nerves). In our studies (Moreano, 1994), the carotid artery was found to be dehiscent in 77 (7.7%) of 1,000 human temporal bones studied. Of these 23.2% were bilateral. Microdehiscences were found in 74 (7.4%), being

bilateral in 12.3% of these paired bones. On the other hand, a thin bony coverage, without the presence of dehiscences or microdehiscences was found in 134 (15.5%) of our temporal bones. Dehiscences tend to decrease with age while microdehiscences tend to increase, thus, suggesting that at birth the carotid canal could, in many cases, be still developing.

Above the carotid canal is the site of opening of the semicanal for the tensor tympani muscle and immediately inferior to this is the tympanic opening of the auditory tube (Eustachian tube), through which the middle ear communicates with the nasopharynx. Strictly speaking, the middle ear is a cavity that is open to the outside (through the Eustachian tube), therefore, is part of the surface of the body (an invaginated part of the surface of the body).

5. *The posterior or mastoid wall* is somewhat of an inverted triangle, with the narrowest portion situated inferiorly, where it

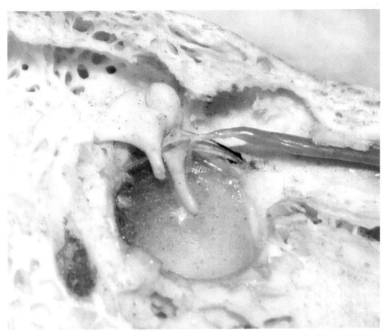

Figure 2 Human temporal bone preparation that shows the lateral wall of the middle ear. The tympanic membrane is seen from the middle ear side. The incus and head of the malleus are seen within the epitympanic space. Posterior to them (posterior wall of the middle ear) is the aditus that connects the middle ear to the mastoid cavity. Superior to them is the tegmen or roof of the middle ear. Superiorly and anteriorly, (anterior wall of the middle ear) is the tendon of the tensor tympani muscle and the muscle itself (the muscle is the only artificial element in this preparation). Inferior to the muscle is the Eustachian tube and inferior to it the carotid canal

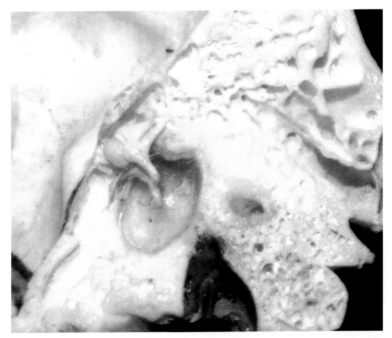

Figure 3 Human temporal bone preparation that shows the lateral wall of the middle ear. The tympanic membrane is seen from the middle ear side. The incus and head of the malleus are seen within the epitympanic space. Inferior to it (in blue) is location of the jugular bulb

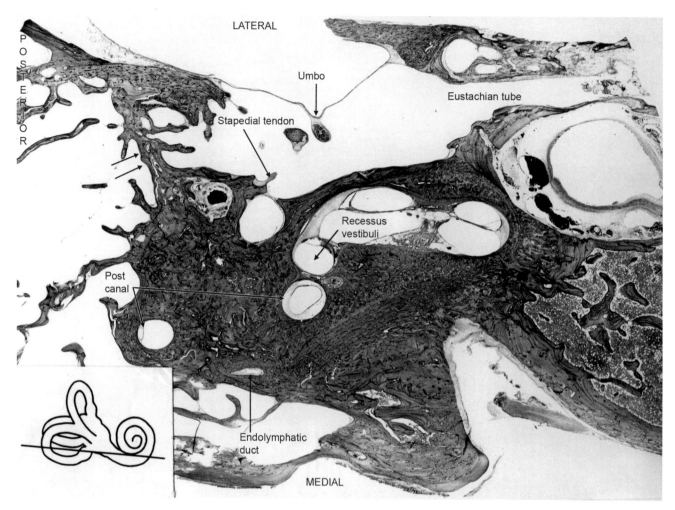

Figure 4 In this section the external ear canal and tympanic membrane can be seen at a lower level. The Eustachian tube is occupying the anterior wall. Note the proximity of the tube to the carotid artery as well as the thin plate of bone that separates both structures

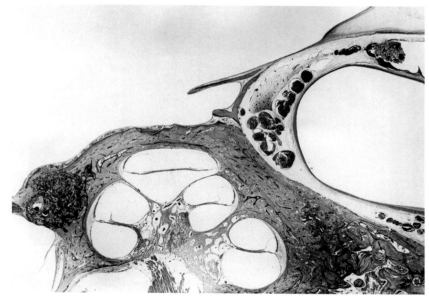

Figure 5 This section shows a focus of otosclerosis, but more importantly a dehiscent carotid artery

is related to a number of tympanic cells (to be remembered when eradicating residual disease). Superiorly, at the level of the epitympanic recess, the posterior wall is deficient (has an opening), forming the aditus, an opening through which the cavity communicates with the mastoid air cells (Figure 6). The posterior wall features can also be seen in detail in horizontal temporal bone sections.

Salient features of the posterior wall include the following:

- The pyramidal eminence, located just below the aditus. The tendon of the stapedius muscle exits at the apex of this eminence and is frequently continuous with the facial canal.
- The iter chordae tympani posterior, a small foramen immediately lateral to the pyramidal eminence. Through this foramen the chorda tympani nerve enters the middle ear.
- The posterior sinus, a small fossa just above the pyramidal eminence.
- The fossa of the incus, which is the point of attachment of the posterior ligament of the incus, situated just above the posterior sinus.

6. *The medial or labyrinthine wall*, which separates the middle ear cavity from the inner ear, is the most complex of the middle ear boundaries. Its major features are shown in Figure 7. The medial wall features can also be seen in detail in Horizontal temporal bone sections.

- The promontory, a slight elevation formed by the basal turn of the cochlea of the inner ear. Within the mucoperiosteum of its wall runs the parasympathetic plexus (Jacobson´s nerve). Extending inferiorly and posteriorly

from the promontory is a slight ridge, the subiculum. More superiorly, running from the posterior aspect of the promontory toward the pyramidal eminence, is a second ridge, the ponticulus. The subiculum and the ponticulus create three small depressions on the posterior part of the tympanic sinus and the fossa of the oval window.

- Posteroinferior to the promontory is the fossula fenestrae cochleae (cochlear fossa or round window niche). This is the lowest of the three depressions of the medial wall. It is bounded superiorly by the subiculum and is the site of the round window in which the membrane is located. The membrane may or may not be visible depending on the size and configuration of the promontory and subiculum. Anteroinferior to the round window niche is located an air cell of variable size, which when well developed can be confused with the round window niche. This can result in problems when trying to insert cochlear implant electrodes.
- The tympanic sinus occupies the middle depression formed by the subiculum and the ponticulus. The extent of the sinus is variable; it may extend far enough into the petrous portion of the temporal bone to bring it into close relationship with the ampullary end of the posterior semicircular canal and the posterior end of the lateral canal.
- The fossula fenestra vestibuli (oval window or "stapes niche"), lying in the superior depression above the ponticulus. It contains the vestibular (oval) window, into which fits the footplate of the stapes that is surrounded by the annular ligament.

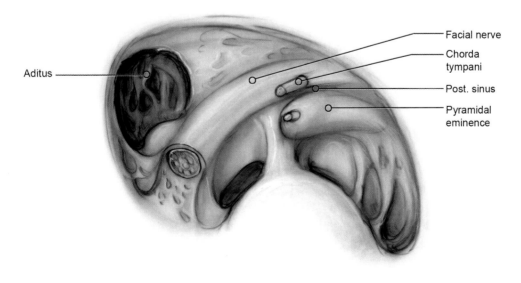

Figure 6 Posterior or mastoid wall (shape is somewhat of as inverted triangle)

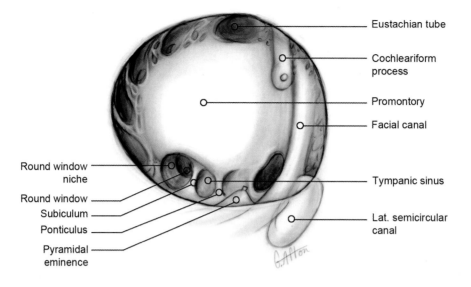

Eustachian tube

Cochleariform process

Promontory

Facial canal

Tympanic sinus

Lat. semicircular canal

Round window niche

Round window

Subiculum

Ponticulus

Pyramidal eminence

Figure 7 Medial or labyrinthine wall

• A slight bony ridge, the prominence of the lateral semi-circular canal, which lies on the posterior aspect of the medial wall in the region of the aditus and marks the anterior end of this canal.

• The prominence of the facial canal, lying above the posterior edge of the promontory and the oval window, immediately below and parallel to the prominence of the lateral (horizontal semicircular canal). This canal (through which the facial nerve courses) runs almost horizontally across the posterior half of the medial wall, then turns to enter the posterior wall. The prominence of the horizontal (lateral) semicircular canal within the aditus marks the anterior end of the facial canal. This relationship is very important to have in mind while doing a mastoidectomy. When the antrum is exposed, the surgeon must identify first and foremost the promi-nence of the horizontal (lateral) semicircular canal. This anatomical landmark will provide the position of the facial canal (which lies immediately below). "As long as you are working above the horizontal canal you are away from the facial nerve (congenital anomalies are an exception)."

• The cochleariform process, located anterosuperiorly on the medial wall. It represents the curved end of the bony semicanal of the tensor tympani muscle. It is also in close proximity to the facial canal. In this area the facial canal is dehiscent in 11.6 % of temporal bones. This is an impor-tant consideration in middle ear surgery since damage

of a dehiscent facial nerve in this area is a real possibility if the surgeon is unaware of this anatomical fact.

THE OSSICLES

" The first an Hammer call´d, whose out-growth sides
Lie on the drumme; but with his swelling end
Fixt in the hollow Stithe, there fast abides:
The Stithes short foot doth on the drumme depend,
His longer in the Stirrup surely plac´t;
But his broad base ti´d to a little window fast."

Phineas Fletcher (1633).

The first recorded descriptions of the malleus and incus are credited to Berengaris da Carpi (1522), the same year in which the city of Santiago, Chile was founded.

Bolz (1971) attributes the first description to Alessandro Achillini of Bologna. O´Malley (1961) stated that it seems pos-sible that they had been initially described by Achillini; since although no record is found it is mentioned in statements of anatomists of the sixteenth century. The first to give an accurate description of the malleus and incus was Vesalius (1543) who gave them the names of hammer and anvil.

It is interesting, and rather perplexing that the Greek fathers of anatomy did not mention the ossicles in spite of their careful dissections and accurate description. On the other hand, the stapes was not described until 1603 by Gian Filippo Ingrassia (he had recognized its existence in 1546 but did not publish his book until 1603). Ingrassia described the stapes as being two

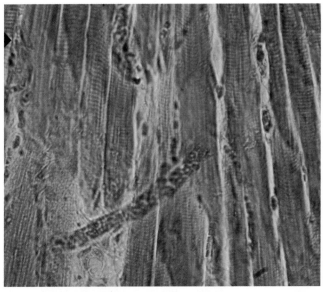

Figure 15 Striated muscle fibers of the tensor tympani

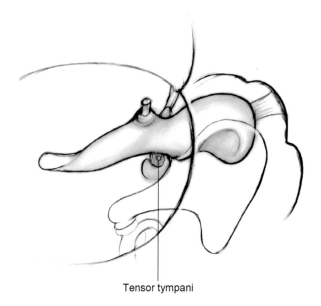

Tensor tympani

Figure 17 Tensor tympani insertion in manubrium of the malleus

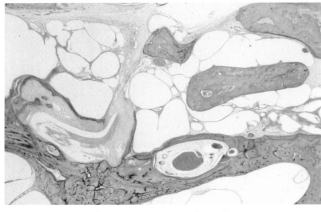

Figure 16 Insertion of the tensor tympani in the malleus

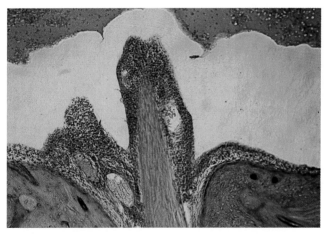

Figure 18 Stapedius muscle—striated muscle fibers—exiting toward the stapes (in a bone with otitis media)

Stapedius (Figures 18 to 20): It originates in a bony canal posteriorly and inserts on the posterior surface of the neck and posterior leg of the stapes. It is innervated by the stapedial branch of the facial nerve. This muscle serves a protective function by preventing excessive excursion of the footplate.

Microscopic Anatomy of the Auditory Ossicles, Joints and Muscles

The ossicles extend throughout the tympanic cavity in a chain-like fashion, connecting functionally the external and internal ear by uniting the tympanic membrane and the oval window.

Their structures have similarities and differences with that of other long bones in the body. They have Haversian systems, interstitial lamellae, Haversian and Volkmann canals as in compact bones, and bone marrow spaces centrally located as in long bones. They also have periosteum or fibrous connective tissue sheath. Some of the differences are that the adult size is obtained in early infancy and that they are isolated in their position in the space of the middle ear cavity, suspended by ligaments and joints, and only attached by two muscles, being

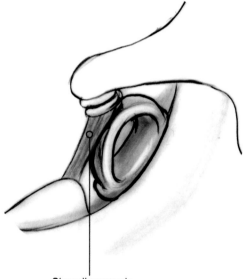

Stapedius muscle

Figure 19 Insertion of stapedius on the posterior surface of the neck and posterior leg of the stapes

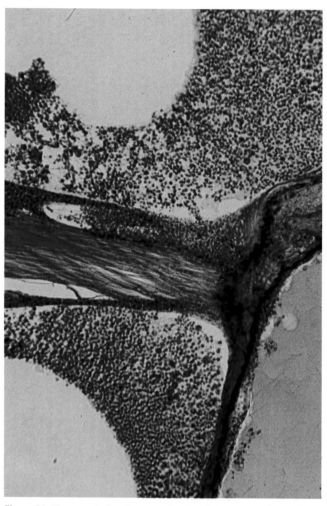

Figure 20 Photograph showing stapedius muscle insertion in the stapes (in a bone with otitis media)

thus devoid of antagonistic muscle forces. This requires special structural features (to be described).

Another unique feature of the ossicles is their complete envelopment by mucosa continuous with the middle ear. The epithelium is almost entirely squamous. Taller ciliated cells are rarely found. The connective tissue is similar to that of the middle ear mucosa. The blood supply comes from the nutrient artery (branch of the middle meningeal) that penetrates the tegmen tympani, spreading its terminals as end arteries.

The facing surfaces of the articulating portion are covered by hyaline cartilage and most of the times have a small interarticular disc. Synovial membrane folds are a rarity in these joints.

Joints are enclosed by a proportionally thick capsule. Another unique feature is the constant activity of these joints. These are perhaps phylogenetically and embryologically the oldest joints together with the vertebrals. This could partially explain the fact that elastic fibers are a prominent feature in the joints of the ossicles. It also helps us to understand the fact that there are no synchronized agonistic and antagonistic muscle forces to maintain position and correct displacements in the absence of muscle tonus. Elastic fibers could also aid in dampening vibration of the ossicles and permit the muscle pull to be more gradual and even.

MUCOSAL LINING

The tympanic cavity is lined throughout by a thin, transparent membrane (of endodermal origin) that is continuous with that of the auditory tube anteriorly and the tympanic antrum and mastoid cells posteriorly. Strictly speaking, this lining is part of the surface of the body since it is an invagination into a cavity. The purpose of this mucosa is to maintain an air filled cavity so that the middle ear can perform its function of sound transmission and amplification. That is the purpose and none other. From time to time, publications describing the gas exchange function of the middle ear mucosa appear in the literature. By evaluating the structure and microanatomy of the middle ear and mastoid, one can accept that gas diffusion must obviously occur, however, if gas exchange would be a function, the good Lord would have provided the mucosa with a different structure.

In biology, cells are built according to a plan and form part of tissues that are conformed for specific purposes. Structurally, this mucosa is not a gas exchange mucosa. The membrane is tightly bound to the periosteum, and also invests the ossicles and their associated ligaments. In reflecting from the walls of the cavity to the ossicles and their ligaments, the mucous lining forms various folds and pouches; the most important of these are the superior pouch (Prussak's pouch), situated medial to the pars flaccida of the tympanic membrane, and the anterior and posterior pouches (of von Troltsch), which are related to the anterior and posterior ligaments of malleus respectively.

This lining or mucoperiosteum consists of epithelium, connective tissue and periosteum proper (Figures 21A to C):

Epithelium

The epithelium is continuous and the distribution of the type of epithelial cells depends on their location in the mucosal lining of the middle ear and mastoid (Figures 22 to 26).

Anteriorly, towards the tympanic orifice (Eustachian tube opening) there is a respiratory epithelium (Figures 27A to E). As it turns back towards the promontory, it gradually becomes cuboidal, with occasional glands (Figures 28 to 30). The hypotympanum has tall ciliated columnar cells with some goblet cells and underlying basal cells, whereas the epitympanum has cuboidal ciliated cells with interposed small numbers of nonciliated cells. Towards the posterior wall, and aditus and antrum the epithelium consists of flat nonciliated cells devoid of glands or goblet cells. The mastoid cavity is covered by simple squamous epithelium with occasionally scattered ciliated (Figures 26A to D). Ossicles are almost entirely lined by flat nonciliated cells.

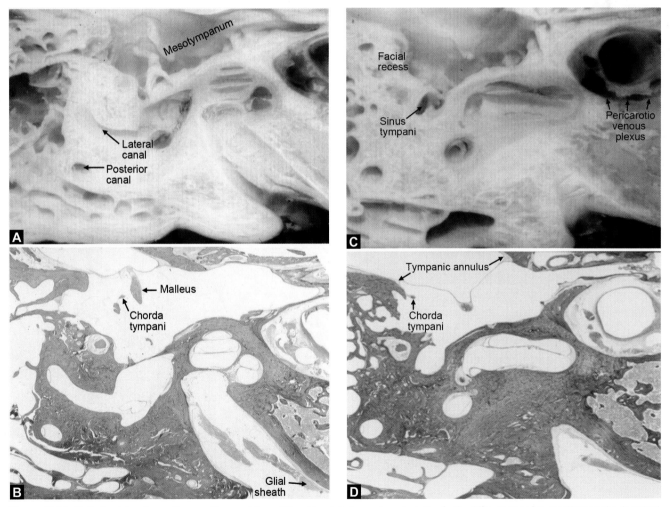

Figures 21A to D Horizontal sections of temporal bones at three different levels; to be used as orientation for the different sites of mucosal lining to be described

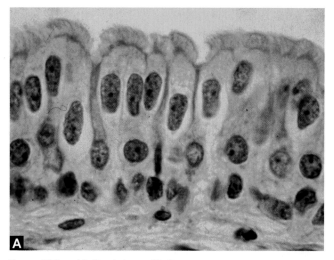

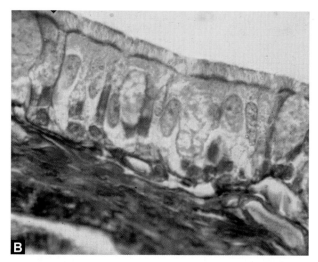

Figures 22A and B Respiratory epithelium

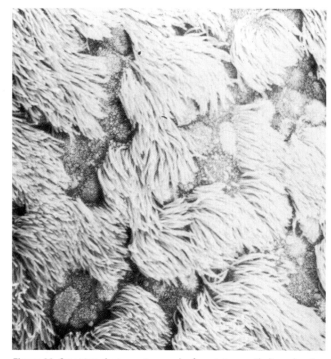

Figure 23 Scanning electron micrograph of respiratory epithelium showing its abundant cilia

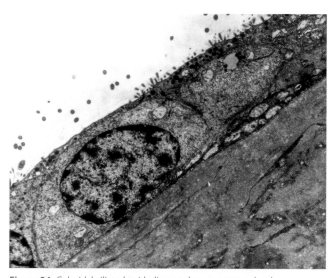

Figure 24 Cuboidal ciliated epithelium at the promontory level

Respiratory epithelium (Figures 27A to E) refers to a ciliated, pseudostratified columnar epithelium with goblet cells. Pseudostratified means that all cells are in contact with the basal lamina. This epithelium provides a moist surface because of mucus production (that is constantly renewed) and a movement of the mucus towards the nasopharynx via the Eustachian tube (mucociliary transport system).

The cells that constitute this epithelium are: ciliated, goblet (mucus secreting cells) intermediate and basal cells. These cells have a polar organization in which three surfaces of their plasma membrane have to be considered: (1) An apical surface

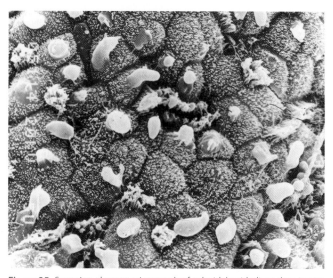

Figure 25 Scanning electron micrograph of cuboidal epithelium showing its cilia which are not as abundant as those of the respiratory epithelium

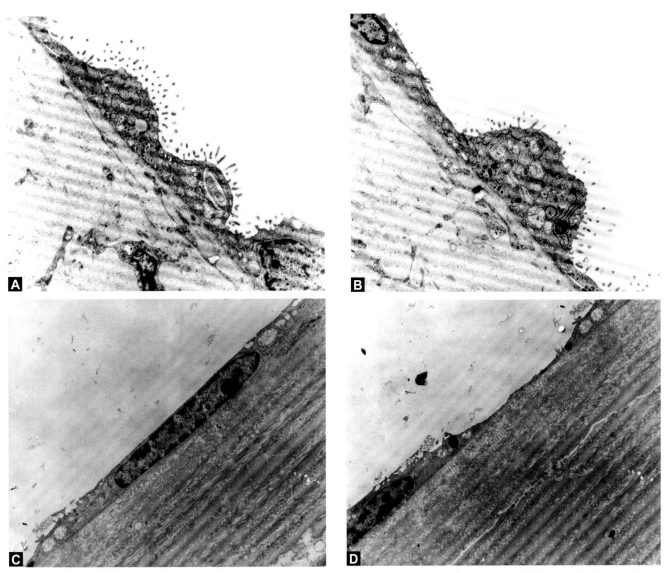

Figures 26A to D Gradual flattening of the epithelium with occasional ciliated cells initially, to become simple squamous epithelium towards the mastoid

in contact with the lumen; (2) Basal surface in contact with the basement membrane (basal lamina), and (3) Lateral surface in contact with neighboring cells (cell junctions).

The different cells of this epithelium have specific purposes. Ciliated cells have cilia that displace mucus towards the nasopharynx. Goblet cells provide the mucus with its secretory contents. Intermediate cells are not fully differentiated but capable of transforming into ciliated or goblet cells. Finally, the basal cell is the stem cell from which the other cells develop.

The basic secreting elements are (Figures 31A and B and 32A to E): glands, goblet cells and ordinary epithelial cells that show intracellular droplets. Three types of secreting cells:

(1) Mucus secretory cells with light granules (most common), (2) Dark granulated, and (3) Mixed granulated have been described. Different types represent different contents. Their discussion is beyond the scope of this Atlas.

Connective Tissue

The connective tissue of the middle ear and mastoid is continuous. In fact, the connective tissue of the entire body is continuous. Of mesodermal origin; the mesenchyme (mesos: middle; enchyma: infusion) joins mechanically the different elements of the mucoperiosteum, establishes a fluid space, and contains vessels, nerves and cells (Figures 33 to 36).

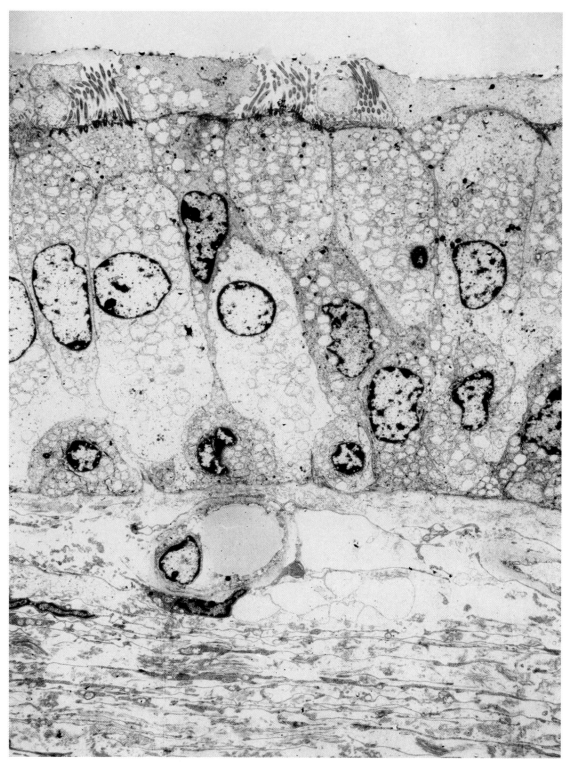

Figure 27A

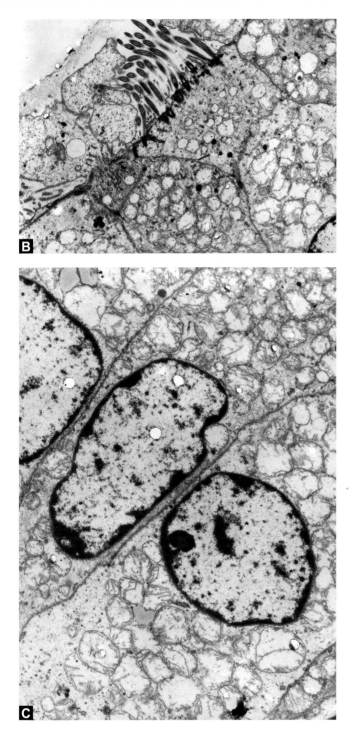

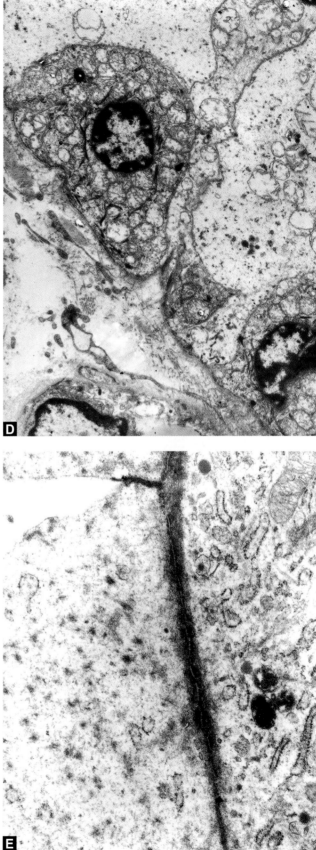

Figures 27B to E

Figures 27A to E (A) Electron micrograph of respiratory epithelium; (B) Ciliated cell; (C) Secretory cell; (D) Basal cell; (E) Cell junction

The most common cells are the fibroblasts (that maintain the fiber system and are seemingly capable of performing other functions) and the cells of the defense system (lymphocytes, neutrophils, plasma cells and mast cells) (Figures 34A and 35).

Macrophages are also present. Mast cells containing histamine and serotonin suggest vasoactive substances that could influence and increase permeability of vessels (Figure 36). Furthermore, macrophages, plasma cells and lymphocytes suggest immunological involvement of the middle ear (immunological aspects will be described in the otitis media section).

Capillaries are also found in this layer. Forming a definite layer around the endothelium are the basement membrane and pericytes. There are nerve fibers (myelinated and unmyelinated) and towards the labyrinthine capsule, a layer of osteoblasts. The stroma is a loose connective tissue with scattered bundles of collagen fibers and few elastic fibers (Figure 34B).

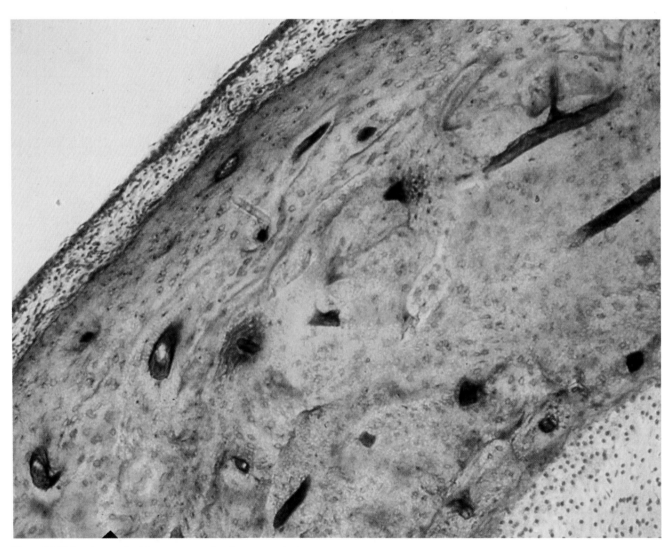

Figure 28 Light micrograph of the promontory lined by mucoperiosteum

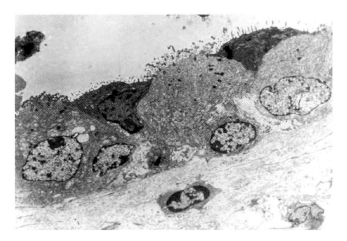

Figure 29 Electron micrograph of promontory epithelium with light and dark cells

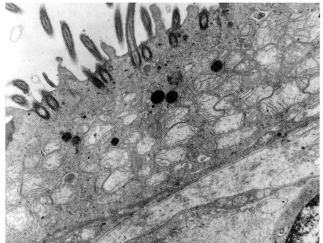

Figure 30 Ciliated cell of the promontory

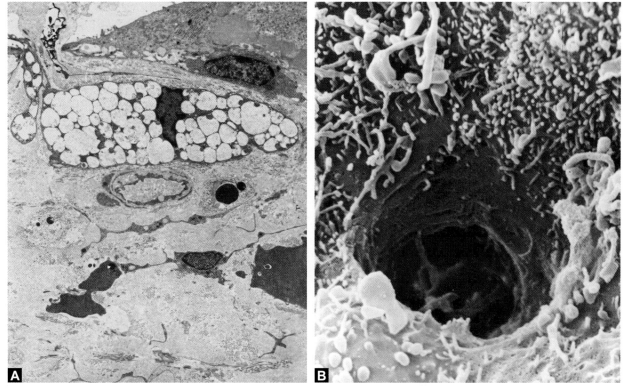

Figures 31A and B (A) Gland; (B) Scanning electron micrograph showing gland opening toward the surface

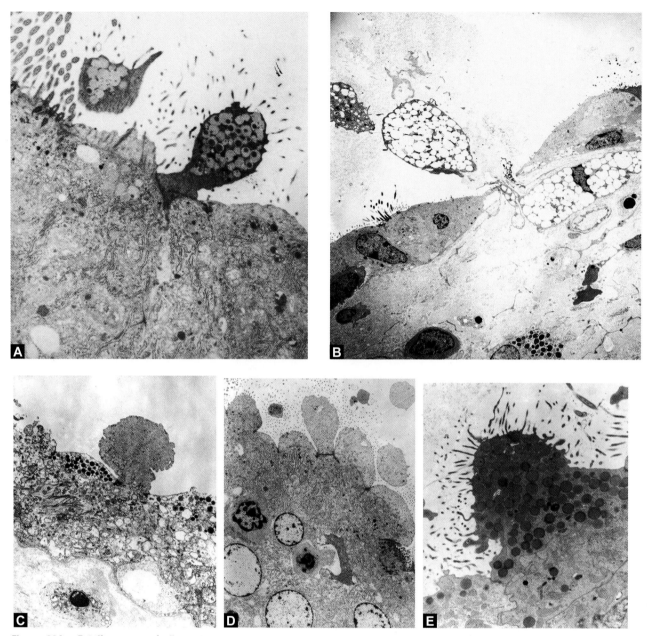

Figures 32A to E Different types of cell secretion

Periosteum

With the exception of the tympanic membrane, Eustachian tube, and round window membrane, the middle ear and mastoid are surrounded by bone which is periosteum, facing the connective tissue layer.

Eustachian Tube—The Auditory (Pharyngotympanic or Eustachian) Tube

The auditory tube extends from its tympanic ostium within the anterior wall of the middle ear cavity to its pharyngeal ostium within the nasopharynx. The latter is situated just posterior to the dorsal end of the inferior nasal concha. In the adult the tube is between 30 mm and 40 mm in length, and has a slight S-shaped configuration as it passes obliquely downward, medial and anterior from the middle ear to the pharynx.

The tympanic ostium is roughly 25 mm higher than the pharyngeal ostium in the adult. There are some basic and sig-nificant morphologic differences between the auditory tube of the child and that of the adult; in the child the tube is shorter and relatively wider and more horizontally situated.

Structurally, the auditory tube consists of both cartilaginous and bony components. The bony portion makes up approximately two-thirds of the tube; it is widest at the tympanic orifice

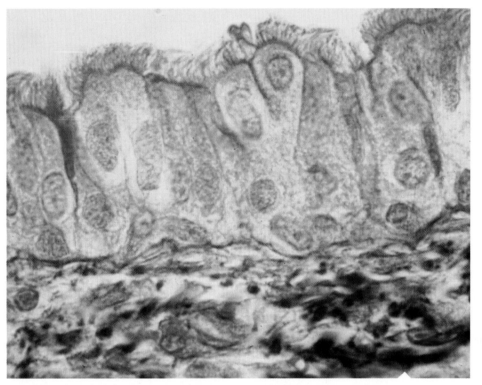

Figure 33 Collagen fibers in the connective tissue layer stained blue with Azan

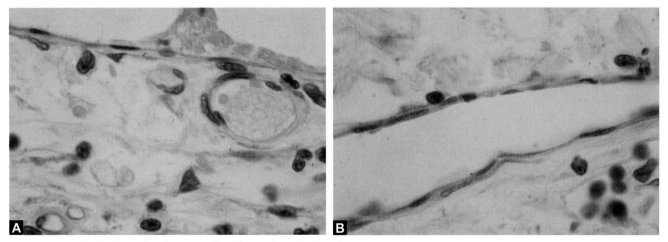

Figures 34A and B Blood vessels with pericytes, fibroblasts and round cells in the connective tissue

and gradually narrows throughout its length, with its anterior extremity (the isthmus) the most constricted portion of the entire tube (Figure 37). In its course the bony tube is lateral to the carotid canal and superior to the jugular fossa. The cartilaginous portion of the tube extends from the isthmus to the nasopharynx. It is not totally cartilaginous, however; its lower lateral and inferior walls consist of fibrous connective tissue overlying the tensor and levator veli palatini muscles.

The lumen of the auditory tube, in the resting state, is a closed, slit-like cavity. The pharyngeal end of the tube strongly resists passage of air from the pharynx to the middle ear. Passage from the tympanic cavity to the pharynx is much easier.

The Eustachian tube is lined by respiratory epithelium and in addition to the opening function of the tensor veli palatine muscle there is seemingly some role of a surfactant (Figure 38). The respiratory epithelium with its cilia and mucus secretion constitute the mucociliary transport system of the middle ear (Figure 39).

VASCULAR ELEMENTS OF THE MIDDLE EAR

The middle ear receives blood via a number of small arteries (Figures 40A and B), which with one exception are derived from the external carotid or its branches. They include:

- The anterior tympanic, a branch of the maxillary artery. It is distributed to the anterior part of the cavity, including the medial surface of the tympanic membrane and enters the middle ear by passing through the petrotympanic fissure.
- The stylomastoid branch of either the posterior auricular or occipital artery. This artery enters the facial canal and gives rise to the posterior tympanic artery, which then enters the middle ear in company with the chorda tympani nerve.
- The inferior tympanic artery, derived from the ascending pharyngeal branch of the external carotid. It accompanies

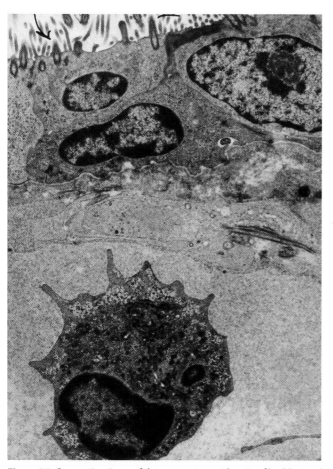

Figure 35 Connective tissue of the promontory with active fibroblast and polymorphonuclear cell

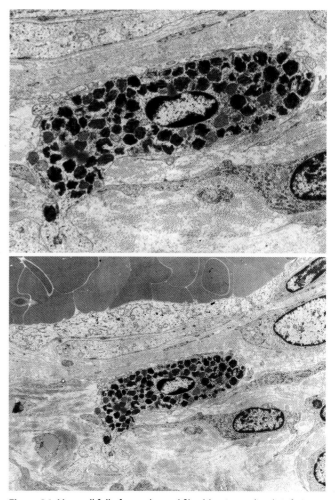

Figure 36 Mast cell full of granules and fibroblast immediately inferior to it. Connective tissue layer of promontory mucoperiosteum

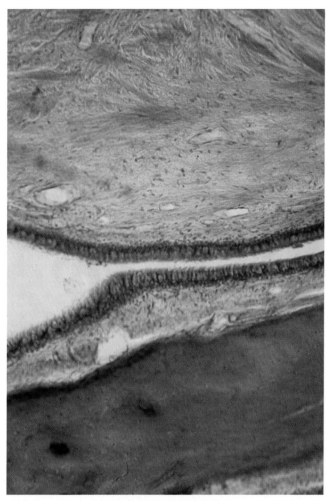

Figure 37 Middle ear opening of the Eustachian tube

the tympanic branch of nerve IX through the tympanic canaliculus to gain the middle ear cavity.

- The superficial petrosal and superior tympanic arteries, which are both branches of the middle meningeal artery. The former runs through the facial canal for a short distance, and then pierces the tegmen tympani to enter the middle ear; the latter enters through the petrosquamous fissure.
- The caroticotympanic arteries arise from the internal carotid as it passes through the carotid canal and enter the middle ear by passing through the thin bony lamina separating the carotid canal from the middle ear.

Although there is an embryonic stapedial artery that usually disappears at the third month of gestation, in some cases it persists and this has importance because of potential injury during surgical procedures, especially in cases of stapedectomy (Figure 41).

In our studies of 1,045 human temporal bones we found a prevalence of five cases (0.48%), all of them unilateral.

The veins of the middle ear parallel the arteries. They are tributary to the superior petrosal dural sinus and the pterygoid plexus of veins.

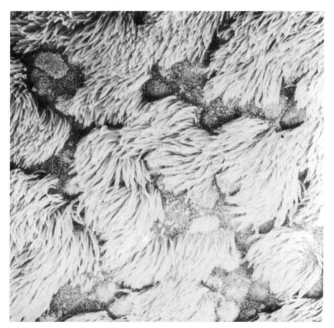

Figure 39 Scanning electron micrograph of cilia of the Eustachian tube

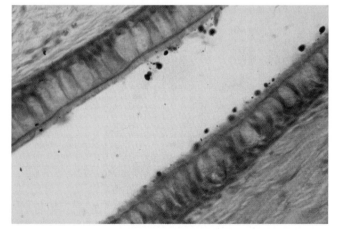

Figure 38 Mid portion of the tube lined by respiratory epithelium

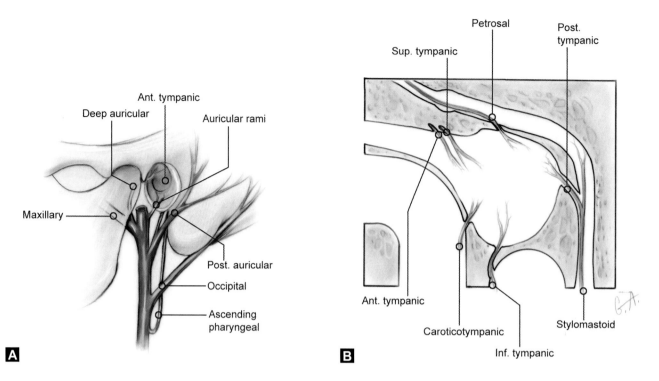

A

B

Figures 40A and B Blood supply of the middle ear

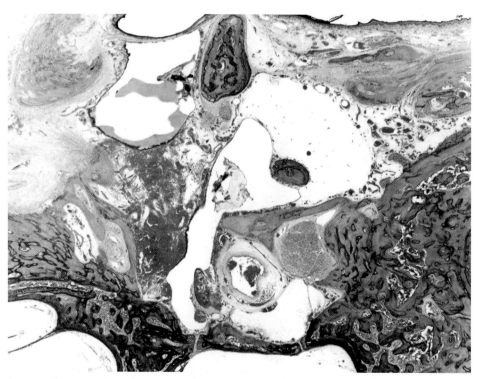

Figure 41 This section shows the presence of a persistent stapedial artery immediately medial to the footplate in a middle ear with thickened mucosa and a dehiscent facial nerve. This persistence (representing persistence of the embryonal artery) is rare and should not be confused with a normal small arterial branch that crosses the footplate. Adequate visualization and careful dissection are crucial when exploring an ear with chronic disease

NERVES OF THE MIDDLE EAR

The major nerve of the middle ear is the tympanic branch of the glossopharyngeal nerve (Jacobson's nerve) (Figure 42). Arising from the inferior ganglion of the parent trunk, the tympanic nerve enters the tympanic canaliculus through a small foramen located on the crest of the thin plate of bone separating the jugular foramen and the external orifice of the carotid canal. Once in the middle ear, the nerve forms the tympanic plexus within the mucosa overlying the promontory. There are two modalities represented in the tympanic nerve/plexus. The great majority of the fibers are sensory; these are distributed to the mucosa of the middle ear, the mastoid air cells and the auditory tube. The remaining fibers are parasympathetic and have no function in the middle ear. Instead, they emerge from the upper border of the plexus to pierce the tegmen tympani and run forward on the floor of the middle cranial fossa as the lesser petrosal nerve; ultimately they leave the skull to run with the auriculotemporal branch of V3 and supply the parotid gland. The middle ear receives sympathetic fibers derived from the internal carotid plexus. These fibers, which enter the middle ear along with the caroticotympanic arteries, are primarily associated with the vessels of the cavity and have a vasoconstrictive effect.

The chorda tympani branch of the facial nerve enters the middle ear through the iter chordae posterius, passes forward and down between the manubrium of the malleus and the long process of the incus, then leaves the cavity by passing through the petrotympanic suture. The chorda tympani has no function in the middle ear. It contains both parasympathetic fibers supplying the submandibular and sublingual glands, and taste fibers for the anterior two-thirds of the tongue. After leaving the middle ear it joins the lingual branch of V3 to be distributed with that nerve.

Although they do not enter the middle ear, the nerves to the muscles associated with the ossicles must be mentioned since they are vital to normal function. The nerve to the stapedius muscle is a branch of the facial nerve and arises from the parent trunk as it descends through the vertical portion of the osseous facial canal. The nerve to the tensor tympani is a branch of the mandibular division of the trigeminal nerve.

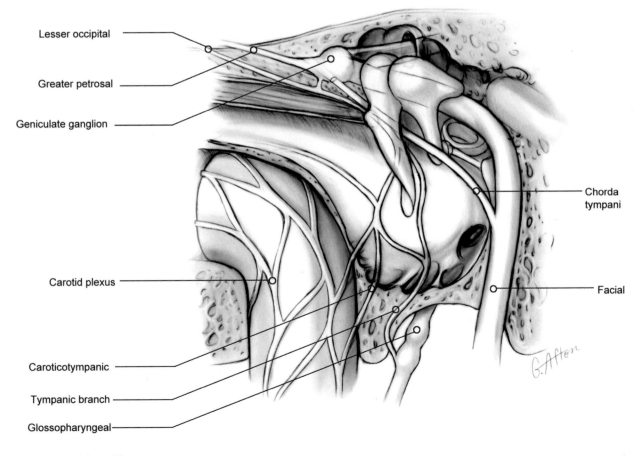

Lesser occipital

Greater petrosal

Geniculate ganglion

Chorda tympani

Carotid plexus

Facial

Caroticotympanic

Tympanic branch

Glossopharyngeal

Figure 42 Nerves of the middle ear

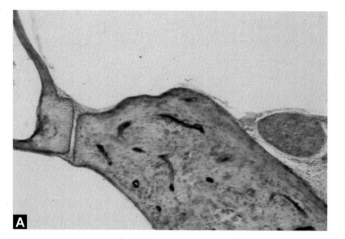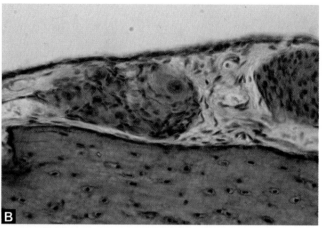

Figures 43A and B Ganglion cells anterior to the stapes

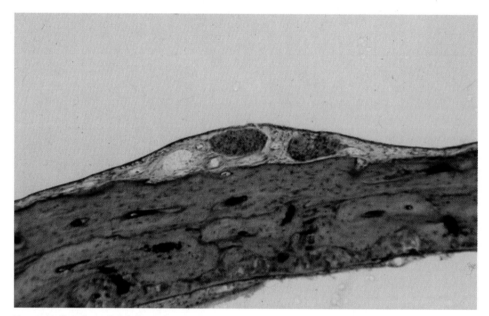

Figure 44 Ganglion cells inferior to the stapes

Ganglia and Ganglion Cells in the Middle Ear

Ganglia and ganglion cells are not isolated findings in the middle ear. Gasser has reported ganglion cells in the promontory of humans both anterior to the stapes and below (Figures 43 and 44). We have confirmed these findings in our studies of temporal bones, as well as the finding of ganglion cells in the course of the lesser superficial petrosal nerve and in the perimysium of the tensor tympani. In addition we described for the first time, the presence of ganglion cells proximal and lateral to the muscle fibers of the tensor tympani (Figures 45A and B). This rich innervation leaves a number of interesting possibilities concerning the pathophysiology and treatment of effusions where these nerve elements could be playing key roles. Interestingly, ganglion cells have also been reported in the vertical portion of the facial nerve (Figures 46A to C). Despite the fact that their functional significance has not been established, these structures are mentioned and described because eventually their knowledge and understanding could be important for treatment.

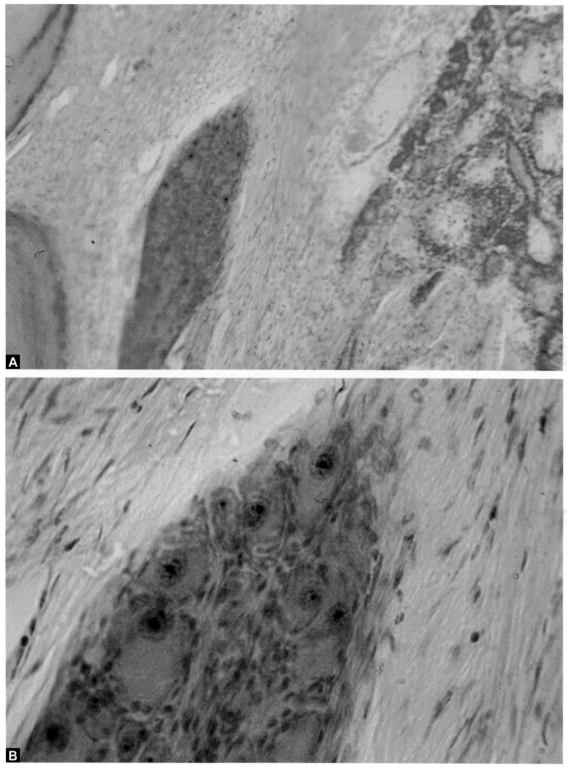

Figures 45A and B Ganglion cells proximal to the muscle fibers of the tensor tympani

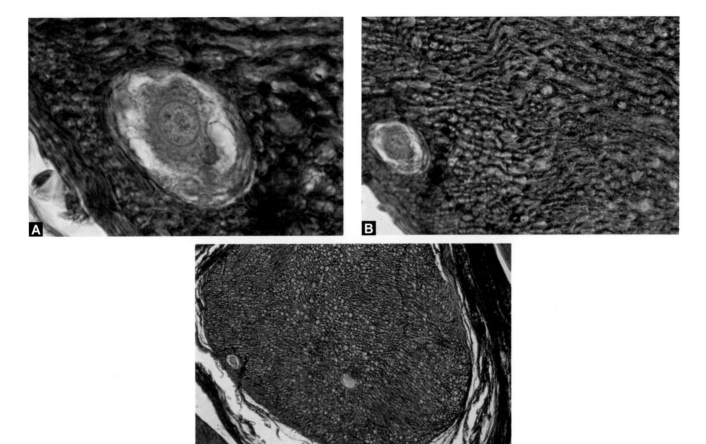

Figures 46A to C Ganglion cells in the vertical portion of the facial nerve

PNEUMATIZATION OF THE TEMPORAL BONE

The temporal bone exhibits varying degrees of pneumatization. Due to intimate relationship of the middle ear to these areas, a basic appreciation of the location and extent of pneumatized areas is desirable.

Since the mastoid process develops from both petrous and squamous portions of the temporal bone, there is a sutural line between the two components that is normally obliterated with growth. Occasionally, however, a heavy plate of bone persists between the two portions, forming what has been designated Korner's septum or the "false bottom." The existence of this septum can cause confusion in surgical approaches through the mastoid process.

The mastoid process is rather consistently pneumatized (80%), the process usually being completed by the third or fourth year. There is, however, considerable variation both in its extent and in the arrangement of the air cells. Due to this variation, several types are described, including the pneuma-

tized, in which the entire process is occupied by air cells; the diploic, in which the process is occupied by bone marrow instead of air cells; the mixed type, consisting of a combination of the pneumatized and diploic types; and the sclerotic or non-pneumatized/nondiploic process. Owing to the considerable variation in the extent and location of the mastoid cells, several terminologies have been used. The position of the sigmoid sinus in the posterior cranial fossa will influence markedly the position or occurrence of all types.

Mastoid air cells may invade adjacent areas of the temporal bone. Some of the more frequent extensions form the hypotympanic cells, which lie in the plate of bone separating the middle ear cavity from the jugular bulb and the epitympanic cells, which are extensions into the roof of the middle ear. The latter group may be extensive enough to include cells that will invade the root of the zygomatic arch and the squamous portion of the temporal bone.

The petrous apex of the temporal bone (i.e. that part of the petrous portion anterior to the labyrinth) may also be pneumatized, particularly by outgrowths from the tympanic cavity.

These cells, the petrous apex cells, are necessarily related to the auditory tube and the carotid canal.

THE FACIAL NERVE IN THE TEMPORAL BONE

The surgical anatomy of the facial nerve will be described in detail in the section related to facial nerve surgery and also in the section dedicated to temporal bone procedures. This section is only dedicated to overall gross anatomy and histology. After traversing the internal acoustic meatus and passing through the lateral end of that structure, the facial nerve enters the bony facial canal (Fallopian canal). This canal continues laterally for a short distance and brings the facial nerve to just above the base of the cochlea, where it makes a sharp turn (the external genu) to run posteriorly. The genu is also the site of the geniculate ganglion of the nerve, which contains the cell bodies of the nerve's sensory components. The genu and the ganglion are anterolateral to the superior semicircular canal and between the vestibule of the inner ear and the cochlea, and can be easily localized from the middle ear as a point situated just medial to the tip of the cochleariform process. Continuing posteriorly with a slight inferolateral inclination, the bony canal forms the prominence of the facial canal on the medial wall of the middle ear. This prominence may be large enough to partially cover the oval window and the base of the stapes. The lateral wall of the canal in this part is extremely thin and may be dehiscent (to be described).

In our studies of 1,000 human temporal bones belonging to the temporal bone laboratory (Moreano 1994; Edwin Moreano was a senior medical student rotating with me at the laboratory at that time) we found a prevalence of at least one facial canal dehiscence in 560 (56%) bones and there was a 76.3% bilaterality of this canal gap. Just as was in the case of carotid canal dehiscences, there is predominance in younger population, supporting the concept that the facial canal itself is still forming at birth (Nager 1982, Anson 1963). There were nine cases (0.9%) in which the entire horizontal segment of the facial canal was dehiscent. The most common site of dehiscence was the oval window area (73.5%) (Figures 47 to 50). Behind the base of the pyramidal eminence the canal makes a broad turn to descend vertically and somewhat laterally through the mastoid process. In this descending or vertical portion the nerve may have a slight anterior concavity. Relative to the exterior of the skull, the canal normally lies deep to the sutural groove between the tympanic and mastoid portions of the temporal bone. It should be remembered that there may be marked deviation from this "normal" position, in which case the canal is usually situated more posteriorly.

In its course from the brainstem through the facial canal the facial nerve is supplied with blood by small arteries derived from the anteroinferior cerebellar branch of the basilar artery, the stylomastoid or occipital branches of the external carotid and the petrosal arteries. There are apparently no anastomoses between the labyrinthine blood supply and these arteries, which seem to anastomose freely with one another. Insufficiency of the vascular supply to the facial nerve, from whatever cause, is regarded by some as one of the primary causes of Bell's palsy.

The tensor tympani area was the site of dehiscence in 11.6%, at the genu it was 12%, and at the rest of the horizontal and vertical segment was 1.4% and 1.6% respectively. Bilaterality was 76.3%, constituting the rule rather than the exception. All these observations have important implications in relationship to surgical procedures in the oval window area (stapedectomy and otitis media procedures) and also in cases of chronic otitis media in the area of the tensor tympani where cholesteatomas usually lodge. This area is the most commonly injured (traumatic iatrogenic facial nerve paralysis) in chronic otitis media surgery. Facial nerve dehiscences also explain cases of facial paralysis associated with acute otitis media (which require drainage and NOT observation) and also explain these cases at times when a local anesthetic is injected and traverses towards the middle ear. In these cases one has to wait until the effect wears off (hours). Unfortunately, at times, the anesthetic also reaches the round window membrane, traverses to the inner ear and results in severe vertigo which, at times, require an overnight stay. Finally, the finding that bilaterality occurs in 76.3% of cases provides a clear warning in cases of dehiscence when a second ear is also to be explored.

ROUND WINDOW MEMBRANE

The structure, function and permeability of the round window membrane will be described in Section VI in relationship to middle and inner ear interaction and surgery for cochlear implants.

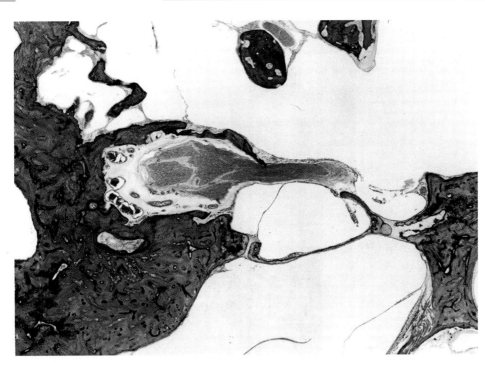

Figure 47 This section at the level of the footplate shows a dehiscent and bulging facial nerve over the stapes crura (the most common area of dehiscence). This photomicrograph serves as a reminder of the importance of thorough visualization before any drastic procedures are performed. The facial nerve can be dehiscent in other areas as well, such as adjacent to the tensor tympani, in the facial recess and in the medial wall of the anterior epitympanic recess. A dehiscent nerve can result in facial paresis or paralysis in cases of acute otitis media, and represents a potential complication in otologic surgical procedures

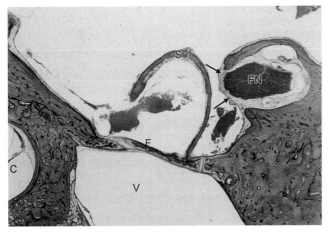

Figure 48 Facial nerve dehiscence at the level of the oval window

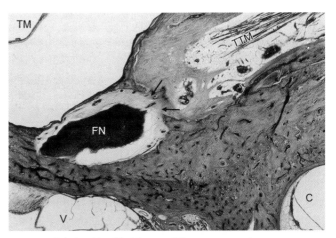

Figure 49 Relationship of facial nerve with tensor tympani

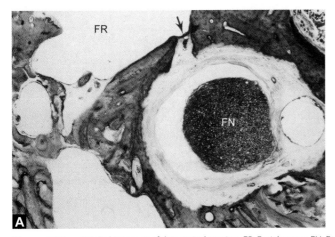

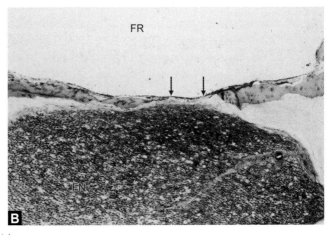

Figures 50A and B Dehiscences of the vertical portion. FR: Facial recess; FN: Facial nerve

BIBLIOGRAPHY

1. Anson BJ, Donaldson JA. Surgical anatomy of the temporal bone and ear. Philadelphia: WB Saunders Co.; 1973.

2. Anson BJ, Harper DG, Warpeha RL. Surgical anatomy of the facial canal and facial nerve. Ann Otol Rhinol Laryngol. 1963;72:713-34.

3. Gasser RF. The development of the facial nerve in man. Ann Chir Cervicofac. 1967;76:37-41.

4. Goycoolea MV. Pathogenesis of Otitis Media. Dissertations Abst Int. 1978;39(6):132-210.

5. Goycoolea MV, Paparella MM, Carpenter AM. Ganglia and ganglion cell in the middle ear of the cat. Archives Otol. 1980;106:269-71.

6. Goycoolea MV, Paparella MM, Juhn SK, et al. The cells involved in the middle ear defence system. Ann Otol. 1980;68(Suppl 89):121-8.

7. Goycoolea MV, Paparella MM, Carpenter AM. Ganglia and ganglion cells in the middle ear of the human and of the cat. Archives Otol. 1982;108:276-8.

8. Goycoolea MV. Pertinent histology in surgical otology. Atlas of Otologic Surgery. In: Goycoolea MV, Paparella MM (Eds). Philadelphia: WB Saunders Co; 1989. pp. 23-7.

9. Goycoolea MV. The normal mucosal lining of the middle ear cavity. Proceedings Upper Respiratory Tract Mucosa. Tromso, Norway; 1994.

10. Goycoolea MV, Larrea R. Embryology of the ear. In: De Souza C, Goycoolea MV, Ruah CB (Eds). Textbook of the Ear, Nose and Throat. Madras, India: Orient Longman Co; 1995. pp. 1-3.

11. Goycoolea MV, Martinez G, Martinez G. Anatomy of the ear. In: De Souza C, Goycoolea MV, Ruah CB (Eds). Textbook of the Ear, Nose and Throat. Madras, India: Orient Longman Co; 1995. pp. 4-19.

12. Goycoolea MV, Aburto R, Hess JC, et al. Neuroanatomy And physiology of the ear. In: De Souza C, Goycoolea MV, Ruah CB (Eds). Textbook of the Ear Nose and Throat. Madras, India: Orient Longman Co; 1995. pp. 19-23.

13. Hentzer E. Ultrastructure of the noremal mucosa in the human middle ear, mastoid cavities and Eustachian tube. Ann Otol. 1972;79:825-33.

14. Holmgren G. Recherches experimentales sur les functions de la trompe dÉustache. Communication prealable. Acta Otol. 1934;20:381-7.

15. Lim DJ, Shimada T. Secretory activity of normal middle ear epithelium. Ann Otol. 1971;80:319-29.

16. Lim DJ. Functional morphology of the mucosa of the middle ear and Eustachian tube. Ann Otol. 1976;85(Suppl 25):36-43.

17. Mogi G. Secretory IgA and antibody activities in middle ear effusions. Ann Otol. 1976;65:97-102.

18. Moreano E, Paparella MM, Zelterman D, Goycoolea MV. Prevalence of facial canal dehiscence and of persistent stapedial artery in the human middle ear: a report of 1000 temporal. Laryngoscope. 1994;104:309-20.

19. Moreano E, Paparella MM, Zelterman D, Goycoolea MV. Prevalence of carotid canal dehiscence in the human middle ear: a report of 1000 temporal bones. Laryngoscope. 1994;104:612-8.

20. Nager GT, Proctor B. Anatomical variations and anomalies involving the facial canal. Ann Otolrhinol Laryngol. 1982;91(Suppl 93):61-77.

21. Paparella MM, Lamey S, Goycoolea MV. Histology and pathology of the ear. In: Paparella MM, Shumrick DA (Eds). Otolaryngology. Philadelphia: WB Saunders Co; 1991. pp. 419-38.

22. Proctor B. Surgical anatomy of the ear and temporal bone. New York: Thieme; 1989.

23. Sade J, Alufa I. Middle ear mucosa. Arch Otol. 1966;84:137-43.

24. Sade J. Ciliary activity and middle ear clearance. Arch Otol. 1967;86:128-35.

25. Scuknecht HF. Pathology of the Ear. Philadelphia: Lea and Febiger; 1993.

26. Tos M, Bak-Pedersen. Goblet cell density in Eustachian tube of children. Arch Otol. 1976;102:20-6.

27. Tos M. Production of mucus in the middle ear and Eustachian tube. Ann Otol. 1974;83:44-58.

1.5.1
Inner Ear Structure

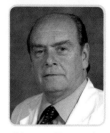

Marcos Goycoolea

The inner ear containing the essential cochlear and vestibular mechanisms, lies within the petrous portion of the temporal bone, the hardest bone in the body. The labyrinth of the inner ear is surrounded by the bony otic capsule, which is a unique structure for several reasons. It is formed from 14 separate centers of ossification that fuse, leaving no sutural lines. These centers, though formed from cartilage, retain no areas of chondral growth. In addition, the bone of the capsule retains its fetal character, that is, a typical Haversian system never develops. Finally, the capsule's maximum dimensions are attained by the fifth week of intrauterine life.

The labyrinth of the inner ear is divided into osseous and membranous components. The osseous labyrinth, a system of bony canals within the otic capsule, consists of three parts:

1. The vestibule, which forms the central portion of the labyrinth; it is relatively large, ovoid space approximately 4 mm in diameter. Its characteristic features include the following:
   - The elliptical recess, located on the floor of the vestibule. It receives the anterior end of the utricular portion of the membranous labyrinth.
   - The spherical recess, located anterior and slightly inferior to the elliptical recess. It is the site of the saccular portion of the membranous labyrinth.
   - The vestibular window, within the lateral wall of the vestibule.
   - Small orifices for the passage of nerves to the vestibular portion of the inner ear. These are found on the medial wall and adjacent floor, where the vestibule abuts on the lateral end of the internal acoustic meatus.

2. The semicircular canals, which are continuous with the vestibule. The anterior (superior) canal forms the arcuate eminence on the bony floor of the middle cranial fossa. The posterior canal has no externally located landmarks associated with it. The lateral canal, as mentioned above, creates a prominence in the region of the aditus of the middle ear. As will be seen, this is an important pointer in mastoid surgery. All of the semicircular canals communicate with the vesti-

bule through both of their crura. There are only five openings into the vestibule, however, since the posterior crus of the anterior canal and the superior crus of the posterior canal unite to form a single crus.

The canals have very definite planes of orientation. The anterior is situated in the vertical plane at an angle of 45° with respect to the sagittal plane of the skull, the posterior crura being more medial. The posterior canal is also in the vertical plane, at 45° with respect to the sagittal plane of the skull (that is, at 90° with respect to the plane of the anterior canal). The lateral canal forms an angle of approximately 30° with the horizontal plane, its anterior end being highest, and is situated in the angle between the anterior and posterior canals.

3. The cochlea, a cone-shaped, hollow, bony spiral of about two and three quarters turns with a relatively broad base and a pointed apex or cupula. Its base lies against the anteromedial surface of the vestibule and the lateral end of the internal auditory meatus. Part of the basal turn of the cochlea forms the promontory of the middle ear. From its base the axis of the cochlea is directed anterolaterally and slightly upward.

The central bony core of the cochlea is the modiolus, through which nerves and vessels travel to attain the structures of the cochlea. From the outer surface of the modiolus the osseous spiral lamina projects into the cavity of the cochlea, partially subdividing the duct. It terminates at the cupular end of the cochlea by projecting slightly beyond the apex of the modiolus. This projecting bony process of the lamina is the hamulus.

By convention, and for ease of reference and description, the cochlea is described as if it were sitting on its base with the apex pointing directly up. Viewed in this orientation, it can be seen that the spiral lamina is initiating the division of the cochlear duct into an upper chamber, the scala vestibuli and a lower chamber, the scala tympani. Only the scala vestibuli communicates with the vestibule of the inner ear; it also communicates with the scala tympani at the apex of the duct. The scala tympani ends blindly at the round window (secondary tympanic membrane) of the middle ear.

The osseous labyrinth is not a closed chamber; there are several areas of communication with the exterior. These include the following:

- The vestibular aqueduct, extending through the otic capsule from the vestibule to the posterior cranial fossa. Its cranial end lies lateral to the internal acoustic meatus on the posterior surface of the petrous portion of the temporal bone, where it is usually overlaid by a scale of bone. This aqueduct transmits the endolymphatic duct and an accompanying vein.
- The cochlear aqueduct, which begins in the scala tympani of the basal coil of the cochlea near the round window. This small canal terminates on the inferior surface of the petrous pyramid, between the jugular fossa and the external orifice of the carotid canal. In the human it is not patent, being filled with connective tissue.
- The oval window, which is closed by the footplate of the stapes and the associated annular ligament.
- The round window, closed by the secondary tympanic membrane.
- The fissula ante fenestram and the fossula post fenestram, small clefts related to the vestibular window of the lateral wall. The fissula ante fenestram usually extends completely through the bony lateral wall of the vestibule, while the fossula does so in only about 25% of all individuals. Normally both are filled with connective tissue. The fissula is important because of its predilection for otosclerotic bone formation.
- The orifices of the nerves and vessels attaining the inner ear.

Lining the entire osseous labyrinth is a layer of periosteum or endosteum, which is continuous with the periosteum of the cranium through various apertures and lies in close apposition to the walls of the osseous labyrinth. The areas of modification

that merit further description occur within the cochlea. At the free edge of the osseous spiral lamina the endosteum is thickened to form the limbus, which then divides into vestibular and tympanic lips separated by a groove, the internal spiral sulcus. The vestibular lip is confluent with the vestibular membrane. The tympanic lip extends from the edge of the osseous spiral lamina across the lumen of the cochlea to the opposing peripheral wall, forming the fibrous basilar membrane. It attaches peripherally to the crest of the spiral ligament, which in turn is an area of thickened, modified endosteum overlying the lateral wall of the cochlea. While the basilar membrane divides the lumen of the cochlea, it does not extend all the way to the cupula but terminates just before it, leaving a small area of communication termed the helicotrema between the scala vestibuli and the scala tympani.

The membranous labyrinth is a system of delicate, epithelium-lined channels surrounded by connective tissue and lying within the osseous labyrinth (Figure 1). Like its osseous counterpart, the membranous labyrinth has vestibular, semicircular and cochlear components that communicate with one another. The membranous labyrinth exhibits certain general features:

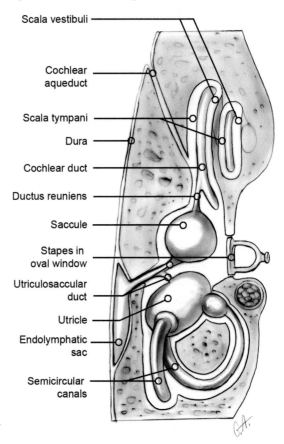

Scala vestibuli

Cochlear aqueduct

Scala tympani

Dura

Cochlear duct

Ductus reuniens

Saccule

Stapes in oval window

Utriculosaccular duct

Utricle

Endolymphatic sac

Semicircular canals

Figure 1 Diagram of the membranous labyrinth

- Its luminal capacity is much less than that of the osseous labyrinth.
- The membranous labyrinth tends to be placed peripherally within the osseous labyrinth; it is surrounded by the perilymphatic space (and perilymph). In most locations this space is traversed by numerous delicate trabeculae extending from the endosteum to the membranous labyrinth. The exception to this is in the cochlea, where the trabeculae are very much reduced or absent.
- The membranous labyrinth contains the receptors for hearing and equilibration.
- It is a self-contained system with no patent communication with other areas.
- The membranous labyrinth contains endolymph.

INDIVIDUAL COMPONENTS OF THE MEMBRANOUS LABYRINTH

The vestibular portion of the membranous labyrinth is characterized by two large dilatations, the utricle and saccule. The utricle, located in the posterior portion of the osseous vestibule, receives the crura of the three-membranous semicircular canals. From its anterior end arises the minute utricular duct through which it communicates with both the endolymphatic duct and the saccule. Situated within the utricle on its floor and lower lateral wall is the macula, one of the receptor sites of the vestibular system. The saccule is located anteromedial to the utricle within the osseous vestibule. From its posterior aspect arises the small saccular duct that is continuous with the utricular duct (hence, utriculosaccular) and the endolymphatic duct. Anteriorly, the saccule is continuous with the cochlear duct through the extremely small ductus reuniens. The saccule has a macula located on its lateral wall.

The endolymphatic duct arises from the union of the utricular and saccular ducts, and passes through the vestibular aqueduct to terminate in a blind dilatation, the endolymphatic sac, within a dural cleft on the medial surface of the petrous portion of the temporal bone. Within the sac are extensive folds of epithelium with cores of vascular connective tissue, which would seem to indicate that this particular site is the region of greatest physiologic activity.

The membranous semicircular canals conform closely to the configuration of their osseous counterparts. At the anterior ends of the anterior and lateral canals, and at the posterior (inferior) end of the posterior canal are prominent dilatations or ampullae, which house the receptor sites (cristae).

The cochlear portion of the membranous labyrinth is the most highly modified. Situated within the bony cochlea, where

it lies upon the upper surface of the basilar membrane, it is a triangular duct extending the full length of the basilar membrane (but not to the apex of the cochlea). Basally it is continuous with the saccule through the ductus reuniens.

The three basic structural components of the cochlear duct include the following:

1. The vestibular membrane, which forms the roof of the cochlear duct and separates the endolymphatic space of the duct from the perilymphatic space of the scala vestibuli. It is an extremely thin membrane (approximately 0.003 mm).
2. The lateral wall, consisting of the stria vascularis, a highly vascular region situated on the inner surface of the spiral ligament. As its name implies, it is characterized by its highly vascular nature and is generally believed to be the source of endolymph.
3. The floor, consisting of the organ of Corti, which is the sensory organ for hearing.

The Sensory Receptors of the Inner Ear

Within the vestibular portion of the inner ear the receptors consist of the following:

- The cristae, located within the ampullae of the membranous semicircular canals. They consist of thickened epithelium containing neuroepithelial hair cells. Overlying the epithelium and extending to the opposite wall of the ampulla is the gelatinous cupula. The cilia of the hair cells project into the base of the cupula.
- The maculae, which are located in the utricle and saccule, and have similar structures. The hair cells of the neuroepithelium are stiff, nonmotile projections embedded in an overlying gelatinous membrane, the statoconic or otolithic membrane. This membrane is unique in that it contains numerous crystals termed otoliths.

The sensory portion of the cochlear duct, the organ of Corti or spiral organ, has the same basic structure as the cristae and maculae. It lies upon the basilar membrane and consists of supporting cells and hair cells overlaid by a gelatinous tectorial membrane. The supporting cells are of several different types; however, all contain fibrils within their cytoplasm and their free edges form a reticular membrane against which the tectorial membrane rests. The most important of the supporting cells are the phalangeal cells, arranged in a single inner row and an outer group consisting of three to five rows depending on the level of the cochlea under consideration, there being more rows apically than basally. The inner row is associated with a single row of hair cells, while the outer group has phalangeal cells alternating with rows of hair cells. Between the inner and outer group of phalangeal cells is an intercellular space extending the entire length of the spiral organ and termed the tunnel, inner tunnel or canal of Corti. It is bounded by special supporting cells designated the inner and outer pillars (Corti's rods). Together the pillars and the canal form Corti's arch. Peripheral to the phalangeal cells are other supportive elements, the tall cells of Hensen and the shorter, more peripherally located cells of Claudius.

The hair cells of the spiral organ have numerous "hairs" projecting from their reticular surface (40–100 per cell). The innermost of these cells are long and are thought to be the least sensitive to sound. In contrast, the outer hair cells are short, being wedged between the apical portions of the phalangeal cells.

Vascular Supply of the Inner Ear

The primary source of blood to the inner ear is the labyrinthine (internal auditory) artery. This artery, just as the coronary arteries, is a terminal vessel, that is to say, it has no anastomoses. Therefore, any blockage will result in a sudden loss, constituting an emergency which in proportion is equivalent to a coronary artery blockage. While this vessel is usually described as originating from the basilar artery, it probably arises more frequently from the anterior inferior cerebellar artery. In addition, it may be duplicated by terminal branches that arise independently to enter the internal acoustic meatus.

In its course the labyrinthine artery accompanies nerves VII and VIII through the internal acoustic meatus. Its main branches run in the endosteum of the labyrinth and small branches traverse the trabeculae to gain the membranous labyrinth. Apparently there are no functional anastomoses between these two areas of distribution.

The most common first branch of the labyrinthine artery is that which is distributed to the utricle, part of the saccule, and the anterior ends of the anterior and lateral semicircular canals. This branch has been called both the anterior vestibular and vestibular artery. When there is an apparent doubling of the labyrinthine artery, it is this branch that most frequently arises independently. The other two common branches of the labyrinthine artery are the vestibulocochlear (posterior vestibular) artery, which is distributed to the saccule, the posterior semicircular canal and parts of the anterior and lateral canals, part of the utricle, and the entire basal coil of the cochlea; and the cochlear artery, which is distributed to the remaining portion of the cochlea. There is considerable variation in the pattern of branching of the labyrinthine artery. Any one of the normal branches may be missing or may arise via a common trunk with another branch.

Descriptions of the venous drainage of the inner ear conflict. In all probability most are accurate, reflecting a considerable but normal variation. The described patterns include the following:

- A vein of the vestibular aqueduct, draining most of the semicircular canals and emptying into either the sigmoid or the inferior petrosal dural sinus.
- A vein of the cochlear aqueduct, draining the entire cochlea and vestibule. It runs in a long canal paralleling the cochlear aqueduct to enter the superior bulb of the internal jugular vein or the inferior petrosal dural sinus.
- A labyrinthine vein, which seems to be inconsistent. When present, it drains the apical and middle coils of the cochlea, and traverses the internal acoustic meatus to become tributary to the inferior petrosal dural sinus.

Nerves of the Inner Ear

Before describing the innervation of the inner ear, we will consider the fundus of the internal acoustic meatus. The fundus is divided into superior and inferior portions by a horizontal bony ridge termed the transverse crest. Located posteriorly within the smaller superior depression are a number of small foramina that transmit the nerves to the utricle, and the ampullae of the anterior and lateral semicircular canals. This is the superior vestibular area. Anteriorly within the upper depression is a relatively large foramen that transmits the facial nerve. In the larger inferior depression, immediately under the posterior end of the transverse crest, is the inferior vestibular area, which contains small foramina transmitting the nerves to the saccule. Below and slightly posterior to the inferior vestibular area is the foramen singulare, through which nerves pass to gain the ampulla of the posterior semicircular duct. Anteriorly the inferior depression is occupied by the foraminiferous spiral tract, a series of minute foramina arranged in spiral fashion that appose the base of the cochlea and the modiolus. At the center of the spiral is the somewhat larger orifice of the modiolar canal.

The nerve of the inner ear is the vestibulocochlear (statoacoustic, acoustic or auditory) nerve. Functionally, it consists of two divisions:

1. The vestibular division, containing fibers arising from the vestibular ganglion, a sensory ganglion situated at the lateral end of the internal acoustic meatus. These sensory fibers form the superior and inferior vestibular nerves. The superior vestibular nerve supplies the ampullae of the anterior and lateral semicircular canals plus the maculae

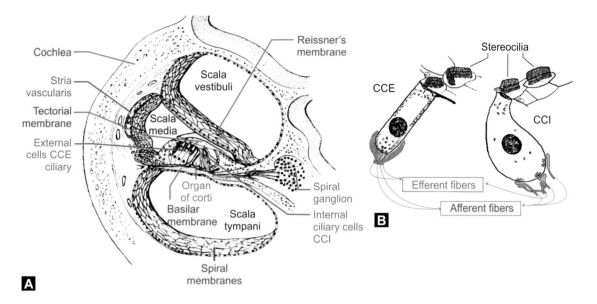

Figures 2A and B (A) The organ of Corti is located in the scala media of the cochlea, over the basilar membrane. The transductors, i.e. the ciliated cells present one row of inner hair cells and three to five rows of outer hair cells. The first bipolar-neuron is located in the ganglion of Corti (spiral ganglion) and its axons project towards the central nervous system as the auditory nerve; (B) The inferior part of the figure shows the two types of ciliated cells with their morphological characteristics and the disposition of the cilia. The distribution of afferent and efferent fibers can also be noted

in the scala vestibuli, ascends to the helicotrema and descends by the scala tympani to end up pushing the round window membrane towards the middle ear cavity. The membranous cochlea is not completely rigid. The basilar membrane is flexible and moves in response to the pressure waves that are generated by sound. This membrane is wider at the apex (five-times more) than at the base of the cochlea and it is more rigid at the base than at the apex (100-times more). G von Bekesy (1960)[5] demonstrated that the movements of the intracochlear fluids generated by sound appear in different directions in both scala, originating movements of the basilar membrane that start at the base and propagate towards the apex forming a "traveling wave" that displaces in the membrane such as a rug that is abruptly shaken.

Until where does this "traveling wave" go? If the frequency is high, the more rigid base of the membrane will vibrate and dissipate the energy, therefore, the wave will not propagate too far. Low frequency sounds generate traveling waves that reach higher areas in order to dissipate the energy, areas where the membrane is less rigid. These characteristics of the basilar membrane allow the discrimination of the component frequencies of sound that distribute along the membrane (tonotopy). Low frequencies are at the apex, high frequencies at the base

and in between all the audible frequencies. In young humans these audible frequencies are between 16 Hz at the apex and 20,000 Hz at the base.

The Cochlear Receptors

There are two types of auditory receptors: (1) The inner hair cells (CCI) which form a single row and are approximately 3,500, and (2) The outer hair cells (CCE) organized in 3–5 rows, totalizing approximately 15,000–20,000 (Figures 2A and B).

The tectorial membrane covers both groups of cells maintaining different relationships with the outer and inner hair cells. The tectorial membrane is fixed to the modiolus, which is the central part of the cochlea. The rest of the organ of Corti, which is fixed to the basilar membrane, can move independently. In this manner, when the basilar membrane is displaced as a consequence of the piston-like movement of the stapes (movement generated by sound), the ciliate cells do so simultaneously against a tectorial membrane that is fixed to the modiolus. This causes a displacement that bends the stereocilia, causing changes in the cilia in relationship to the cell bodies which are fixed by the supporting cells. The stereocilia moves as a unit in one direction or another.

Link for the Video on "Auditory Transduction" of Brandon Pletsch.

Flow Chart 1 Steps of auditory transduction

The sound waves make the tympanic membrane vibrate.
↓
The tympanic membrane makes the ossicles vibrate.
↓
The ossicles move the membrane of the oval window causing
↓
Movements of the cochlear fluids that consequently cause
↓
a relative movement of the cilia with aperture of ionic channels
↓
release of neurotransmitters at the base of the cells with
↓
activation of synapsis with the afferent fibers
↓
generating action potentials in the auditory nerve

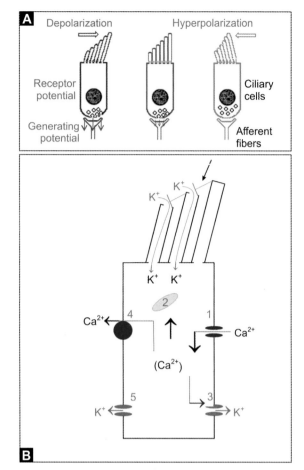

Figures 3A and B Ionic activity of a ciliated cell. (A) The mechanical displacement of a bundle of stereocilia opens the corresponding potassium ionic channels, determining their entrance. They present filaments that unite the stereocilia (arrow) and cause the opening of the channels. When the cilia bend towards the tallest cilia there is depolarization and release of a neurotransmitter. When the cilia bend in the opposite direction, hyperpolarization occurs. During the resting state there is a basal release of neurotransmitter; (B) The depolarization initiates activation (opening) of the calcium channels that are voltage-dependent. The entrance of calcium (1) increases the depolarization of the cell and produces the activation of the potassium-calcium dependent channels (3) and this initiates the release of potassium. Since the base of these cells has an environment that is low in potassium, potassium will tend to exit by the voltage-dependent channels (5) As potassium is released the repolarization starts, diminishing the activation of the calcium channels. In addition, the concentration of calcium diminishes because the mitochondria sequester some calcium and there is an activation of extrusion calcium pumps (4) The intracellular potential returns to its initial state and the cell is now prepared for a new cycle (Hudspeth, 1985)[6]

How are these mechanical changes in the stereocilia converted—transduced—into neural signals? (Hudspeth, 1985).[6] When the stereocilia bends in one direction, the cell becomes hyperpolarized and the reverse occurs when it bends in the other direction (Figure 3A). These changes of polarity produce the receptorial potential, oscillating below and above the resting potential which are of –45 mV in the internal hair cells and of –70 mV in the external cells. The difference in potential that is established between the endolymph (+80 mV) and the inside of the cell (for example –45 mV) is of 125 mV, which being the highest electrical gradient of excitable cells in the body. This assures fast ionic displacements when the channels are opened.

What is the ionic basis for the receptorial potential? (Figure 3B). The influx of potassium ions into the cell through the channels that open up at the tip of the stereocilia is the first event that occurs as a result of the bending of the stereocilia. The displacement in the direction of the taller stereocilia will open the channels mechanically, allowing the entrance of potassium (as a difference with neurons in which potassium exits during activation) while the displacement to the opposite side (away from the taller stereocilia), closes these channels. The entrance of potassium into the cell causes a depolarization that activates the calcium channels that are located in the walls of the ciliated cells. The entrance of calcium increases depolarization and at the same time increases the concentration of intracellular calcium which in turn causes the activation of the potassium channels (dependent on calcium) localized at the base of the ciliated cell. This region is surrounded by an extracellular milieu with low concentration of potassium and this allows the exit of potassium ions. As this occurs, the cell starts to repolarize, diminishing then the entrance of calcium and once the potassium channels that are dependent on calcium start closing, the cell goes back to its initial condition and a new cycle can then start.

The axons that form the auditory nerve have their somas (cell bodies)—first auditory neuron—located in the spiral ganglion of the organ of Corti. This bipolar neuron sends its peripheral extensions (partly myelinized) toward the ciliated cells, while

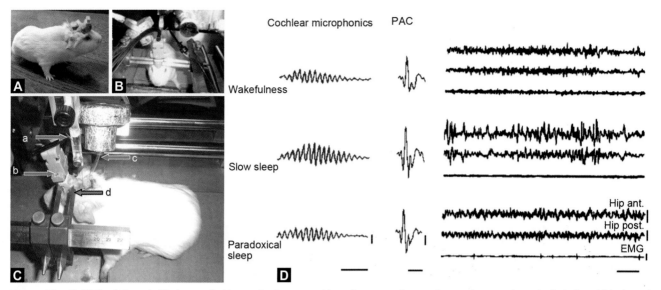

Figures 8A to D (A) The Guinea pig (Cavia porcellus) is completely recovered from the surgery that was done under general anesthesia during which electrodes were implanted. These electrodes were implanted for studying sleep-wakefulness by means of electrograms (of hippocampus) and electromyograms (EMG). An electrode was also placed in the round window; (B) Cochlear potentials can be registered; (C) This experimental model can also be used to register activity of profound nuclei; (D) Cochlear microphonics and compound action potentials of the auditory nerve (PAC) registered in guinea pigs in wakefulness and slow, and paradoxical sleep. Potentials increase when passing from wakefulness to slow sleep and decrease in paradoxical sleep (Velluti, Pedemonte, García-Austt, 1989)[20]

Modifications of the Mechanical Status of the Cochlea

Experimental data providing information on the mechanical effect of the efferent system over the basilar membrane are scarce. The electromotility of outer hair cells modifies the basilar membrane displacement and this modifies the cochlear mechanics and consequently the transduction processes and the receptorial sensibility system termed the "cochlear amplifier". This is the positive feedback process that increases the sensibility to the response of the basilar membrane to low intensity stimuli (Table 1).

Efferent Activity: General Considerations

The discrepancy between the level (dB) of natural ambient noises and the high intensity sounds that are used experimentally to stimulate the medial olivocochlear bundle is evidence that the efferent system is not involved in protection from acoustic trauma of ambient noises (Kirk and Smith, 2003).[21] The

most intense level of a natural continuous sound corresponds to a choir of frogs that can reach levels up to 90 dB SPL (Narins and Hurley, 1982)[22] and is probably close to a waterfall. The efferent system is present in all mammals that have evolved in 170 million years in absolute lack of maintained natural noises of high intensity. The global functions of the efferent system and particularly of the olivocochlear bundle are not well known. The main suggestions are:

- To improve the detection of a signal that is masked by noise.
- To modify the mechanical state of the cochlea by means of controlling the movement of the outer hair cells and their cilia. Therefore, influencing in this manner the activity of inner hair cells and otoacoustic emissions.
- To control (at the beginning of the hearing process) the natural sounds originated in the body which are eliminated from a conscious level by the central nervous system. For example, internal noises such as chewing, breathing, heart beat as well as physiologic noises such as circulation through arteries that are close to the cochlea, etc. (Velluti et al. 1994).[11]

- Actions over the receptor during sleep (Velluti, 1997; Velluti and Pedemonte, 2002; Pedemonte and Velluti, 2005)[23-25] and in habituation and attention phenomena (Buño et al. 1966, Oatman 1971, Délano et al. 2007).[18,19,26]
- As a corollary we have suggested a new hypothesis (Velluti, 2008).[14] Since the efferent system is related to a great diversity of areas related to hearing, this system would have an effect on the entrance and processing at different levels.

This would allow the establishment of a synergy between the auditory system and the functional changes of the central nervous system. This synergy means maintaining reciprocal activity between the central nervous system and the corresponding sensory input. This continuous interaction-adaptation between the central nervous system, the environment and the body can only occur through systems (receptors, afferents and efferents) that are capable

Table 1 Variation of the cochlear potentials under different experimental conditions

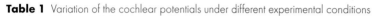

	Experimental conditions	Changes in the compound action potential.	Changes in the cochlear microphonics.
R Galambos (1956)	Anesthesized cats Electrical stimulation in the floor of the IVth ventricle.	⋀⋁ → ⋀⋁	
J Fex (1962)	Anesthesized cats. Electrical stimulation in the floor of the IVth ventricle.		▬▬ → ▬▬
W Buno, R A Valluti, P Handler, E Garcia -Austt (1966)	Awake guinea pig. Habituation to a constant stimulus.	V V ⋀⋁ → ⋀⋁	V V ▬▬ → ▬▬
L C Oatman (1971)	Awake cat without middle ear ossicles. Changes of the compound action potential because of intercurrent visual stimulus.	V V ⋀⋁ → ⋀⋁	

contd...

contd...

R A Velluti, M Pedemonte (1986)	Awake guinea pig with systemic injection of benzodiazepine. Without middle ear ossicle in a closed system of stimulation.	V → SL	V → V
R A Velluti, M Pedemonte, E Garcia Austt (1989)	Guinea pig with controlled sleep and wakefulness. Without middle ear ossicles in a closed system of stimulation.	V → SL	V → SL
M Pedemonte, D G Drexler, R A Veluti (2004) Pavez et al (2006)	Guinea pig with controlled sleep and wakefulness. Without middle ear ossicles in a closed system of stimulation.	V → SL	V → SL
P H Delano, D Elgueda, C M Hamame, I Robles (2005)	Awake chinchill as. Attentional changes of cochlear potentials.	V → V	V → V

of continuously follow the rapid and slow changes of the central nervous system that are constantly occurring.

REFERENCES

1. Bernal B, Altman N. Auditory Functional MR Imaging. Am J Roentgenology. 2001;176:1009-15.
2. Limb CJ, Braun AR. Neural Substrates of Spontaneous Musical Performance: An fMRI Study of Jazz Improvisation. PLoS ONE. 2008;3(2):e1679.
3. Suárez H, Mut F, Lago G, et al. Changes in cerebral blood flow in postlingual cochlear implant users. Stockh: Acta Otolaryngol. 1999;119:239-43.
4. MØller AR. Hearing Anatomy, Physiology and Disorders of the Auditory System. Amsterdam: Academic Press; 2006.
5. Békésy GV. Experiments in Hearing. New York: McGraw-Hill; 1960.
6. Hudspeth AJ. The cellular basis of hearing: the biophysics of hair cells. Science. 1985;230:745-52.
7. Oliver D. Prestin. In: Basbaum AJ, Kaneco A, Sheperd GM, Westheimer G (Eds). The Senses: A Comprehensive Reference. Vol. 3, Audition, Dallos PP, Oertel, D. San Diego: Academic Press; 2008.
8. Kemp DT. Stimulated acoustic emissions from within the human auditory system. J Acoust Soc Am. 1978;64:1386-91.
9. Siegel J. Otoacoustic Emissions. In: Basbaum AJ, Kaneco A, Sheperd GM, Westheimer G (Eds). The Senses: A Comprehensive

Reference. Vol. 3, Audition, Dallos PP, Oertel, D. San Diego: Academic Press; 2008.

10. van Dijk P, Narins PM, Mason MJ. Physiological vulnerability of distortion product otoacoustic emissions from the amphibian ear. J Acoust Soc Am. 2003;114:2044-8.

11. Velluti RA, Peña JL, Pedemonte M, et al. Internally-generated sound stimulates cochlear nucleus units. Hearing Res. 1994;72:19-22.

12. Velluti RA, Platas A, Iglesias L. An adequate head-holder to be used in auditory and posterior cranial fossa research. Acta Neurol Latinoamer. 1980;26:129-31.

13. Robles L, Délano PH. Efferent System. In: Basbaum AJ, Kaneco A, Sheperd GM, Westheimer G (Eds). The Senses: A Comprehensive Reference. Vol. 3, Audition, Dallos PP, Oertel, D. San Diego: Academic Press; 2008.

14. Guinan JJ. Physiology of olivocochlear efferents. In: Dallos P, Popper A, Fay R (Eds). The Cochlea. New York: Springer; 1986.

15. Elgoyhen AB, Vetter DE, Katz E, et al. α10: A determinant of nicotinic cholinergic receptor function in mammalian vestibular and cochlear mechanosensory hair cells. PNAS. 2001;98:3501-6.

16. Galambos R. Suppression of auditory nerve activity by stimulation of efferent fibers to cochlea. J Neurophysiol. 1956;19:424-37.

17. Velluti RA. The Auditory System in Sleep. Amsterdam: Elsevier-Academic Press; 2008.

18. Oatman LC. Role of visual attention on auditory evoked potentials in unanesthetized cats. Exp Neurol. 1971;32:341-56.

19. Délano PH, Elgueda D, Hamame CM, et al. Selective attention to visual stimuli reduces cochlear sensitivity in chinchillas. J Neurosci. 2007;27:4146-53.

20. Velluti RA, Pedemonte M, García-Austt E. Correlative changes of auditory nerve and microphonic potentials throughout sleep. Hearing Res. 1989;39:203-8.

21. Kirk E, Smith DW. Protection from acoustic trauma is not a primary function of the medial olivocochlear efferent system. J Assoc Res. Otolaryngol. 2003;4:445-65.

22. Narins PM, Hurley DD. The relationship between call intensity and function in the Puerto Rican Coqui (Anura: Leptodactylidae). Herpetologica. 1982;38:287-95.

23. Velluti RA. Interactions between sleep and sensory physiology. J Sleep Res. 1997;6:61-77.

24. Velluti RA, Pedemonte M. In vivo approach to the cellular mechanisms for sensory processing in sleep and wakefulness. Cell Mol Neurobiol. 2002;22:501-16.

25. Pedemonte M, Velluti RA. What individual neurons tell us about encoding and sensory processing in sleep. In: Parmeggiani PL, Velluti RA (Eds). The Physiologic Nature of Sleep. London: Imperial College Press; 2005. pp. 489-508.

26. Buño W, Velluti R, Handler P, et al. Neural control of the cochlear input in the wakeful free guinea pig. Physiology Behav. 1966;1:23-35.

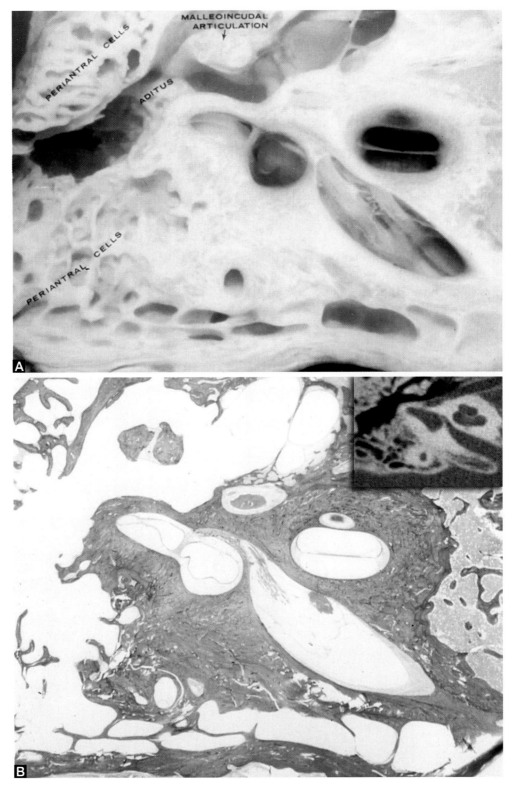

Figures 9A and B

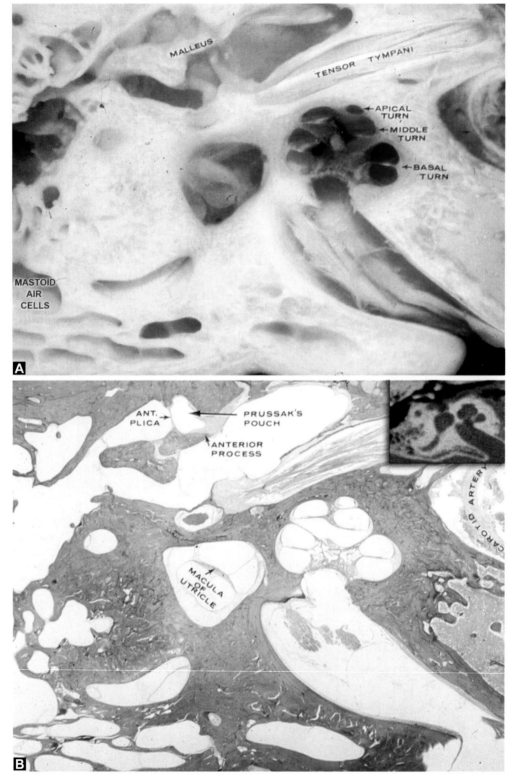

Figures 10A and B

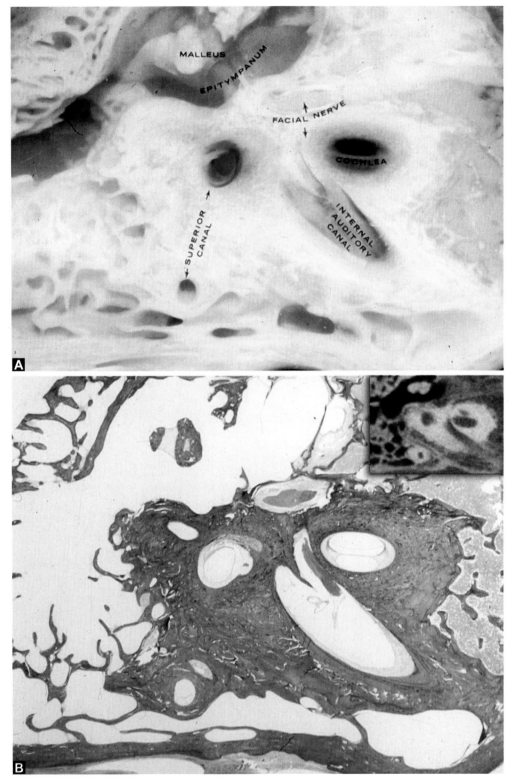

Figures 11A and B

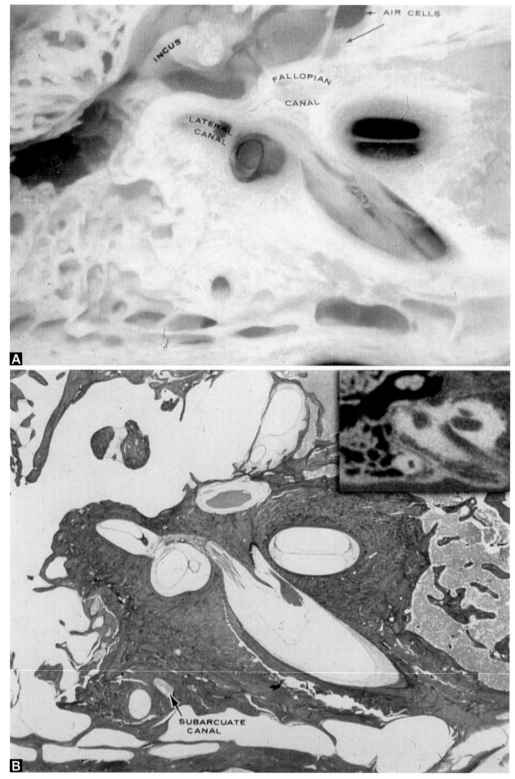

Figures 12A and B

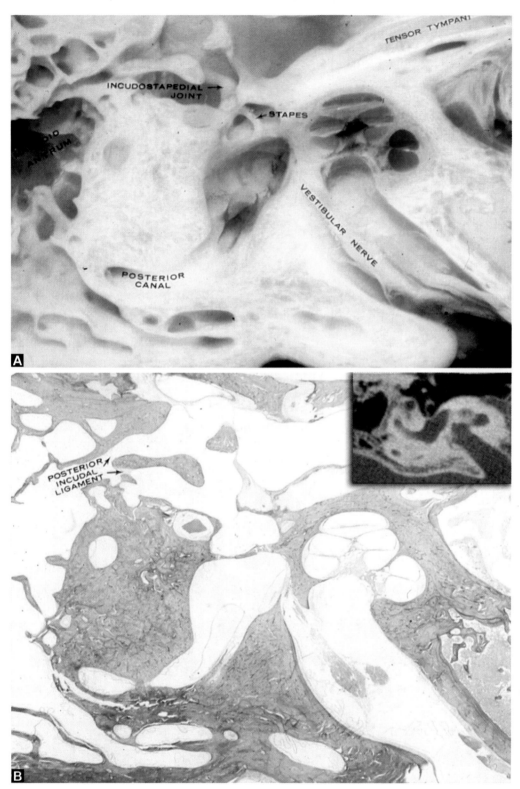

Figures 13A and B

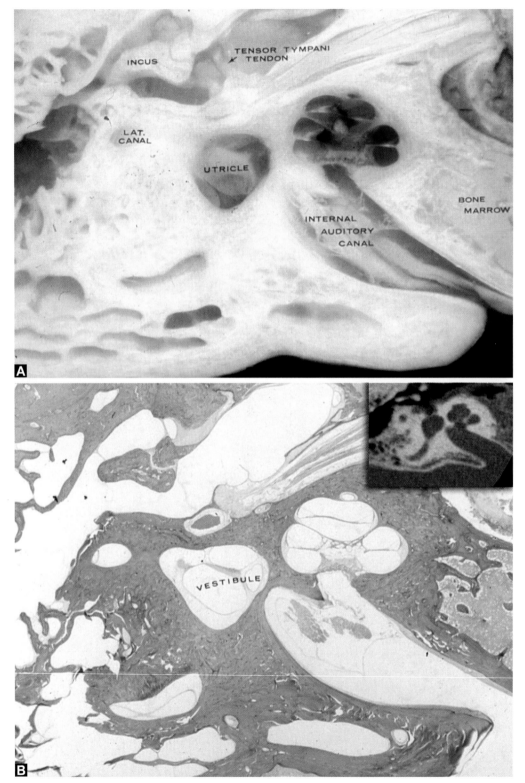

Figures 14A and B

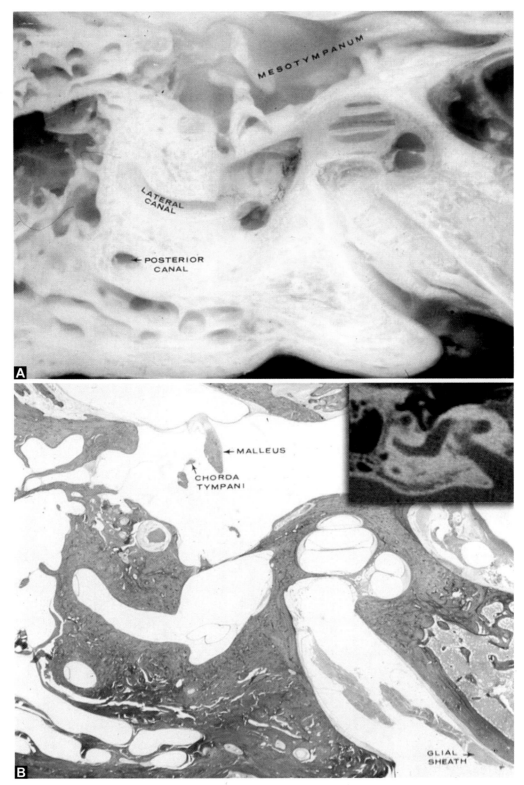

Figures 15A and B

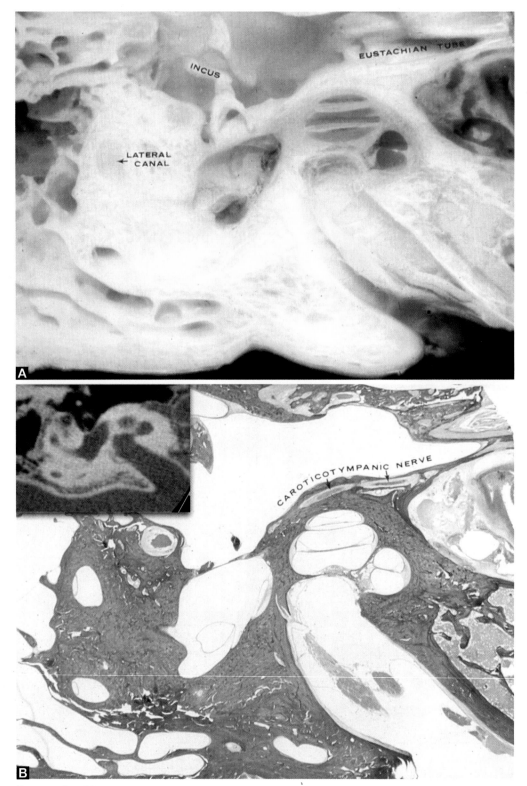

Figures 16A and B

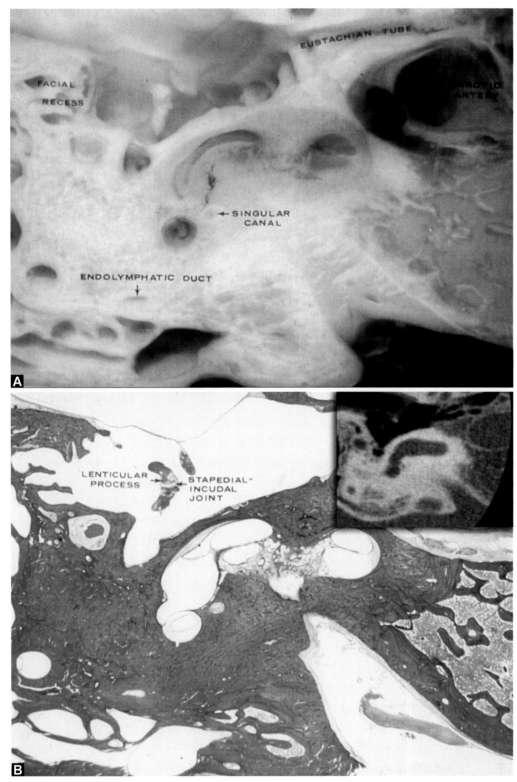

Figures 17A and B

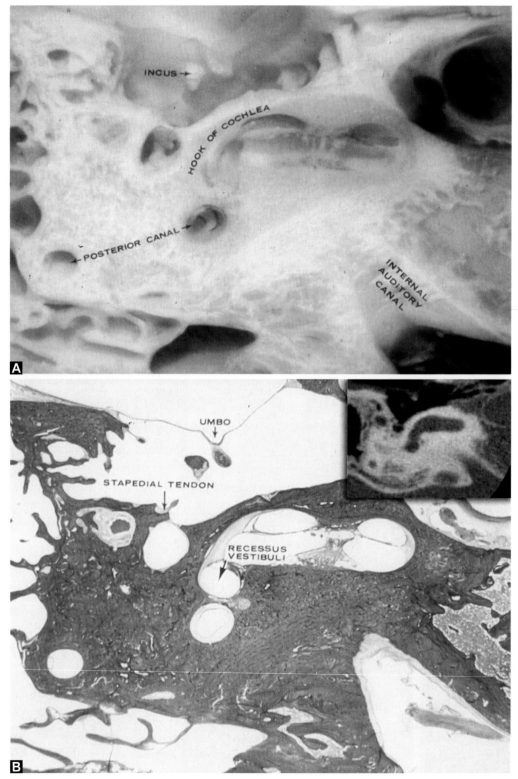

Figures 18A and B

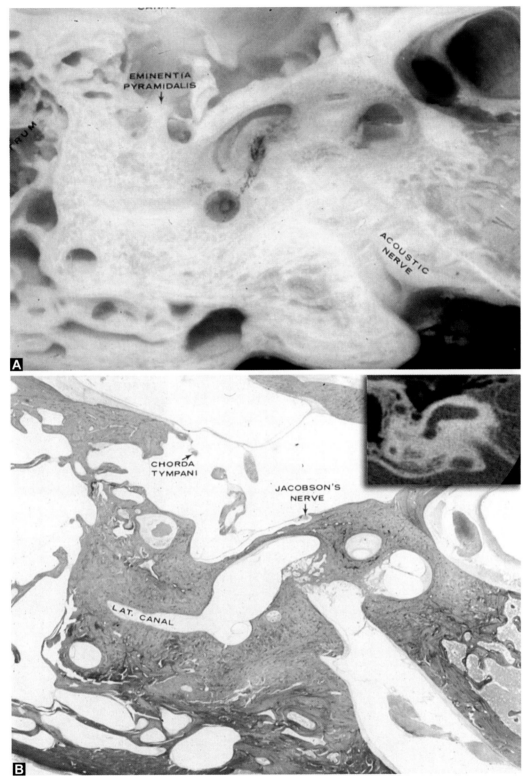

Figures 19A and B

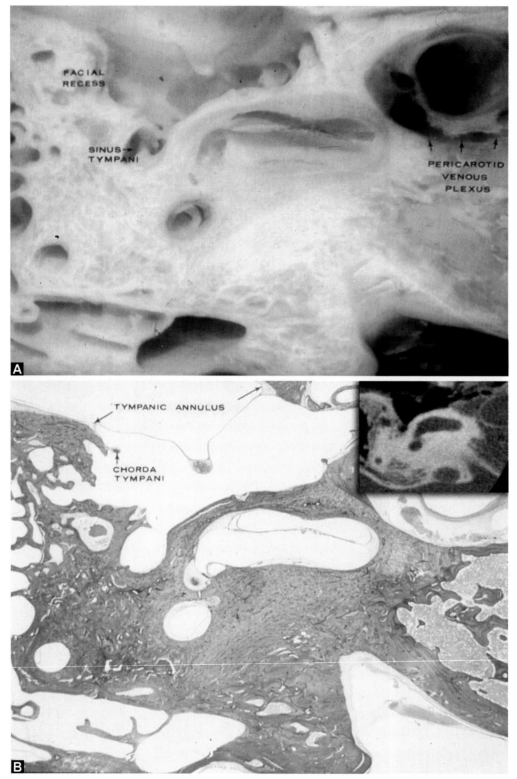

Figures 20A and B

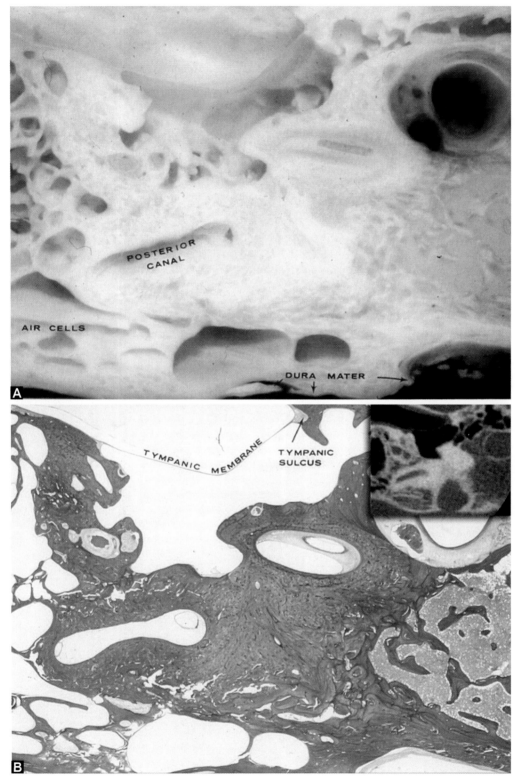

Figures 21A and B

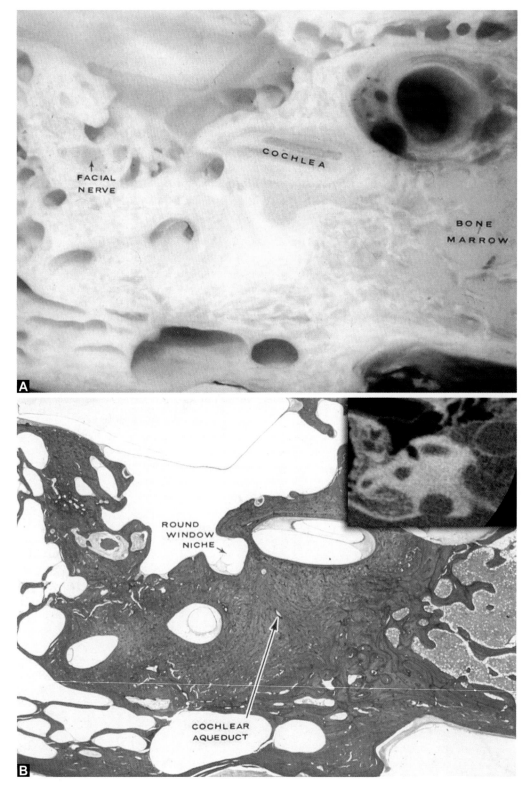

Figures 22A and B

Figures 5A and B to 22A and B Represent serial sections of human temporal bones from superior to inferior. Although some of the structures are labeled, the sections are presented without detailed descriptions. The purpose is that the reader uses them to review the structures that have been described in the previous sections of anatomy and also for anatomical understanding and analysis in the surgical approaches that are described in the following sections

1.8

Imagenology of the Temporal Bone

Miguel Casals

INTRODUCTION

Nuclear magnetic resonance (NMR) and computerized axial tomography (CT scan) have introduced significant changes in the diagnosis of petrous bone pathology.

Continued technical improvements of both examinations have allowed and will continue to allow new ways of visualizing the complex ear anatomy. Each of these diagnostic tools sets new challenges. Today, it is almost impossible to answer the ongoing question "Which of the exams is the best exam?" Each technique used must suit each particular case; hence, there must be a fluent communication between the radiologist and the otolaryngologist, and/or the neurosurgeon treating the patient. Radiology has introduced a progressive and increasing reliance in deciding surgical procedures.

Different pathology and its radiologic findings will be reviewed according to their frequency, and the significance of radiology in their diagnosis and therapeutic decisions.

All radiology exams shown here have been done using a 16-channel, multicut CT scan and a 1.5 tesla nuclear magnetic resonator as well as an open 0.2 tesla, both with an image processor.

Selected topics:
- Normal radiology anatomy
- Cholesteatoma and inflammatory pathology images
- Cerebellopontine angle tumors
- Cochlear implant imaging.

NORMAL RADIOLOGY ANATOMY

A complete knowledge of the complicated ear anatomy is difficult for an outsider.

It is not unusual to see petrous bone radiology examination laying in Radiology Departments waiting to be informed.

A schematic anatomy and its comparison with normal tomography anatomy will be reviewed, aiming to point out the main petrous bone elements seen in Radiology (Figures 1A and B).

It is important to consider the relationship of the petrous bone with other skull base structures (Figure 1A) mainly the sella turcica at the clivus level (1) posterior portion of the cavernous sinus (2) sphenoid sinus (3) and optical chiasma with its relation to the superior aspect of the clivus.

Figure 1B is a lateral view showing the relationship between the clivus with the petrous apex and the posterior segment of the cavernous sinus in relation with the cranial nerves within it. The sphenoidal plane and the crista galli can be seen in the anterior portion.

Figure 2 emphasizes the importance of the anatomic structures adjacent to the petrous bone, such as the parotid gland: there is a close lymphatic relation between the intraparotid lymph nodes and the EAC submucosa with a direct passage between the two structures. When the EAC is involved, X-ray imaging should include at least the superficial lobe of the ipsilateral parotid gland.

A schematic close relationship between the lateral mastoid cells and the retroauricular area can be seen (3).

Figure 3 schematically shows the contents of the middle ear with the cul-de-sac of the EAC with the superior insertion of the tympanic membrane in the scutum (1), Promontory (2) with the stylomastoid canal in it (3), The oval window (4) and horizontal view of the lateral semicircular canal (5).

There is a small space between the promontory and the posterior portion of the posterior wall of the middle ear called

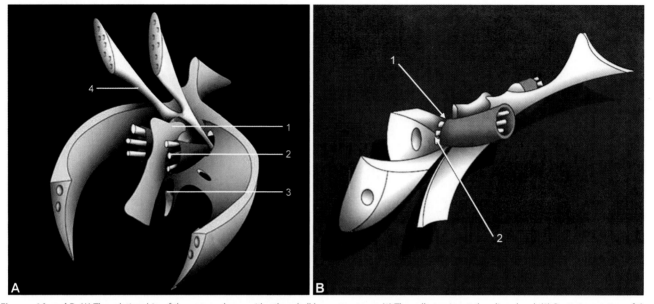

Figures 1A and B (A) The relationship of the petrous bone with other skull base structures: (1) The sella turcica at the clivus level; (2) Posterior portion of the cavernous sinus; (3) Sphenoid sinus; (4) Optical chiasma with its relation to the superior aspect of the clivus. (B) Lateral view showing the relationship between the clivus with the petrous apex and the posterior segment of the cavernous sinus in relation with the cranial nerves within it. The spherical plane and the crista galli can be seen in the anterior portion

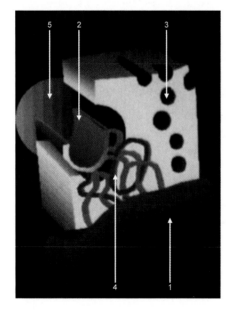

Figure 2 The external auditory canal (EAC) is outlined:
(1) The parotid gland is visualized; (2) EAC; (3) Mastoid cells; (4) Lymphatic channels communicating the parotid gland with the submucous region of the EAC; (5) Tympanic membrane fundus

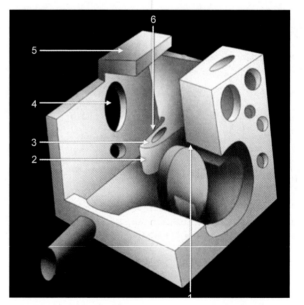

Figure 3 Schematic diagram showing the contents of middle ear:
(1) Scutum; (2) Promotory; (3) Stylomastoid canal; (4) Oval window; (5) Horizontal view of the lateral semicircular canal; (6) Sinus tympani

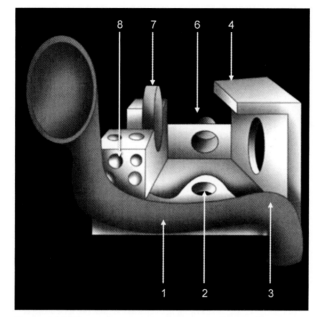

Figure 4 Middle ear after removing the posterior bony wall:
(1) Sigmoid sinus; (2) Stylomastoid canal at the promontory; (3) Jugular
vein; (4) Lateral semicircular canal

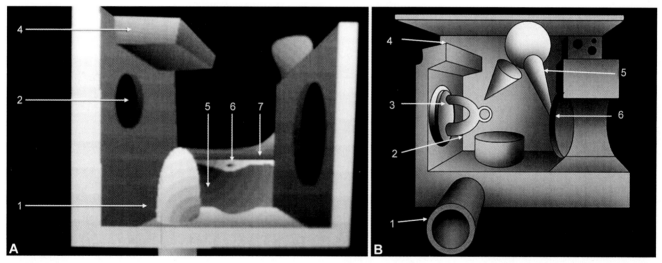

Figures 5A and B Middle ear with anterior wall has been removed: (A) The same anatomical structures are seen, going from anterior to posterior, with a partial resection of the posterior wall. The sigmoid sinus, the promontory and the stylomastoid canal are seen (6); sinus tympani (5); jugular vein protruding into the sinus tympani (1); oval window (2) and horizontal lateral semicircular canal protruding towards the middle ear (4). (B) The ossicular chain is seen; merging of the Eustachian tube (1); sinus tympani (2); stapes footplate (3); lateral projection of the horizontal semicircular canal with the attic above (4); malleus head and handle (5); tympanic membrane (6)

the sinus tympani (6). This is an important radiologic landmark not usually visualized when doing a clinical otoscopy.

The posterior bony wall of the middle ear has been removed (Figure 4). The sigmoid sinus is seen (1). Stylomastoid canal at the promontory (2); the jugular vein (3) protruding into the posteromedial part of the middle ear cavity and its relation

to the sinus tympani; the lateral semicircular canal (4). There is a close relation between the posterior mastoid cells and the sigmoid sinus, immediately behind.

In Figures 5A and B the anterior wall of the middle ear has been removed and in Figure 6 the ossicular chain has been removed.

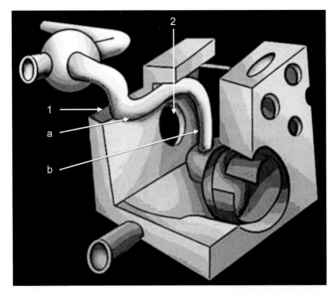

Figure 6 The ossicular chain has been removed visualizing the first segment of the facial nerve (1) the intratympanic, and horizontal portions of the facial nerve and its exit at the stylomastoid foramen (b); oval window (2)

It is important to consider the facial nerve location in its intratympanic portion, immediately above the oval window and below the horizontal semicircular canal (Figures 7A to C).

Structures seen after removing anterior and medial middle ear cavity walls (Figures 8 to 12).

Some cisternal structures can be seen showing that an angle lesion does not necessarily mean an expansive lesion. Not all the anatomical structures in the cerebellopontine angle can easily be seen through images—radiology reconstruction using different levels and planes are needed. These are usually done in T2 sequence NMR (Figures 13 and 14).

RADIOLOGY OF CHOLESTEATOMA AND INFLAMMATORY PROCESS

Purulent inflammatory lesions of the middle ear, with or without associated cholesteatoma, usually follow pathways that can be traced with radiology images. A relevant anatomical

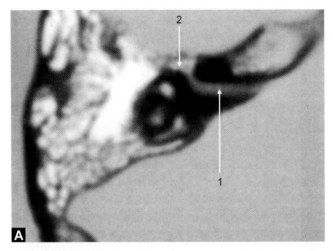

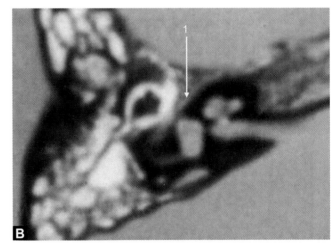

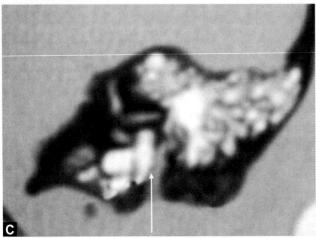

Figures 7A to C (A) CT scan showing the facial nerve emerging from the internal acoustic meatus and extending above the cochlea (1) reaching the ganglion (2); (B) This figure shows a slightly lower axial projection with the horizontal or intratympanic facial nerve segment; (C) Posterior coronal cut of the petrous bone showing the facial nerve merging from the styloid canal. The facial nerve trajectory can be seen. The posterior wall of the middle ear has been removed to have a better idea of the intratympanic projection of the horizontal canal. Facial nerve through the stylomastoid canal and the promontory

reference is the tympanic membrane: it will present inflammatory changes in its inner side. It may become thicker (1), have a perforation (2), retraction pockets (3) and calcifications. A cholesteatoma may disrupture the superior segment of the

annulus eroding the scutum and filling Prussak's space (4) (see Figure 15).

Prussak's space invasion with erosion of the scutum is characteristic of a recently developed cholesteatoma as opposed

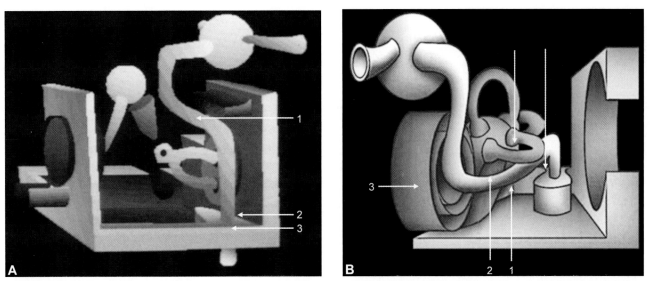

Figure 8A and B The anterior and medial middle ear cavity walls have been removed. A large cavity formed in conjunction by the middle ear and inner ear is seen. Tympanic sinus (1); horizontal portion of the facial nerve (2); cochlea, horizontal semicircular canal projection and exit of the facial nerve (arrows) (3)

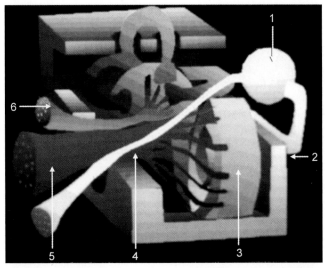

Figure 9 The anterior and medial walls of the middle ear have been removed. The facial nerve ganglion can be seen (1); incipient segment of the horizontal, intratympanic portion of the facial nerve (2); cochlea (3); facial nerve above and anterior to the nerves contained in the internal auditory canal (IAC). The facial nerve is below the cochlear nerve, and behind and posterior to the vestibular branch which may be single or double (4)

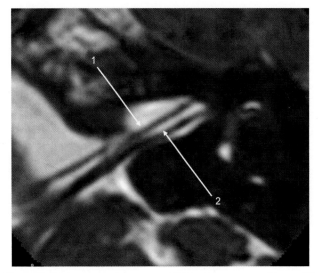

Figure 10 Nuclear magnetic resonance (NMR) with sequence solid-state (SS) reconstruction following the direction of the cranial nerves contained in the internal auditory meatus. As described in Figure 9, the facial nerve is seen in the anterosuperior segment of the IAC (1). The superior vestibular nerve is behind the facial nerve (2)

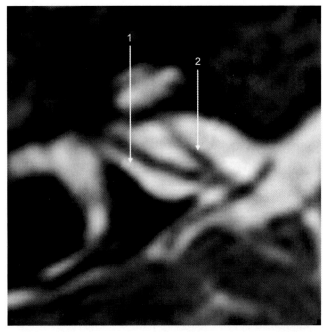

Figure 11 NMR reconstruction in a plane slightly below the one in Figure 10; inferior vestibular nerve (1); cochlear nerve immediately anterior to the inferior vestibular nerve (2)

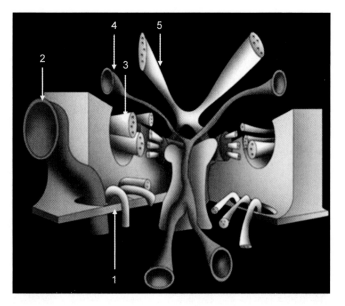

Figure 13 The occipital bone has been removed. The cisterns of the cerebellopontine angle and the posterior fossa nervous structures can be seen. The clivus is in depth and in the first plane are the vertebrobasilar vessels with the posterosuperior cerebellar arteries. Jugular foramen with its pars nervosa and its pars vascularis; the jugular bulb is emerging (2); internal auditory canal (3); posterosuperior cerebellar arteries (4); optical chiasm over the posterosuperior cerebellar arteries (5); bilateral cranial nerves III, IV and VI at the petrous vertex are seen in proximity with the lateral wall of the cavernous sinus

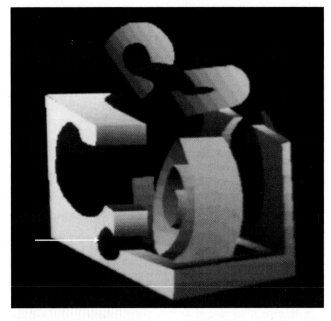

Figure 12 The IAC at the level of the internal acoustic meatus is seen. Right below is the cochlear aqueduct connecting the subarachnoid space with the perilymph. The cochlear aqueduct lumen varies from narrow enough not to be identified, up to a width similar to that of the EAC. Perilymphatic hypertension can fixate the stapes footplate giving a "conductive" hearing loss

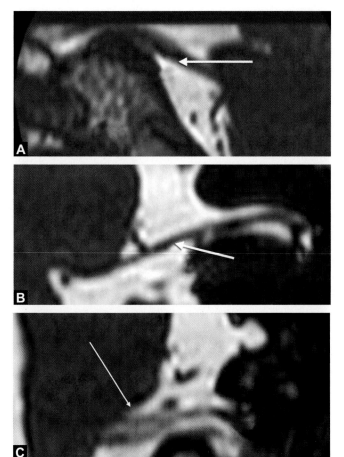

Figures 14A to C NMR multiplane reconstruction using T2 sequence. (A) The course of the cisternal portion of the trigeminal nerve is singled; (B) Coronal view of the cochlear nerve: cisternal and intracanal segment; (C) Hypoglossal and glossopharyngeal nerves at the level of the jugular foramen, Oblique coronal cut

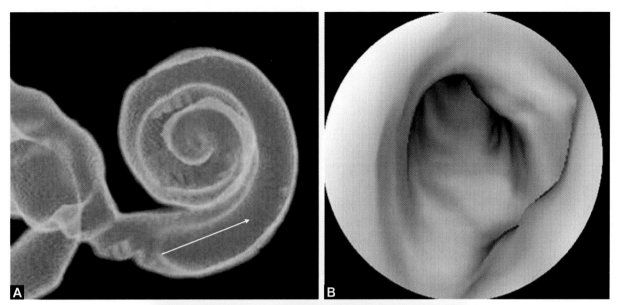

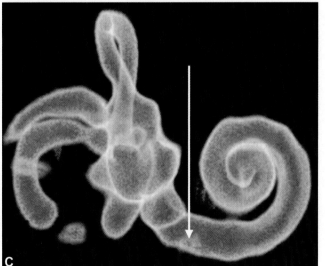

Figures 27A to C Different types of intracochlear stenosis probably secondary to postmeningitis fibrosis presenting a relative obstructive difficulty when inserting the cochlear implant electrode

Congenital VIII cranial nerve absence is usually easy to diagnose. It is generally bilateral with a filiform canal. Cochlear nerve absence is an absolute contraindication for cochlear implant in the ipsilateral ear. Figure 31 shows bilateral VIII nerve absence with filiform internal auditory canal and bilateral normal cochlea.

Oval Window Patency

In spite of not being essential for surgical decision, oval window visualization is important in certain types of surgery. The oval window should be studied bilaterally using under one millimeter CT scan cuts with MIP reconstruction following the cochlear basal turn axis (Figure 32). This same technique is useful for visualizing eventual intracochlear calcifications not seen in NMR.

Associated Anomalies Study

CT scan allows an anatomical map of the future surgical pathway avoiding, therefore, eventual difficulties such as sigmoid sinus lateralization, an abnormal carotid artery or an occupied middle ear (Figures 33 to 36).

The previous examples underline the importance of a thorough preoperative radiology evaluation with both CT scan and

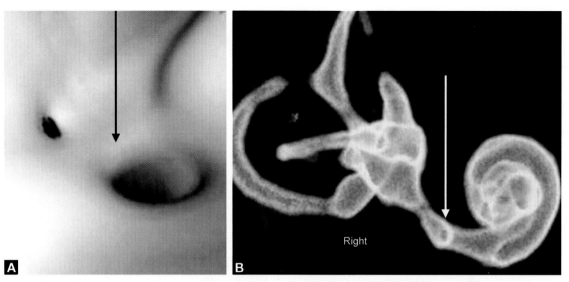

Figures 28A and B Incomplete cochlea and an absent vestibule in a deaf infant is shown with a significant stenosis of the basal turn

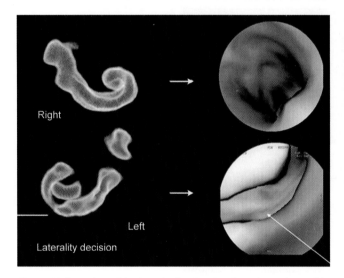

Figure 29 Stenotic cochlea in a deaf patient in whom it was impossible to insert an electrode; there was intraoperative cochlear bleeding and the electrode insertion was aborted. NMR later showed absence of cochlear signal due to blood flooding as well as a magnetic artifact in the cul-de-sac of the internal acoustic canal

Figures 30A to D Solid-state (SS) sequence, being a volumetric acquisition, allows variable thickness and angles when studying the course of the cranial nerves, both intracanal and in the cistern

NMR for differential diagnosis as well as avoiding difficulties and/or complications during surgery.

Central Nervous System Evaluation

Children with neurological deficit or seizures need a clinical and neurological work up.

Radiology evaluation should include at least one FLAIR NMR sequence as well as coronal cuts to evaluate the cortex and the white substance which may be damaged due to perinatal hypoxia.

Cortex damage per se is neither a contraindication for cochlear implants nor does it make the surgical procedure more difficult, but it might help to choose the side. In preschool and school children we have seen neurologic improvement after being implanted.

ADULT COCHLEAR IMPLANT IMAGES

Cochlear implant images in adults are different from children.

The deaf adult patient usually has pericochlear and perivestibular bone changes like otospongiosis with or without

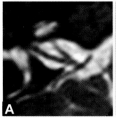
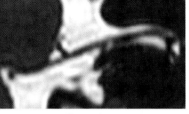

Axial | Coronal

Figures 31A and B Bilateral VIII nerve absence with filiform internal auditory canal and bilateral normal cochlea

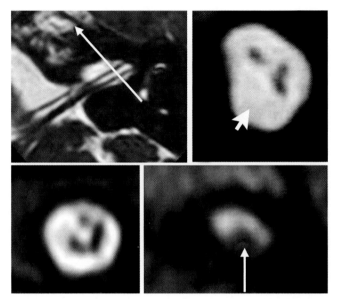

Figure 32 The oval window should be studied bilaterally using under one millimeter CT scan cuts with MIP reconstruction following the cochlear basal turn axis

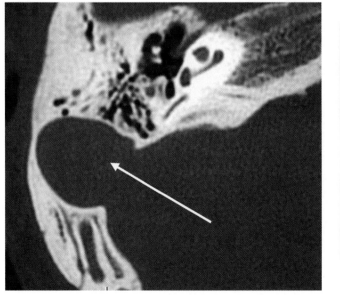

Figure 33 Anatomical variation with sigmoid sinus lateralization

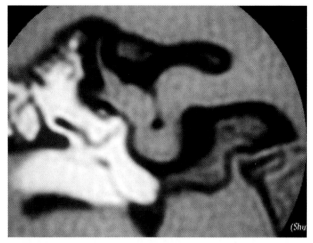

Figure 34 Internal ear congenital malformation with an internal auditory canal open to the basal portion of the cochlea

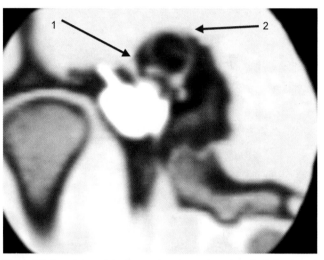

Figure 35 Superior semicircular canal erosion with perilymphatic fistula and tegmen dehiscence

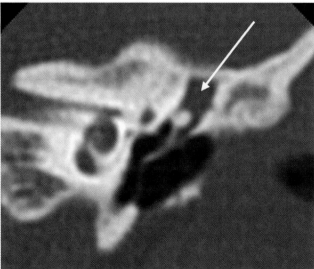

Figure 36 Fibroadhesive attic tissue with absence of oval window permeability

window involvement. The bony reaction can involve the basal turn of the cochlea impeding electrode implantation (Figure 37).

Intracochlear bleeding, either due to trauma or to autoimmune disease, can cause an obstruction in some segment of the cochlea (Figure 38).

Radiology evaluation in adult candidates for an implant is aimed towards ruling out acquired inflammatory, traumatic, tumor or degenerative pathology.

POSTOPERATIVE FOLLOW-UP

Implanted patients cannot have a NMR done. The magnetic field irreversibly damages the implant. Postoperative follow-up must be done with CT scan intending to visualize:

- Electrode position and its eventual migration (Figures 39A to C)
- Electrode indemnity (Figure 40)
- Inflammatory reaction of the middle ear.

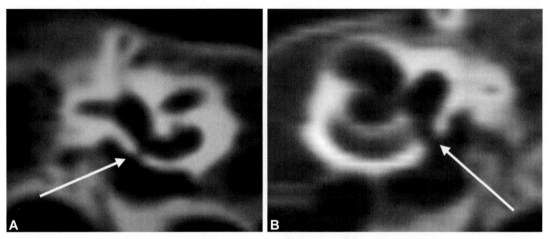

Figures 37A and B Otospongiosis with or without window involvement. The bony reaction can involve the basal turn of the cochlea impeding electrode implantation

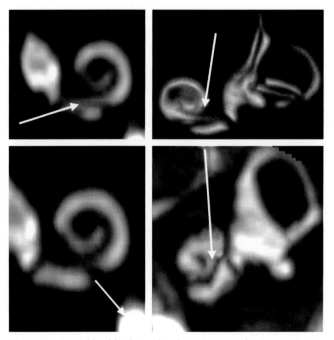

Figure 38 Intracochlear bleeding, either due to trauma or due to autoimmune disease, can cause an obstruction in some segment of the cochlea

Table 1 Stimulation with pure tones. Percent of cortical HMPAO in different Brodmann areas

Area Brodmann MAX		Area 7 (Left)	Area 7 (Right)	Area 9 (Left)	Area 9 (Right)	Area 10 (Left)	Area 10 (Right)	Area 17 (Left)	Area 17 (Right)	Area 18 (Left)	Area 18 (Right)	Area 19 (Left)	Area 21 (Left)	Area 21 (Right)	Area 22 (Left)	Area 22 (Right)
Ear Stimulated																
Right	Mean	91.2	90.5	91.4	91.8	94.0	94.2	95.6	96.7	95.5	97.3	90.2	93.4	91.7	94.3	92.5
	SD	5.0	4.9	6.3	6.5	7.2	6.6	3.1	1.9	3.1	2.5	3.1	2.5	4.5	3.3	3.8
Left	Mean	93.2	89.3	92.7	90.8	95.7	95.3	93.7	93.3	94.2	94.6	87.4	90.7	88.7	92.4	92.1
	SD	5.7	4.2	4.9	3.8	5.2	5.7	4.3	4.4	5.0	4.2	3.9	5.5	5.0	4.3	4.4
Bilateral	Mean	87.83	86.78	87.15	86.54	87.82	87.95	90.86	90.93	91.23	91.23	88.53	87.55	87.33	88.20	87.73
	SD	2.25	3.73	3.33	2.67	2.35	1.66	1.53	1.44	1.21	1.21	1.53	2.22	1.68	1.76	1.97

Area Brodmann MAX		Area 31 (Left)	Area 31 (Right)	Area 32 (Left)	Area 32 (Right)	Area 39 (Left)	Area 39 (Right)	Area 40 (Left)	Area 40 (Right)	Area 46 (Left)	Area 46 (Right)	Caudate Nucleus (Left)	Caudate Nucleus (Right)	Putamen (Left)	Putamen (Right)	Thalamus (Left)	Thalamus (Right)
Ear Stimulated																	
Right	Mean	96.3	96.1	90.9	87.3	91.9	88.1	93.5	92.1	90.0	90.8	91.2	91.7	92.7	92.5	100.1	97.2
	SD	3.1	2.3	6.8	4.8	4.7	4.5	5.4	4.4	5.8	6.1	2.7	5.0	3.8	2.2	2.2	4.0
Left	Mean	95.4	92.7	91.8	85.2	90.1	86.1	93.1	90.7	91.7	92.4	90.2	91.8	92.5	90.8	97.3	95.7
	SD	3.5	5.1	6.9	5.8	4.1	3.4	5.0	5.6	5.8	3.3	3.0	5.3	2.9	6.3	4.1	4.2
Bilateral	Mean	91.23	91.23	89.09	90.63	88.01	86.87	87.95	87.55	86.88	87.28	85.88	84.74	88.60	87.86	91.23	90.06
	SD	1.21	1.21	4.56	1.85	1.99	2.18	2.10	2.06	2.28	1.78	5.64	3.67	2.89	2.53	1.21	3.24

normal range is depicted in gray color and corresponds to 2 SD above and below the normal mean for this age group.

There is also intense and statistically significant stimulation in the right posterior parietal lobe corresponding to the projection of areas 39 and 40 of Brodmann respectively. Finally, we also see significant diminution of perfusion in the left lateral temporal lobe and in the medial aspects of these lobes. The statistical significance is 2 SD and 3 SD below the normal mean for the age of the patient and is depicted by colors light blue and dark blue respectively (Figures 2A and B).

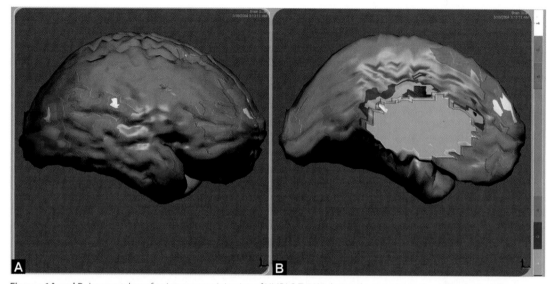

Figures 1A and B Images taken after intravenous injection of HMPAO Tc99M during the pure tone stimulation in the left ear: a very intense stimulation of frontal lobes at 2, 3 and 4 SDs above the normal mean gathered during basal state—colored red, pink and white respectively; the normal range is depicted in color gray corresponds to 2 SD above and below the normal mean for this age group

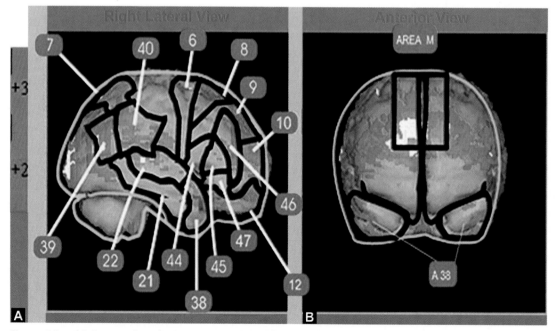

Figures 2A and B Images taken after intravenous injection of HMPAO Tc99M during the pure tone stimulation in the left ear, showing intense and statistically significant stimulation corresponding to the projection of different areas of Brodmann. (A) Right lateral view; (B) Anterior view

Results of stimulation in the right ear demonstrate less intense activation of both frontal lobes, predominantly at the level of the intermediate gyrus. There is also activation in the right posterior parietal lobe corresponding to areas 39 and 40 of Brodmann, however, with less intensity than the observed when the left ear was stimulated.

On the other hand, in this patient it is clear that the deactivation of the temporal lobes are more intense when the right ear is stimulated than the left ear, and this deactivation is observed bilaterally extending in both lateral aspect and both medial aspects of the temporal lobes. There is also deactivation in the limbic system at the level of the intermediate gyrus. In the projection of the Brodmann areas on the neuroSPECT data, one can see that the activation of the executive frontal area in this patient corresponds to area 9, 10, 46 and 47. Also in the posterior parietal lobe there is activation in the area 40, 39 and 7 of Brodmann. While at the level of temporal lobes, there is deactivation at the area 38, 21 and 22 of Brodmann (Figure 3). At the level of basal ganglia there is diminution of the right caudate nucleus as shown in the Figure 4.

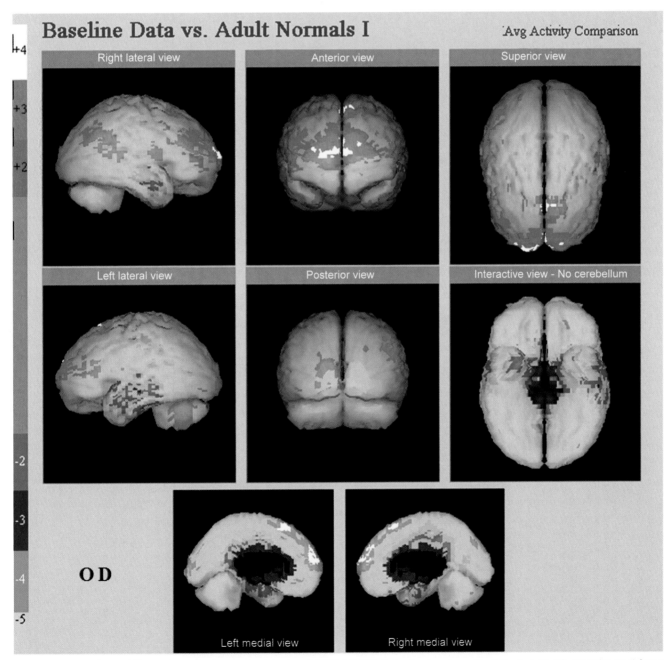

Figure 3 Images taken in different views after intravenous injection of HMPAO Tc99M during the pure tone stimulation in both left and right ear, showing average activity comparison when the right ear is stimulated than the left ear

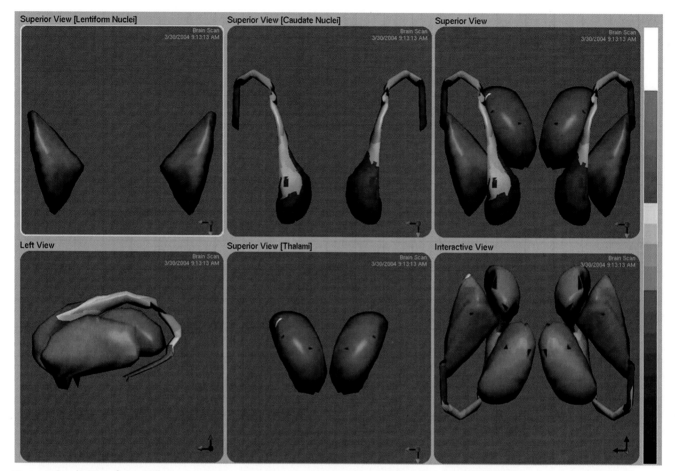

Figure 4 Ganglia 3D perfusion (different views): Diminution of the right caudate nucleus is seen at the level of basal ganglia

Bilateral Pure Tone Activation[9]

During bilateral pure tone activation in the soundproof room in six normal volunteers, we observed activation of both frontal lobes at the level of the intermediate gyrus, but less extensively and intensively than in the unilateral pure tone activation (Figure 5).

On contrast, there is also, in this patient, less activation of the posterior parietal lobes lateralized in this case to the left side which is distinctively more active than the right hemisphere. The deactivation of the temporal lobes appears very significant in both lateral aspects and extends also in the inferior gyrus bilaterally and finally, at the level at the limbic system, there is diminution of perfusion in anterior, intermediate and posterior cingulate gyri.

The analysis of perfusion in the basal ganglia demonstrate increased perfusion above 2 SD of the normal mean (color white), located bilaterally in the ventral aspect, intermediate section of the thalami and also in both lentiform nuclei at the level of the projection of the globus pallidus (white color), while the perfusion of caudate nuclei appears to be increased in the ventral view of the left caudate (Figure 6).

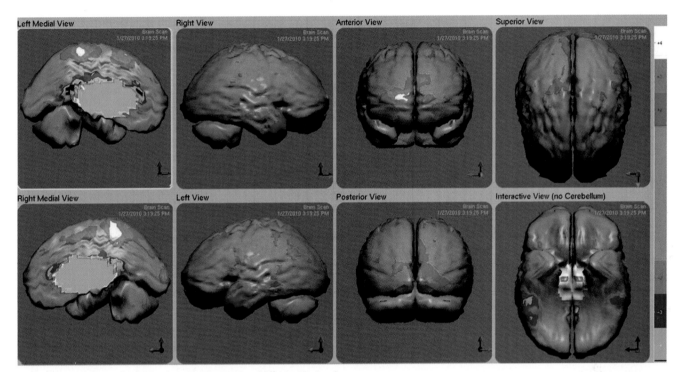

Figure 5 Images taken after bilateral pure tone activation (different 3D views)

Autoevocation of Music[5]

The patient described in Figures 7 and 8 is representative of a group of six normal individuals during the process of autoevocation of music and the characteristic response gathered in the soundproof room is again an activation of both frontal lobes at the level of the intermediate gyrus. There is also increased function in both posterior parietal lobes, more marked and extensive in the right hemisphere and activation in both inferior frontal lobes and the anterior pole of the right temporal lobe in the projection of the amygdale. In this patient, there is also the mild deactivation of both temporal lobes more significant in the left hemisphere and in the projection of the area 38 of Brodmann, the anterior pole of the left temporal lobe (Figure 7).

At the level of the basal ganglia there is activation of both thalami in the ventral aspects of the anterior aspects of these nuclei. There is also activation in the lentiform nucleus in the ventral aspects of both inferior sections, while perfusion in caudate nuclei appear normal (Figure 8).

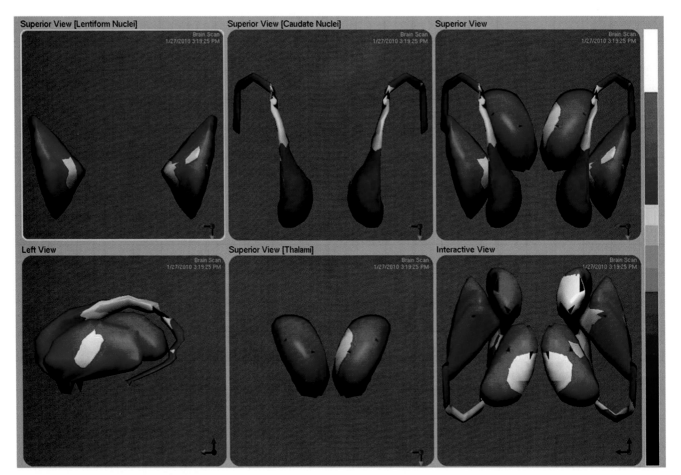

Figure 6 Analysis of perfusion at the level of basal ganglia

Auditory Hallucinations[2,4]

The patient described in Figures 9 and 10 who presented with auditory hallucinations, after abruptly becoming deaf, presents with activation of both frontal lobes at the level of the intermediate gyrus with extension to the orbital frontal aspects of the frontal lobe predominantly in the right hemisphere (Figure 9).

The statistical significance of these findings fluctuate between 2 SD and 4 SD above the normal mean of the normal range, namely red, pink and white colors (at 2, 3 and 4 SD) respectively. In this patient of note, there is no activation in the posterior parietal lobes, but there are signs of deactivations in the lateral aspects of temporal lobes more significant in the right hemisphere, light and dark blue colors, at 2 and 3 SD below the normal mean respectively.

At the level of the basal ganglia in this patient, experimenting auditory hallucinations, there is very intense activation of both lentiform nuclei predominantly in the inferior aspects, while perfusion in both thalami and both caudate nuclei appear normal (Figure 10).

Of note, there is also increased perfusion in areas of association of the visual cortex mainly areas 17, 18 and 19 of Brodmann, in the three groups of studies, mainly, stimulation of the right ear, stimulation of the left ear and bilateral stimulation. There is also increased perfusion in areas 7 (posterior parietal area), predominantly in unilateral stimulation (area 7 is an area of

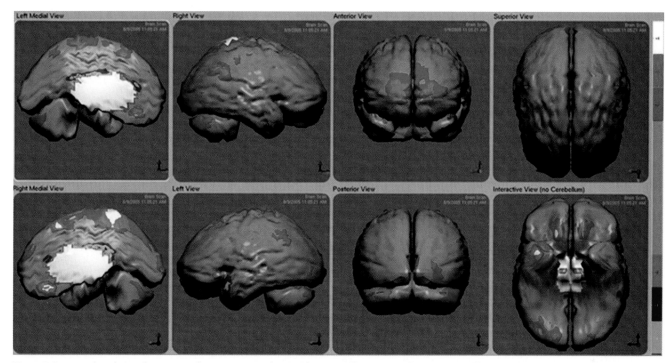

Figure 7 Images taken during the process of autoevocation of music (showing different areas of activation in different 3D views)

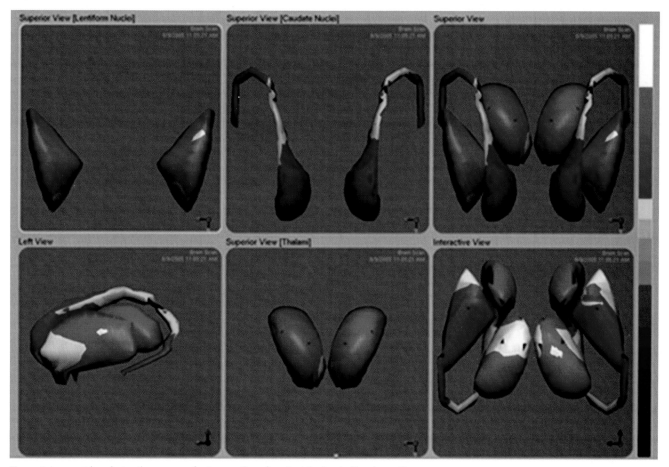

Figure 8 Images taken during the process of autoevocation of music at the level of basal ganglia

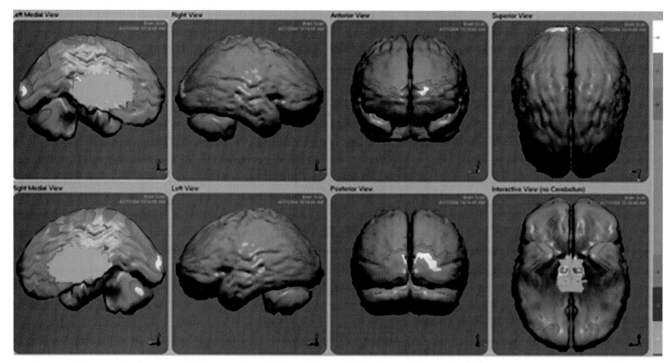

Figure 9 Images taken in a deaf patient, presenting with auditory hallucinations

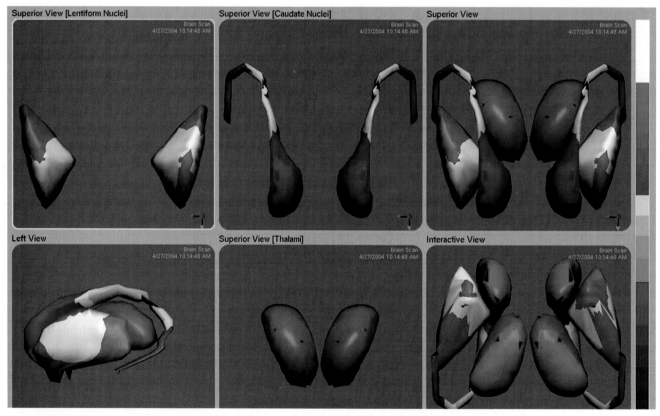

Figure 10 Images taken at the level of basal ganglia in deaf patient, presenting with auditory hallucinations

visual auditory association), and at the level of the thalamus, there is markedly increased function in both unilateral stimulations and less so in the bilateral stimulation, please see Table 1.

DISCUSSION

The analysis of the group of patients that have been reported demonstrate a remarkable reproducibility of results among the four populations, thus validating the accuracy of their functional imaging technique. The reconstruction process in the Oasis NeuroGam software is automatic, thus rendering it a highly reproducible image processing technique. We equate brain perfusion with brain function, as there is in the brain 1:1 relationship among these phenomena. The brain tracer Tc99m HMPAO evaluates primarily brain perfusion in the presence of intact blood-brain-barrier, which is a condition for the accurate analysis of these experiments.

Furthermore, we were impressed by the constant activation of frontal lobes during perception of unilateral sound, bilateral sound, autoevocation of sound and musical hallucinations. This phenomenon also occurs in normal individuals during frontal activation with the Wisconsin card sorting test and in pathological conditions in bipolar mood disorder, obsessive compulsive disorder, attention deficit disorder and schizophrenia with hallucinogenic activity.[1,6,7] One wonders if this phenomenon is a manifestation of frontal lobe normal control and modulation of sensory perception and it is more intense if the sensations are abnormal as in the comparison unilateral versus bilateral audition. In the former, frontal activation is more intense than in the later.

These studies also point out that the site of storage of the audition phenomenon appear to be areas 39 and 40 of Brodmann in the posterior parietal lobes, in the left hemisphere adjacent to the Wernike's area. Other cortical areas that participate in the audition phenomenon are areas of visual-auditory association, such as area 7 of Brodmann, also posterior parietal lobes and visual association areas 17 and 18, and audio-visual areas, area 19 of Brodmann. During all these cortical activation processes, there is temporal inhibition in particular of area 38 of Brodmann in the anterior pole of the temporal lobes. Area 38 of Brodmann is a modulatory region of impulses generated in the surrounding environment, therefore, sensory information. Furthermore, the auditory process activates intensely both thalami with intense activity in the anterior dorsoventral area.

All these findings are present in the four groups studied with variable intensities and cortical extensions that are characteristic for each group.

In activation of the left ear, Figure 1 depicts the very intense and extensive frontal activation; Figure 2 demonstrates intense activation also of areas 39 and 40 of Brodmann, while there is deactivation of the temporal lobes in areas 38, 21 and 22 of Brodmann, also area 7 appears very active. Something similar appears for activation of the right ear, with lack of thalamic activation in Figures 3 and 4. While in Bilateral pure tone activation, there is a much milder frontal activation and also posterior parietal, with marked temporal deactivation and thalamic activation (Figures 5 and 6).

A very interesting phenomenon occurs among musicians and music composers, namely autoevocation of music. This is well-known for the great music composers, such as Beethoven, Mozart, Brahms, etc. they had the capacity to hear their compositions, edit them and create new music while auto evoking it. Figures 7 and 8 demonstrate the functional changes occurring during this phenomenon, namely significant bilateral frontal and posterior bilateral parietal activation, with activation also of the anterior temporal lobe in the projection of the amygdala, while there is temporal deactivation and strong thalamic increased perfusion. In auditory hallucinations, there is weak frontal activation, markedly increased lentiform nucleus activation and also activation in the medial aspects of the cerebellum, while there is mild deactivation of the temporal lobes.

In summary these experiments demonstrate a complex cortical structure involved in the process of audition involving in their storage and modulation, frontal, parietal, temporal and subcortical structures that intervene with different intensities and extensions in the four modalities of audition tested in these experiments.

REFERENCES

1. Mena I, Correa R, Nader A, et al. Bipolar affective disorders: Assessment of functional brain changes by means of Tc99m HMPAO NeuroSPECT. Alasbimn Journal 6(23);2004. [online] Alasbimn Journal website. Available from www2.alasbimnjournal. cl/alasbimn/CDA/sec_b/0,1206,SCID%253D7485,00.html. [Accessed June, 2011].

2. Goycoolea M, Mena I, Neubauer S. Fuctional studies of the human auditory cortex, auditory memory and musical hallucinations. Alasbimn Journal 6(25);2004. [online] Alasbimn 134 Journal website. Available from www2.alasbimnjournal. cl/alasbimn/CDA/sec_b/0,1206,SCID%253D11173,00.html. [Accessed June, 2011].

3. Goycoolea M, Mena I, Neubauer S. Functional studies of the human auditory pathway alter monaural stimulation with pure

tones. Establishing a normal database. Acta Oto-Laryngologica. 2005;125:513-9.

4. Goycoolea M, Mena I, Neubauer S. Spontaneous musical auditory perceptions in patients who develop abrupt bilateral sensorineuronal hearing loss. An uninhibition syndrome. Acta Oto-Laryngologica. 2006;126:368-74.

5. Goycoolea M, Mena I, Neubauer S, et al. Musical Brains: a study of spontaneous and evoked musical sensations without external auditory stimuli. Acta Oto-Laryngologica. 2007;127:711-31.

6. Mena I. Editorial: El Futuro de NeuroSPECT. Alasbimn Journal. 2008;10 (40).

7. Mena G, Ismael. NeuroSPECT applications in Psychiatry. Alasbimn Journal 2009;11(45). Article N° AJ45-1. [online] Alasbimn journal website. Available from www.alasbimnjournal.cl/. [Accessed June, 2011].

8. Goycoolea M, Mena I, Neubauer S. Is there a difference in activation or in inhibition of cortical auditory centers depending on the ear that is stimulated? Acta Oto-Laryngologica. 2009;129(4):348-53.

9. Goycoolea M, Mena I, Neubauer S. Functional studies (NeuroSPECT) of the human auditory pathway after stimulating binaurally with pure tones. Acta Oto-Laryngologica. 2011;131(4):371-6.

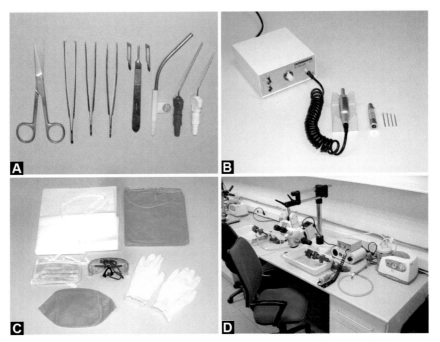

Figures 3A to D Instruments used for dissecting and obtaining a temporal bone by drilling

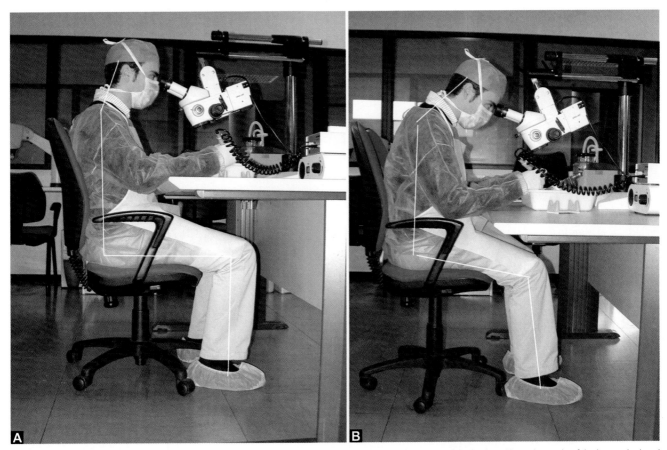

Figures 4A and B (A) Ergonomic position for dissection. Notice the resting position of the back, the angle of the back and legs, the angle of the knees, the head position and the leaning of the hands. (B) Also notice the nonfatiguing position on the right, with the neck slightly flexed, and the legs extended because of the correct height and position of the chair

Surgical Instruments and Drilling and Suction

A standard set on microsurgical instruments including a drill as well as instrumentation for temporal bone removal are a basic requirement. Cutting, as well as diamond burrs are required. Suction irrigation systems must be in working conditions and must have the capability of being regulated. Suction irrigation tips of different sizes are to be available.

Microscope

An operating microscope in working order and with an adjusted interpupillary distance is required. The usual focal distance is 200 mm.

Para-axial Work

It is very important to avoid that the axis of illumination of the microscope coincides with the axis of the surgical instruments because this makes vision and illumination inadequate, causing either poor illumination or appearance of shadows. Instruments that are used in cavities should have angles as open as possible. At times in narrow cavities such as the ear canal, focal distances of 250 mm can be useful (Figures 5A and B).

Drilling Technique

Drilling should be firm and slow, and it should be adapted to the underlying surface that is being drilled, depending on its consistency and hardness. Compact areas of bone require long movements and pneumatized areas short ones. Larger burrs are safer, however, size will depend on the area that is being drilled. Large burrs in the mastoid cortex and smaller ones in the attic or in posterior tympanectomy (to be described). Diamond burrs should be preferably used in areas like the labyrinth or near the facial nerve.

The Reference Points

Another important principle is that of following a series of reference anatomical points. These are natural anatomical structures that are to be used in a step-by-step manner in order to have

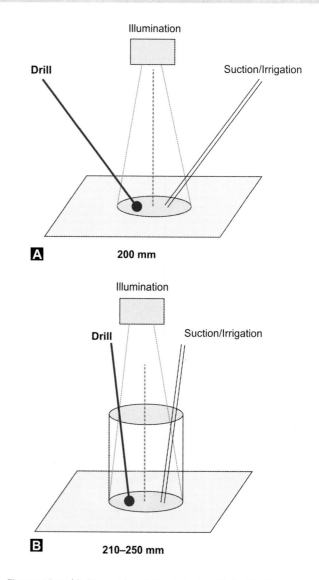

Figures 5A and B Para-axial work: the student avoids that the instruments cause a shadowing effect

a safe drilling procedure. For example, in mastoidectomy, MC Ewen area, the horizontal semicircular canal and the body of the incus are essential points to be identified (to be described in the following sections).

OBTAINING CADAVER SPECIMENS

Temporal bones can be obtained fresh or can be fixed after removal. They can also be obtained from archeological sites.[4]

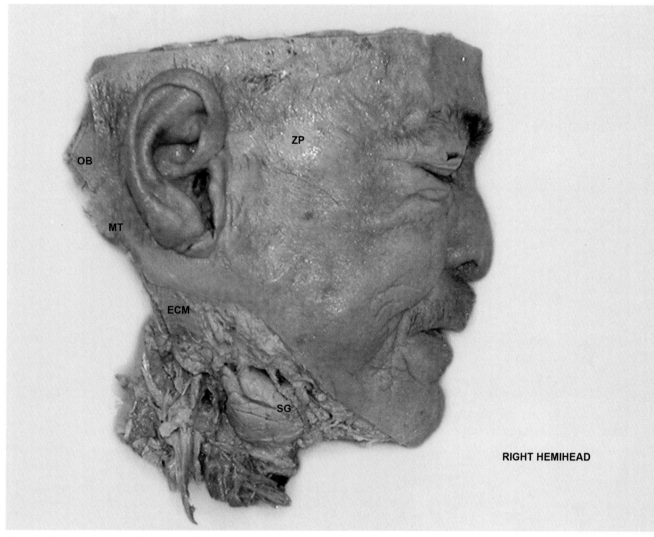

Figure 6 The head is positioned for temporal bone removal

Due to the current difficulties in obtaining human temporal bones (ethical, legal, practical, economic, etc.) temporal bones made of artificial materials that simulate human temporal bones have become available and are also useful as well as computerized 3D reproductions that allow surgical simulation using a computer.

In order to obtain a temporal bone from a cadaver, reference points are to be identified in the external as well as in the endocranial aspect (Figures 6 and 7). Having done this, the soft tissues are dissected and a saw is used (Figures 8 and 9). In this manner a block is obtained which has the squama, the mastoid tip and the root of the zygoma. Endocranially, the petrous and lateral sinuses are included as well as the petrous tip (Figures 10A to D). This is the specimen that is mounted and prepared for surgical dissection (Figure 11). This technique is also described later in this section.

145

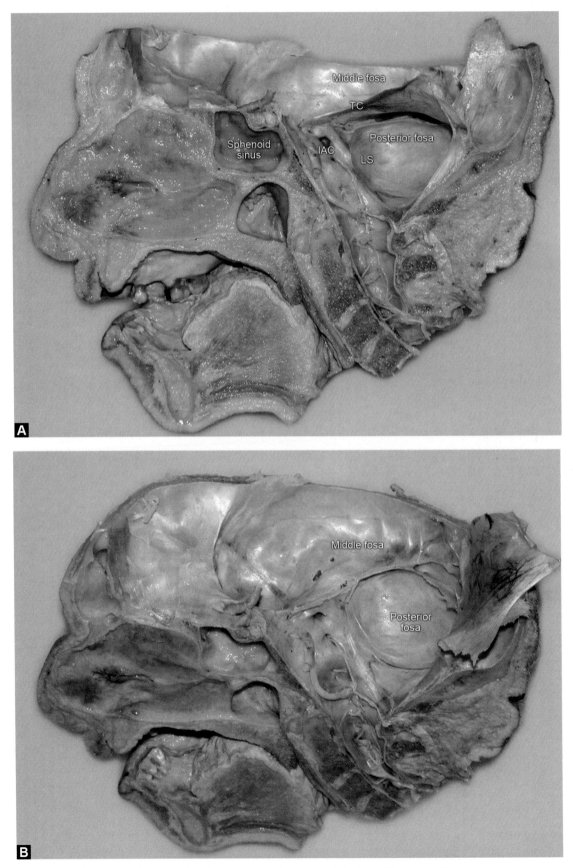

Figures 7A and B Positions that are used to observe intracranial anatomic relationships of the temporal bone

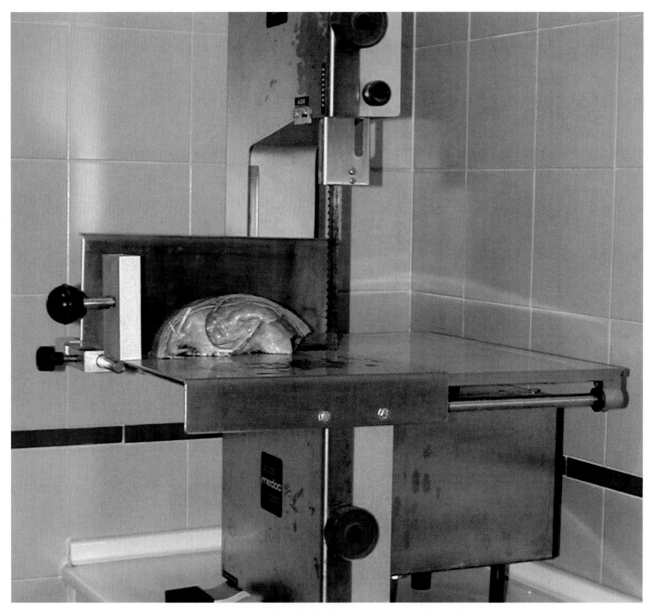

Figure 8 Saw for temporal bone removal

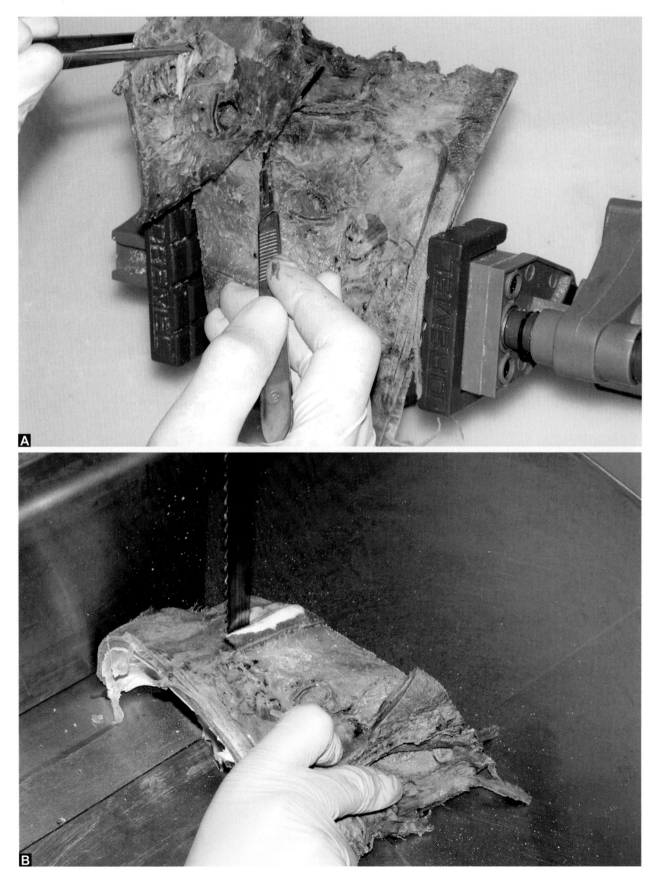

Figures 9A and B (A) Preparation of the soft tissues; (B) Sectioning with the saw

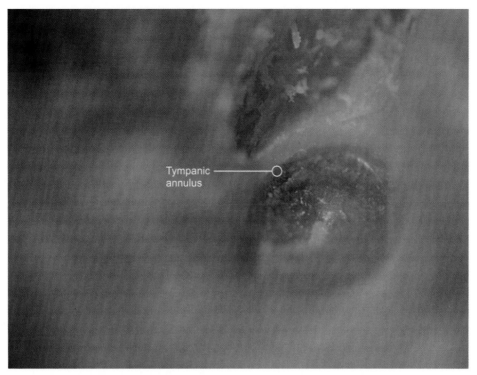

Figure 3 Canalplasty allows seeing the tympanic annulus as it is shown in this anatomic piece

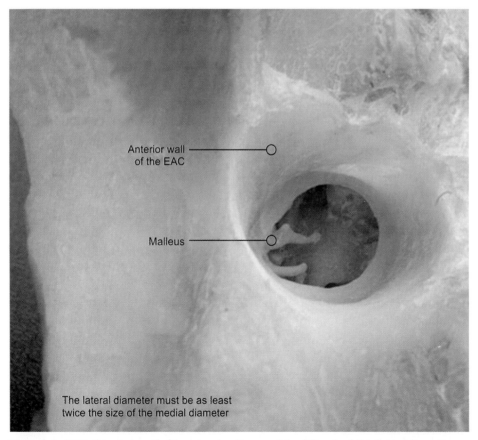

Figure 4 For TMJ in the anterior wall of the external auditory canal, the drilling should be done under continuous suction-irrigation, using diamond burr, to improve the visibility and help to appreciate the change of color in the wall

diamond burr, to improve the visibility and to help appreciate the change of color in the wall; (2) Perform the canalplasty first, before the mastoidectomy, because on the contrary, the posterior wall could be excessively thin, making an appropriated canalplasty difficult.

Creation of the tympanic sulcus (Figure 5): this surgical act is important when there is neither drum nor tympanic annulus. It is not a common situation, but it is critical to create the new sulcus to avoid the lateralization of the fascia. Remember to leave at least 2 mm of the medial flap, between the 2 and 4 (right ear) and the 8 and 10 (left ear), to avoid the blunting of the graft and because this medial flap improves the transmission of the sound. We can perfectly see the tympanic orifice of the Eustachian tube, the semicanal of the malleus muscle and the ossicular chain (Figure 6). This eases the surgical maneuvers, e.g. mastoidectomy with wide exposition of the mastoid, after canalplasty is performed as shown in the Figure 7.

Dissection of the anterior mallear ligament (Figure 8), a very important structure in the pathophysiology of the ossicular chain, because it is often ossified or hyalinized, which reduces the mobility of the ossicles. The intraoperative assessment (Figure 9) of the mobility of the ossicular chain in stapes surgery

is very important, especially when the anterior malleal ligament is fixed or hyalinizated; or when the long process of the incus is missing or atrophic, being malleostapedotomy the best option when it is not possible to perform incus-stapedotomy. Results are the same or even better than those of the incus-stapedotomy. For explanation of this technique, please consult ("Tympanoplasty, Mastoidectomy and Stapes Surgery, Prof Fisch U, May J, Linder T), Verlag T (2008).

Malleostapedotomy technique is not more difficult than an incus-stapedotomy. By removing the incus, one can see the footplate better. The placement of the prosthesis is not so difficult if one widen the loop a little, as the malleus handle is larger than the long process of the incus. Do not detach the drum from the malleus handle more than 1 mm under its short process, because when doing this, the prosthesis can be displaced, as it would lack the drum support (Figure 10).

Beginning of the surgical treatment of otosclerosis (Dr Julius Lempert, 1890–1968) fenestration of the horizontal semicircular canal in one surgical stage time is shown in the Figure 11.

Deciding to choose the closed cavity in a cholesteatoma surgery (Figure 12) depends on the possibility to fully remove the cholesteatoma through this way, without any doubt, and

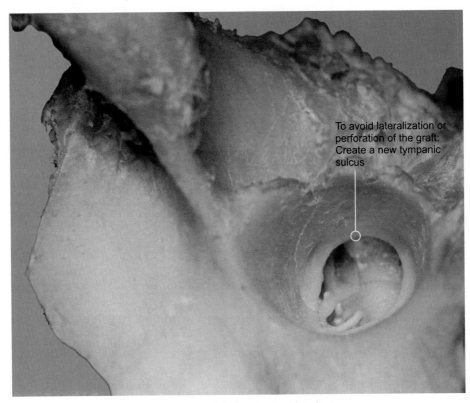

To avoid lateralization or perforation of the graft: Create a new tympanic sulcus

Figure 5 Creation of the tympanic sulcus to avoid the lateralization of the fascia

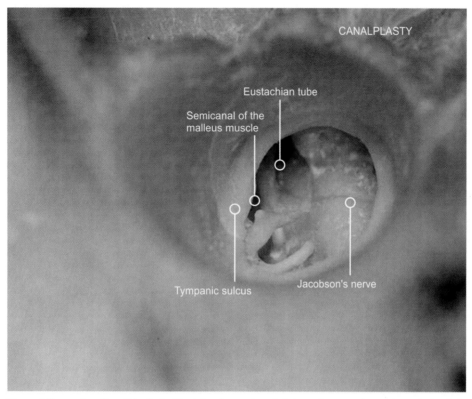

CANALPLASTY

Eustachian tube

Semicanal of the
malleus muscle

Tympanic sulcus

Jacobson's nerve

Figure 6 Tympanic orifice of the Eustachian tube; the semicanal of the malleus muscle and the ossicular chain seen after canalplasty eases the surgical maneuvers

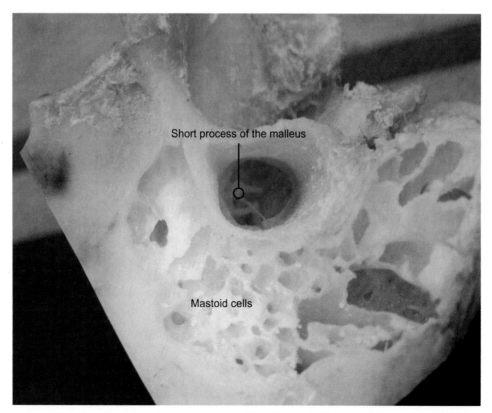

Short process of the malleus

Mastoid cells

Figure 7 Beginning of a mastoidectomy with wide exposition of the mastoid, after canalplasty has been performed

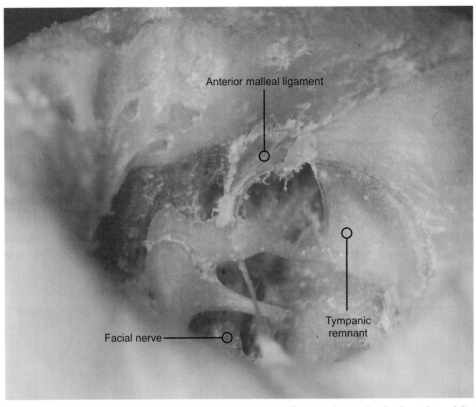

Figure 8 Dissection of the anterior mallear ligament when it gets ossified or hyalinizated and reduces the mobility of the ossicles

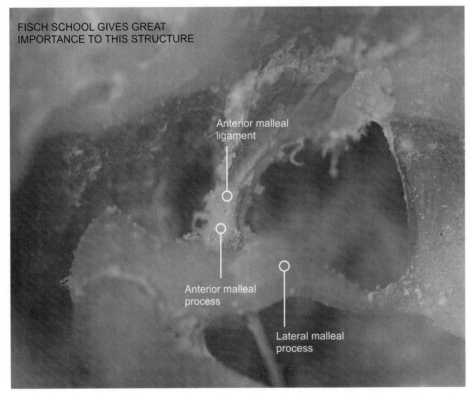

Figure 9 The intraoperative assessment of the mobility of the ossicular chain in stapes surgery is done when the anterior malleal ligament is fixed or hyalinizated; or when the long process of the incus is missing or atrophic

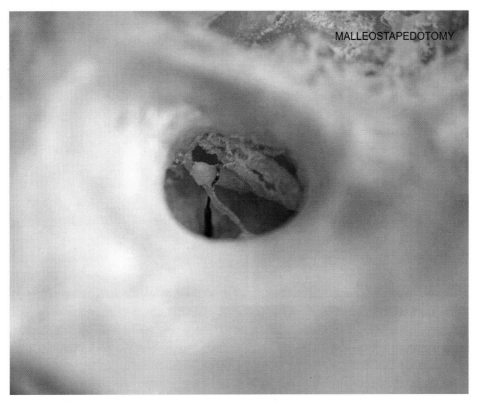

Figure 10 Malleostapedotomy technique

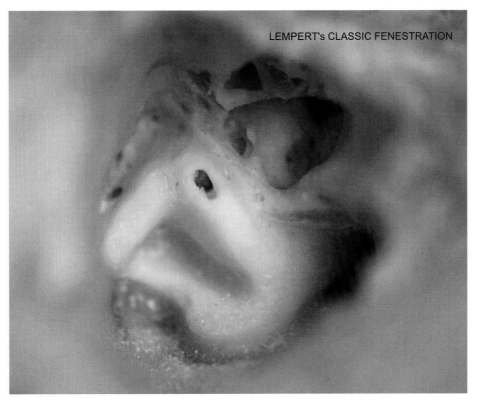

Figure 11 Lempert's classic fenestration

without leaving any pathology (e.g. cholesteatoma, cholesterol granuloma).

Closed cavity technique (Figure 13) is also universally accepted for cochlear implants; in the exploration of the tympanic and mastoid portion of the facial nerve and in tympanic glomus type A (Fisch classification). The principles of: exposition, skeletonization, exenteration and exteriorization are very important in all Fisch's techniques.

Skeletonization means that the structure becomes transparent; leaving only the last shell of bone that protects the structure, as illustrated in Figures 14 and 15.

This surgery was performed for cholesteatoma, early in the 20th Century, when excellent quality microscopic vision was not available; when the instrumental was limited and when there was great fear of injuring the facial nerve. One can see remaining mastoid cells (not exentered at all), the ossicular chain can be intact or partially, or totally destroyed as shown in the Figure 16.

Open cavity indications (Figure 17): Cholesteatoma, that it is not possible to completely remove using the closed cavity technique. This will be explained further in the chapter "Surgical treatment of the Cholesteatoma". Look at how regular and depurated the dissection is, without leaving bony overhangs or irregular surfaces. Keep in the mind that open cavity is the first step of the subtotal petrosectomy (Microsurgery of the Skull

Base: Fisch U, Mattox D, Thieme Verlag, 1988). One can see, in one shot, all the elements of the middle ear and the labyrinth, e.g. sigmoid sinus, semicircular canals, facial nerve, stylomastoid foramen, ossicular chain, Eustachian tube, semicanal of the tensor tympani muscle and round window (Figures 18 and 19).

Exenteration (Figures 20 and 21) means that all the mastoid and perilabyrinthine cells must be removed. One can see here the cochleariform process, a very steady anatomical structure in terms of its position and shape, useful for identification of the tympanic facial nerve.

The anatomical piece shown in Figure 22: a mastoid facial nerve that is perfectly skeletonized, preserving the last shell that protects the structure. Keep in mind that exploring the facial nerve from the stylomastoid foramen reduces the risk of injury to the semicircular canals. Besides, it is a very important and constant anatomic landmark (Figures 23A and B). Dissecting labyrinthine facial nerve is very important because the cholesteatoma is most commonly localized in the medial wall of the attic (supratubal and supralabyrinthine recesses) (Figure 24). It is important to take into account the acute angle formed by the labyrinthine and the tympanic segment of the facial nerve and the fact that the labyrinthine facial nerve runs under the tympanic facial nerve (nonfamiliarity with this anatomical feature creates a high-risk situation).

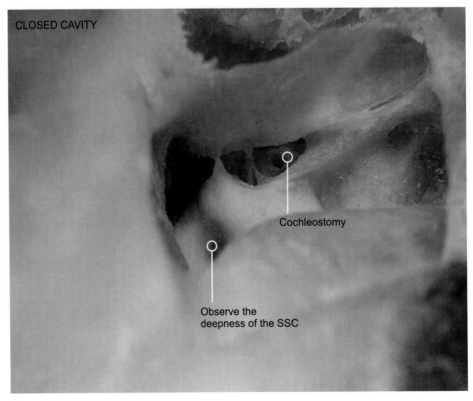

Figure 12 Cholesteatoma surgery

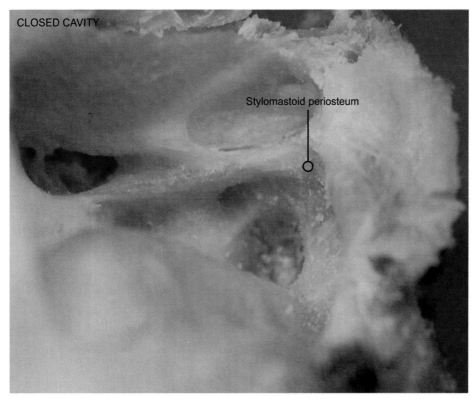

CLOSED CAVITY

Stylomastoid periosteum

Figure 13 Closed cavity technique for cochlear implants

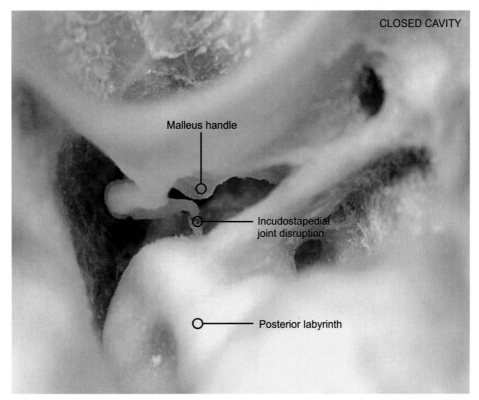

CLOSED CAVITY

Malleus handle

Incudostapedial
joint disruption

Posterior labyrinth

Figure 14 Skeletonization means that the structure become transparent; leaving only the last shell of bone that protects the structure

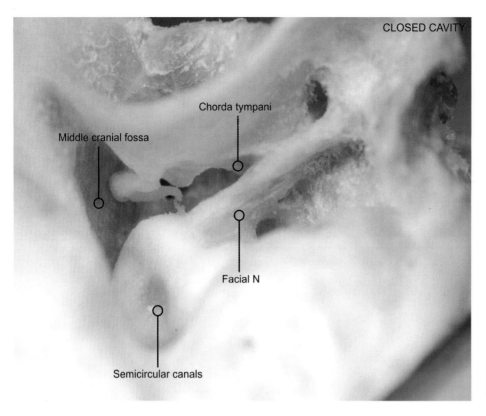

CLOSED CAVITY

Chorda tympani

Middle cranial fossa

Facial N

Semicircular canals

Figure 15 Skeletonization of the structures: middle cranial fossa, semicircular canals, facial nerve and chorda tympani

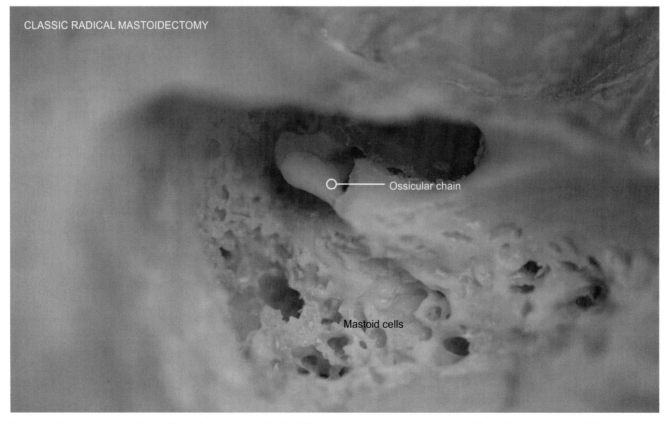

CLASSIC RADICAL MASTOIDECTOMY

Ossicular chain

Mastoid cells

Figure 16 This surgery was performed for cholesteatoma early in the 20th Century, one can see remaining mastoid cells (not exenterated at all), the ossicular chain can be intact, or can be partially or totally destroyed

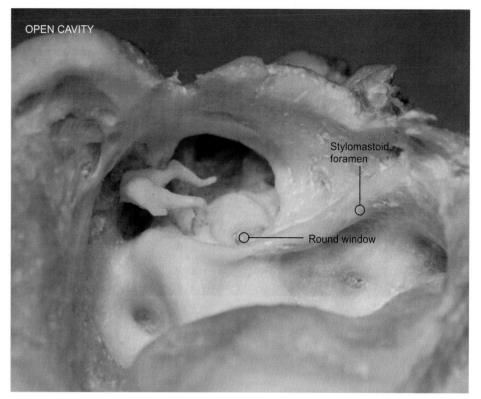

Figure 17 Open cavity technique is indicated in cholesteatoma, that it is not possible to completely remove using the closed cavity technique

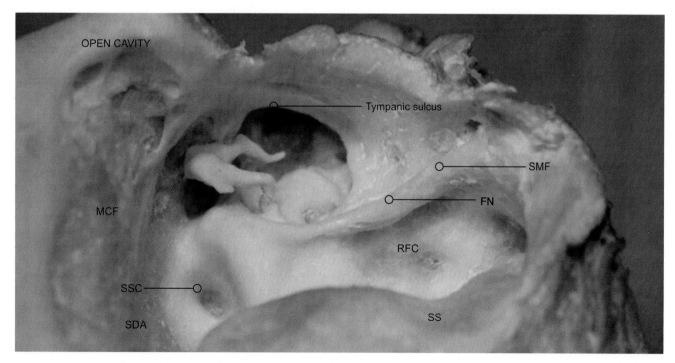

Figure 18 Open cavity technique: one can see, in one shot, all the elements of the middle ear and the labyrinth; FN: Facial nerve, MCF: Middle craneal fossa, RFC: Retrofacial cells, SMF: Stylomastoid foramen, SS: Sigmoid sinus, SSC: Superior semicircular canal

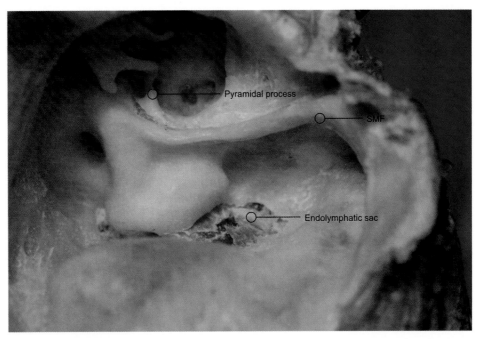

Figure 19 Open cavity technique: the principle is to see all anatomical structures with one position of the microscope
SMF: Stylomastoid foramen

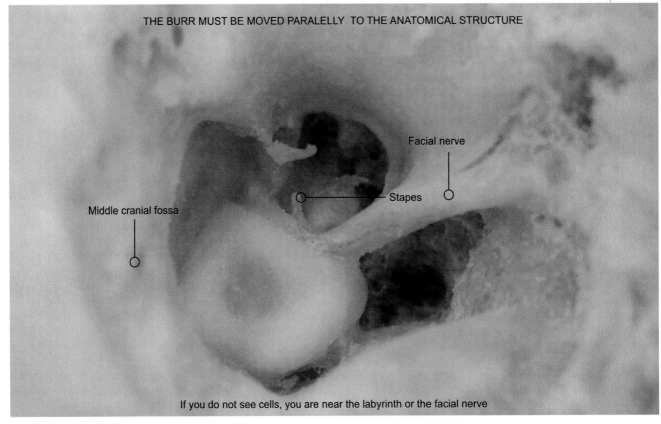

THE BURR MUST BE MOVED PARALELLY TO THE ANATOMICAL STRUCTURE

If you do not see cells, you are near the labyrinth or the facial nerve

Figure 20 Exenteration: all the mastoid and perilabyrinthine cells are removed

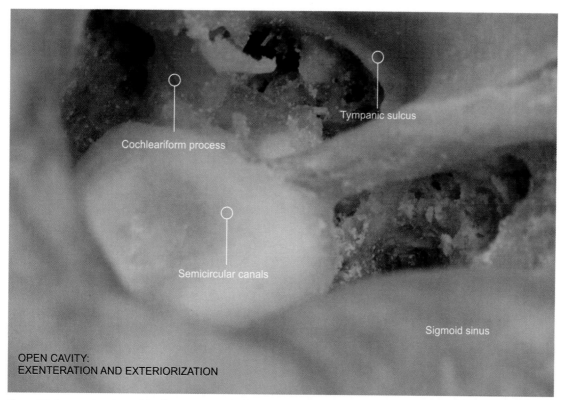

Figure 21 Exenteration: the cochleariform process in the figure, is a very steady anatomical structure in terms of its position and shape, useful for identification of the tympanic facial nerve

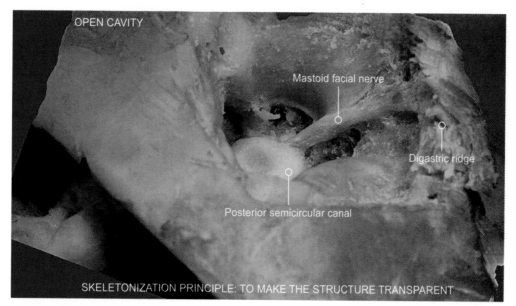

Figure 22 This anatomical piece shows a mastoid facial nerve that is perfectly skeletonized, preserving the last shell that protects the structure

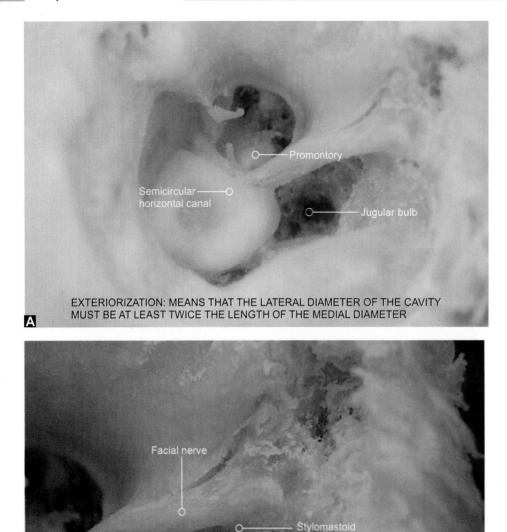

Figures 23A and B (A) Exteriorization with lateral diameter of the cavity must be at least twice the length of the medial diameter; (B) Exploring the facial nerve from the stylomastoid foramen

Skeletonization of facial nerve, semicircular canals and chorda tympani, with epitympanectomy: removal of malleus and incus head, with visualization of the chorda tympani, through the tympanic cavity (Figure 25), one can observe the anterior maleollar ligament. Remember that in the Fisch technique, the epitympanectomy is a fundamental principle of the cholesteatoma removal. Take this into account that in the cholesteatoma surgery, it is critical to remove the pathology and not only to improve the hearing temporarily, which would leave a pathology that would require future additional surgeries.

Figure 26 is showing the beginning of the labyrinthectomy with exposition of the mastoid facial nerve and the jugular bulb. Skeletonization of the internal carotid artery, jugular bulb, modiolus, semicircular canals and facial nerve, as shown

THIS IS A VERY IMPORTANT DISSECTION

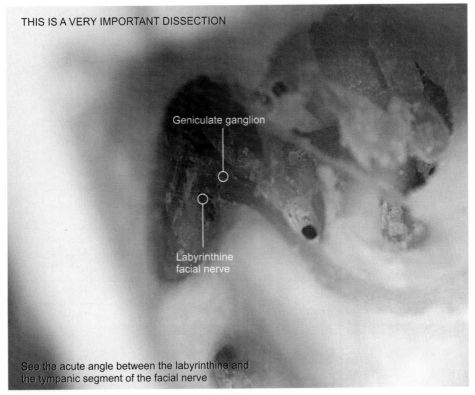

Geniculate ganglion

Labyrinthine
facial nerve

See the acute angle between the labyrinthine and
the tympanic segment of the facial nerve

Figure 24 Dissecting labyrinthine facial nerve is very important because the cholesteatoma is most commonly localized in the medial wall of the attic (supratubal and supralabyrinthine recesses)

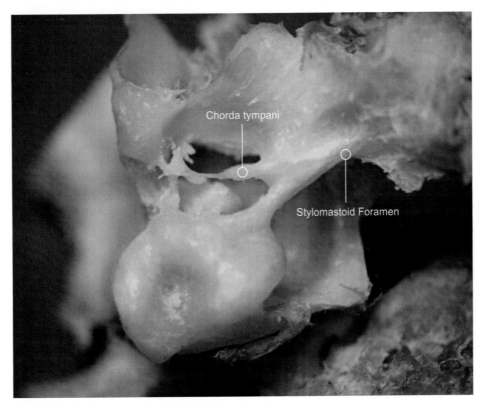

Chorda tympani

Stylomastoid Foramen

Figure 25 Skeletonization of facial nerve, semicircular canals and chorda tympani, with epitympanectomy: removal of malleus and incus head, with visualization of the chorda tympani, through the tympanic cavity one can observe the anterior maleollar ligament

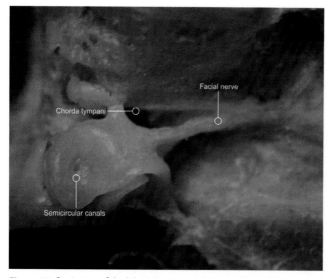

Figure 26 Beginning of the labyrinthectomy with exposition of the mastoid facial nerve and the jugular bulb

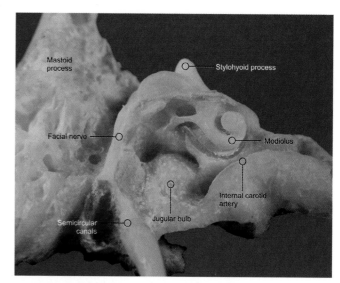

Figure 27 Skeletonization of the internal carotid artery, jugular bulb, modiolus, semicircular canals and facial nerve

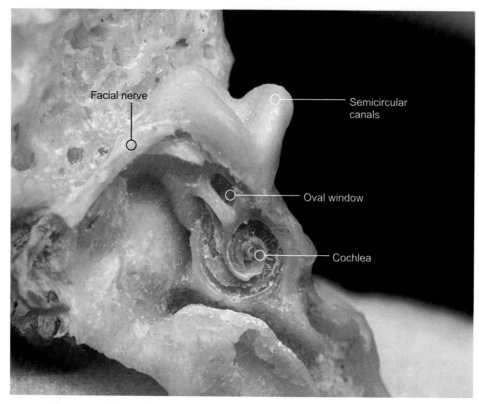

Figure 28 Exposition of the membranous cochlea

in the Figure 27. This is an important dissection to evaluate the structures surrounding the cochlea for cochlear implantation purpose. Exposition of the membranous cochlea is also shown in the Figure 28.

Dissection seen from the anterosuperior wall of the petrous bone, exposing the cochlea, the facial acoustic bundle, the superior vestibular nerve and its entrance to the superior semicircular canal is shown in the Figures 29 and 30(A and B).

One can see how the superior semicircular canal has been skeletonized and thus exposed the endosteum, therefore, helping to find the internal auditory canal with confidence through the "Fisch's angle mark" (a 60° angle constituted by the blue

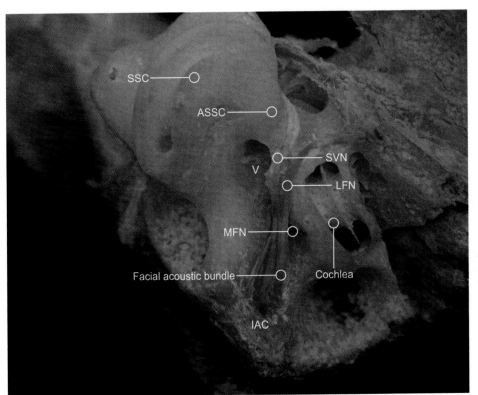

SSC —○

ASSC —○

SVN

V

LFN

MFN —○

Facial acoustic bundle —○

Cochlea

IAC

Figure 29 Dissection seen from the anterosuperior wall of the petrous bone, exposing the cochlea, the facial acoustic bundle, the superior vestibular nerve and its entrance to the superior semicircular canal
ASSC: Anterior superior semicircular canal
IAC: Internal auditory canal
LFN: Labyrynthine facial nerve
MFN: Meatal facial nerve
SSC: Superior semicircular canal
SVN: Superior vestibular nerve; V: Vestibule

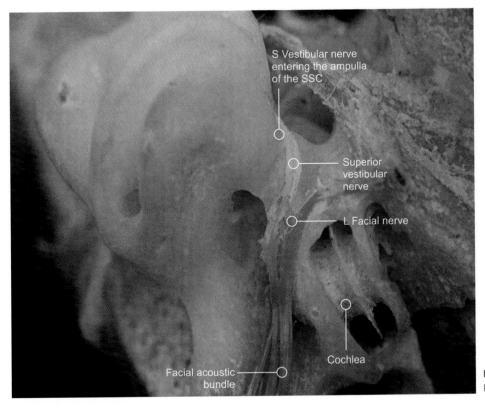

S Vestibular nerve entering the ampulla of the SSC

Superior vestibular nerve

L Facial nerve

Cochlea

Facial acoustic bundle

Figure 30A Closer shot of the same anatomic piece as shown in Figure 29.

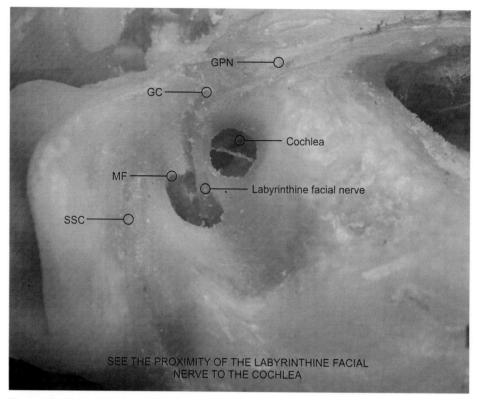

SEE THE PROXIMITY OF THE LABYRINTHINE FACIAL
NERVE TO THE COCHLEA

Figure 30B GC: Geniculate crest; GPN: Greater petrosal nerve; MF: Meatal foramen; SSC: Superior semicircular
canal

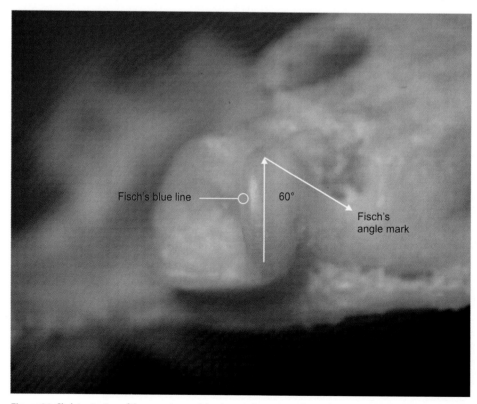

Figure 31 Skeletonization of the superior semicircular canal, exposing the endosteum, therefore, helping to find
the internal auditory canal with confidence through the "Fisch's angle mark" (a 60° angle constituted by the blue
line of the semicircular superior canal and an imaginary line to the internal auditory canal) to avoid injuring the
middle meningeal artery

line of the semicircular superior canal and an imaginary line to the internal auditory canal) avoiding to injure the middle meningeal artery (Figure 31).

Structures identified after drilling the anterosuperior wall of the petrous bone (Figure 32) include greater petrosal nerve, superior vestibular nerve, superior ampullar nerve, tympanic segment of the facial nerve, labyrinthine segment of the facial nerve, geniculate crest (Fisch), meatal foramen (Fisch) and vertical crest (Bill's Barr).

The Bill's Barr separates the labyrinthine facial nerve from the superior vestibular nerve (Figures 33 and 34). The difference between a middle cranial fossa approach (as described by William House), and a transtemporal supralabyrinthine approach (as described by Ugo Fisch) is that according to House, the exposition is obtained by the elevation of the dura and according to Fisch, it is obtained by removing the bone between the dura and the otic capsule which minimizes the lesions to the middle fossa dura.

Dissection of the semicircular canals show that the subarcuate artery, which is usually located between the semicircular canals, in this case is above, or entering into the superior semicircular canal (Figure 35). Unawareness of the minimal variations in the temporal bone anatomy could lead to the destruction of the superior semicircular canal, which results in the patient's total loss of hearing. When revision surgery of chronic ear or cholestomatous ear is performed, it is highly recommended to use a facial nerve monitor, accompanied by the best possible anatomical knowledge.

It is important to locate the cochleariform process, as a landmark to find the tympanic facial nerve (Figure 36). This is another place where the facial nerve is often injured in cholesteatoma surgery.

Superior and posterior semicircular canal joint is shown in the Figure 37. Note the change in color and density of the bone when one is arriving to the labyrinth, on top of the absence of mastoid cells.

One can see the vestibule after opening the semicircular canals. First steps of the labyrinthectomy in cochleovestibular neurectomy or in Fisch transotic approach (Figures 38A to D).

Skeletonization of the internal auditory canal from the anterosuperior wall of the petrosal bone; the cochlea and the attic can be seen [Figures 39 and 40(A to H)].

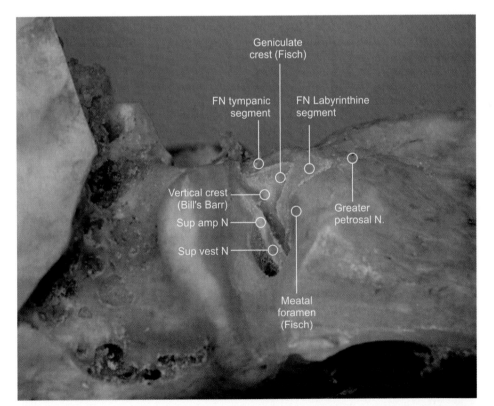

Figure 32 Identification of the structures after drilling the anterosuperior wall of the petrous bone: greater petrosal nerve, superior vestibular nerve, superior ampullar nerve, tympanic segment of the facial nerve, labyrinthine segment of the facial nerve, geniculate crest (Fisch), meatal foramen (Fisch) and vertical crest (Bill's Barr)

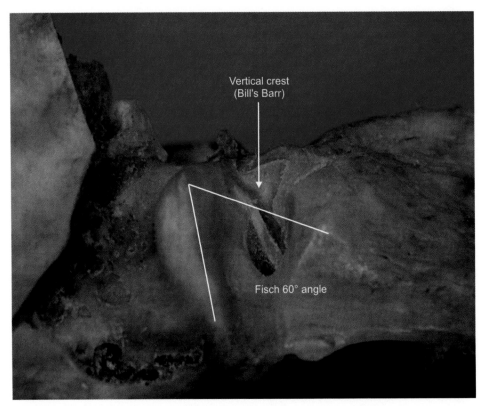

Figure 33 The Bill's Barr separates the labyrinthine facial nerve from the superior vestibular nerve

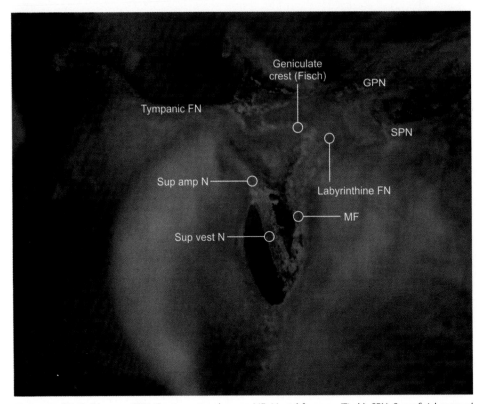

Figure 34 FN: Facial nerve; GPN: Greater petrosal nerve; MF: Meatal foramen (Fisch); SPN: Superficial petrosal nerve

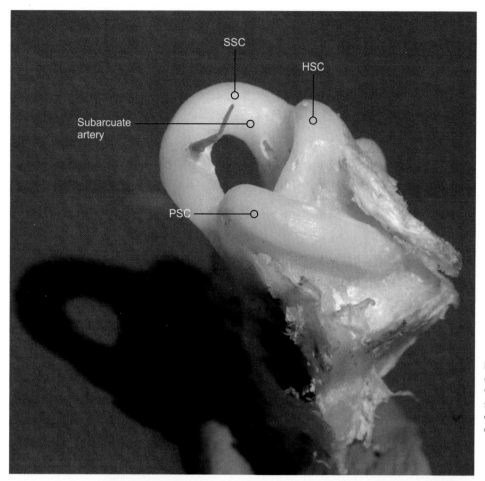

Figure 35 Dissection of the semicircular canals show that the subarcuate artery, which is usually located between the semicircular canals, in this case is above or entering into the superior semicircular canal

HSC: Horizontal semicircular canal
PSC: Posterior semicircular canal
SSC: Superior semicircular canal

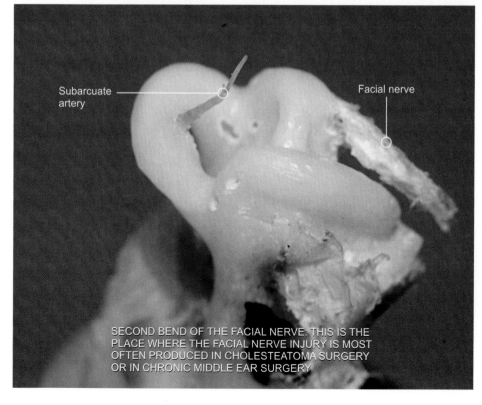

SECOND BEND OF THE FACIAL NERVE: THIS IS THE PLACE WHERE THE FACIAL NERVE INJURY IS MOST OFTEN PRODUCED IN CHOLESTEATOMA SURGERY OR IN CHRONIC MIDDLE EAR SURGERY

Figure 36 Locating the cochleariform process, as a landmark to find the tympanic facial nerve

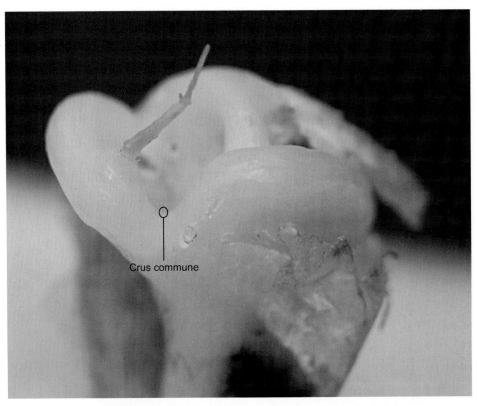

Figure 37 Superior and posterior semicircular canal joint

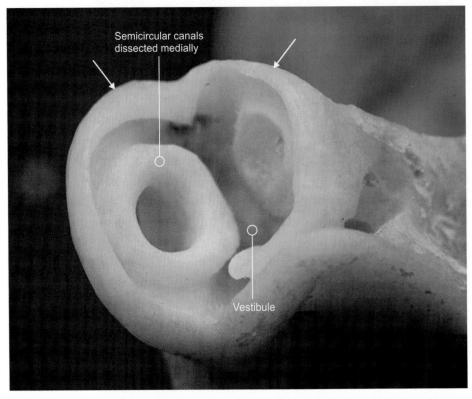

Figure 38A

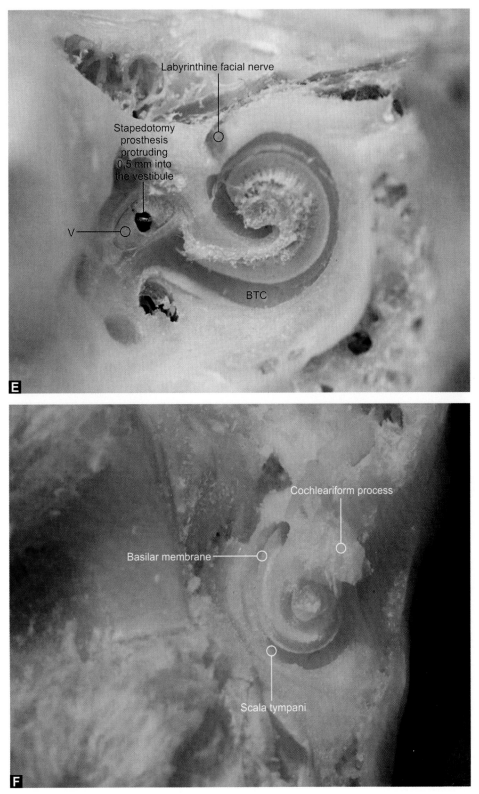

Figures 40E and F

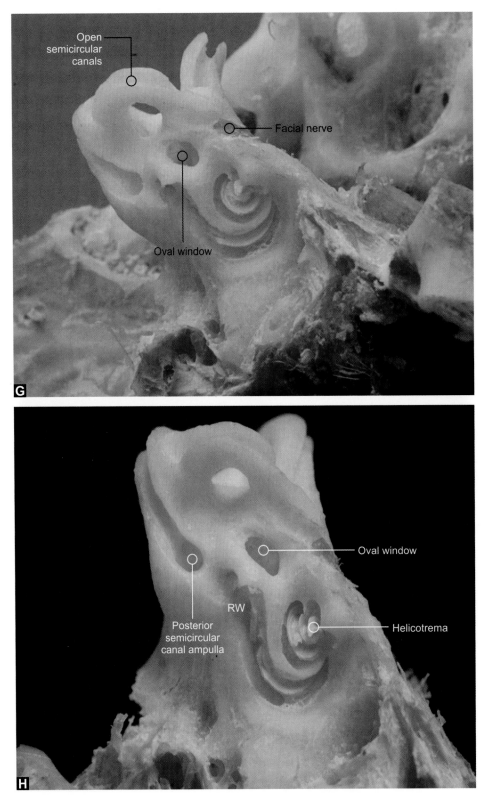

Figures 40G and H

Figures 40A to H Exposition of the internal auditory canal
RW: Round window; SV: Superior vestibule; V: Vestibule; BTC: Basal turn of the cochlea

2.3
Temporal Bone Dissection

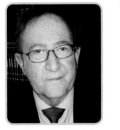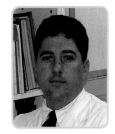

Edgar Chiossone Lares, Juan A Chiossone Kerdal

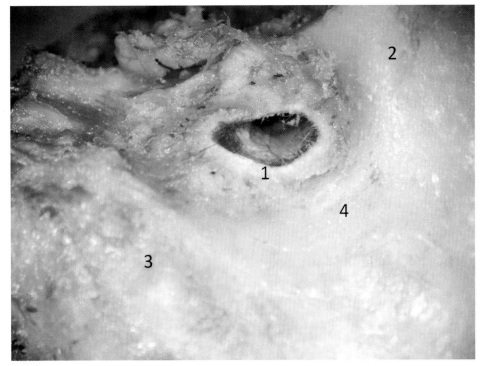

Figure 1 Left temporal bone. 1. External auditory canal (EAC); 2. Zygoma; 3. Mastoid; 4. Spine of Henle

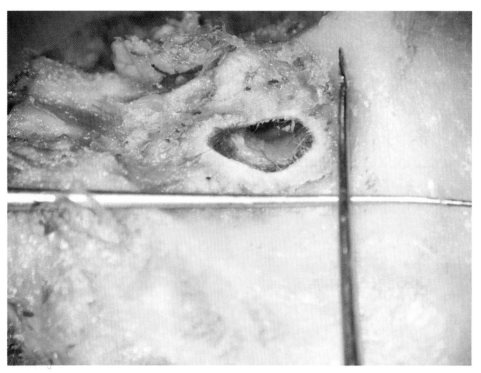

Figure 2 If a line is drawn tangential to the superior wall of the EAC and a second one is drawn by the posterior wall, the point where both lines come together, corresponds (in depth) to the area of the mastoid antrum. This usually coincides in the surface with the area that is posterior to the spine of Henle

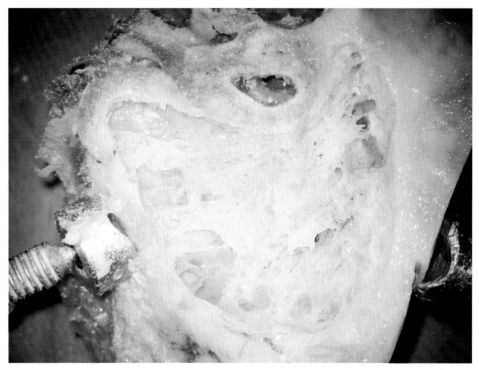

Figure 3A The mastoidectomy should be wide from the very beginning. The temporal bone is the route for the approach of the base of the skull, therefore, the anatomical dissection must involve exanteration of all the mastoid air cells

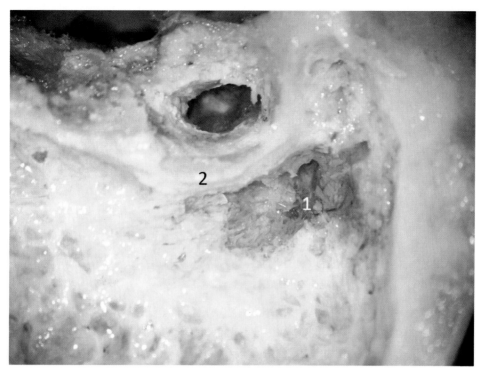

Figure 3B The 1. Mastoid antrum; 2. Posterior wall of EAC

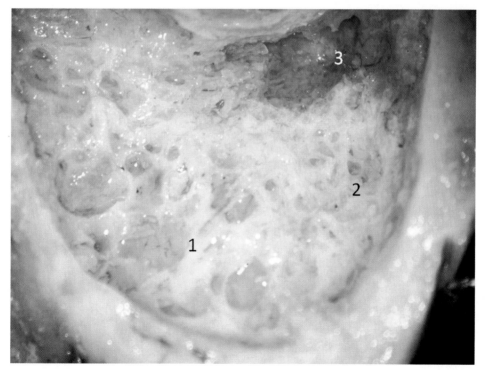

Figure 3C The sigmoid sinus (1) starts to appear gradually and so does the dural plate of the middle cranial fossa (2) and the mastoid antrum (3)

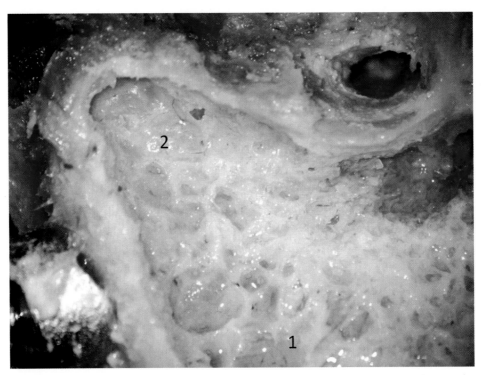

Figure 4 Dissection of the mastoid tip. The sigmoid sinus (1) and the digastric ridge (2) can be seen by transparency

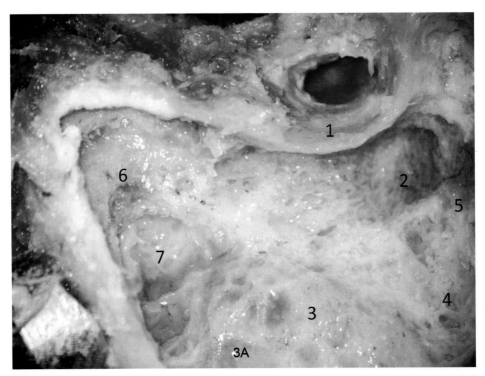

Figure 5 After a wide mastoid dissection the following structures can be observed: 1. Intact posterior wall of the external auditory canal; 2. Horizontal semicircular canal in the mastoid antrum; 3. Sigmoid sinus with its retrosigmoid region (3 A); 4. The sinodural angle; 5. The dural plate of the middle fossa; 6. The digastric ridge; 7. Medial to it, the jugular bulb starts to appear

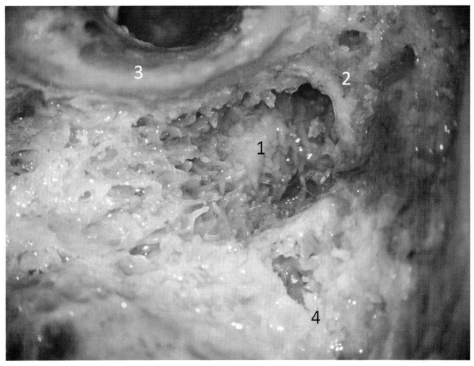

Figure 6 Structures in the mastoid antrum: 1. Horizontal semicircular canal; 2. Osseous wall that forms the lateral wall of the attic; 3. External auditory canal.; 4. Sinodural angle

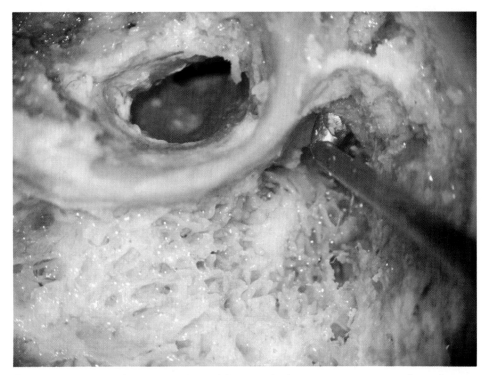

Figure 7 The lateral wall of the attic must be carefully removed with a curette, moving it externally in order not to harm or disarticulate the ossicular chain; in particular the incudomalleolar joint

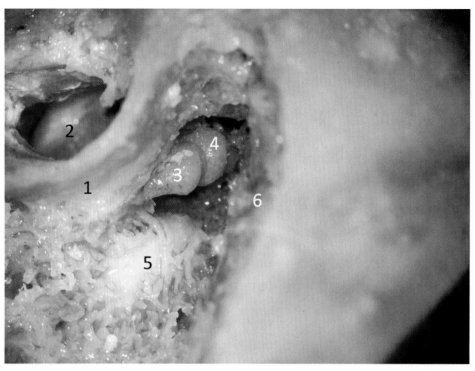

Figure 8 Structures of the mastoid antrum and attic. 1. External auditory canal; 2. Tympanic membrane; 3. Body of the incus; 4. Malleus head; 5. Horizontal semicircular canal; 6. Dural plate of the middle cranial fossa

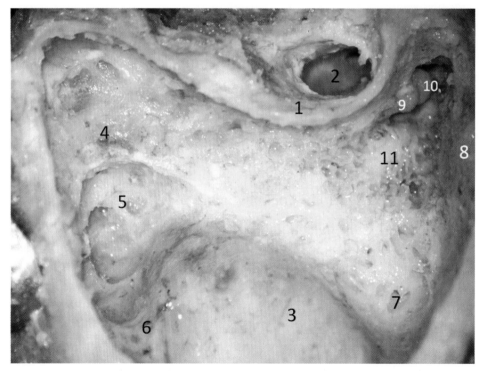

Figure 9 General view after a simple mastoidectomy. 1. External auditory canal; 2. Tympanic membrane; 3. Sigmoid sinus; 4. Area of the digastric ridge; 5. Area of the jugular bulb; 6. Retrosigmoid cells with a posterior emissary vein; 7. Sinodural angle; 8. Dural plate of the middle cranial fossa; 9. Incus; 10. Malleus; 11. Horizontal semicircular canal

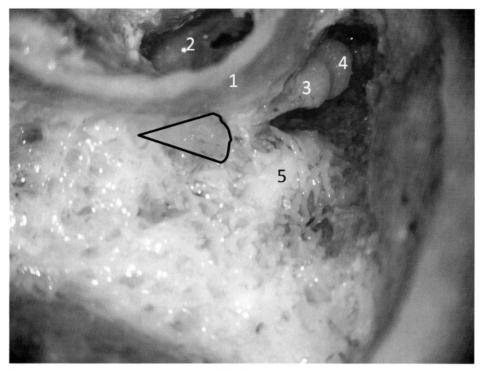

Figure 10A Posterior tympanotomy. Dissection of the facial recess. 1. The external auditory canal is thinned in order to expose the facial recess; 2. Tympanic membrane (at the end of the external auditory canal); 3. Body of the incus; 4. Malleus head; 5.Horizontal semicircular canal

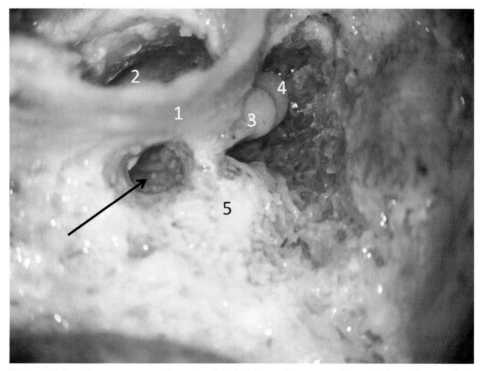

Figure 10B Posterior tympanotomy. Dissection of the facial recess. The arrow in Figure 10B shows the view of the middle ear cavity that is obtained through the posterior tympanotomy. 1. The external auditory canal is thinned in order to expose the facial recess; 2. Tympanic membrane (at the end of the external auditory canal); 3. Body of the incus. 4. Malleus head; 5.Horizontal semicircular canal

185

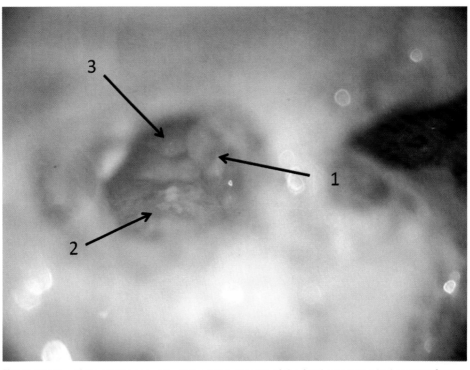

Figure 11 View of the middle ear cavity through the opening of the facial recess at a higher magnification. 1. Incudo stapedial joint; 2. Promontory; 3.Umbo of the tympanic membrane seen from the middle ear side

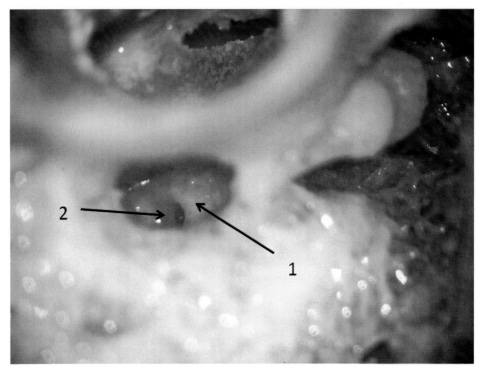

Figure 12 View of the round window niche (1) and the round window (2) as seen through the posterior tympanotomy

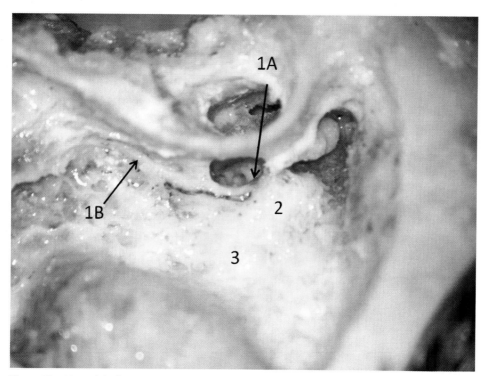

Figure 13 1. View of the facial nerve in its second genu (1 A) and its third or mastoid portion (1 B); 2. Horizontal semicircular canal; 3. Posterior semicircular canal

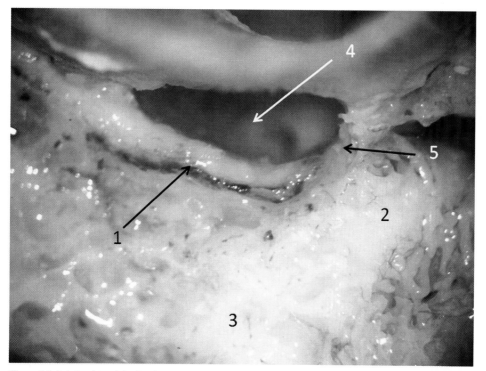

Figure 14 Relationship of the facial nerve (1) with the horizontal semicircular canal (2), the posterior semicircular canal (3), the posterior tympanotomy (4), and the fossa incudis (5)

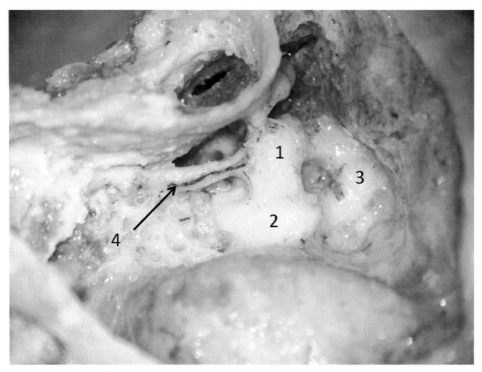

Figure 15 Exposure of the semicircular canals. 1. Horizontal semicircular canal; 2. Posterior semicircular canal; 3. Superior semicircular canal; 4. Facial nerve

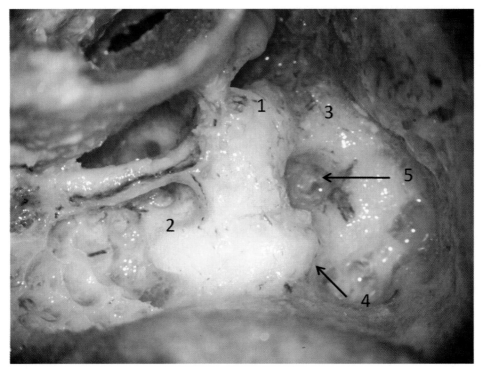

Figure 16 Dissection of the semicircular canals. 1. Ampullary end of the horizontal semicircular canal; 2. Ampullary end of the superior semicircular canal; 3. Area of the crus commune, area where tails of the superior and posterior semicircular canals come together; 4. Area where the subarcuate artery is found

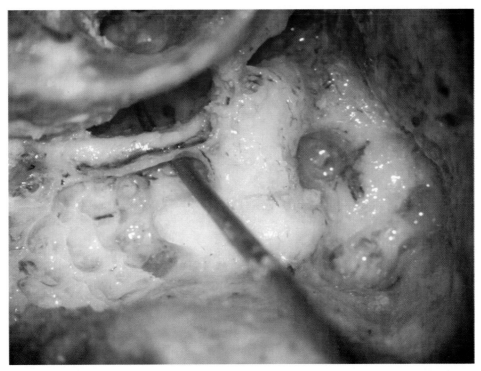

Figure 17 The instrument indicates the access to the middle ear through a retrofacial tympanotomy which allows a middle ear approach through the tympanic sinus

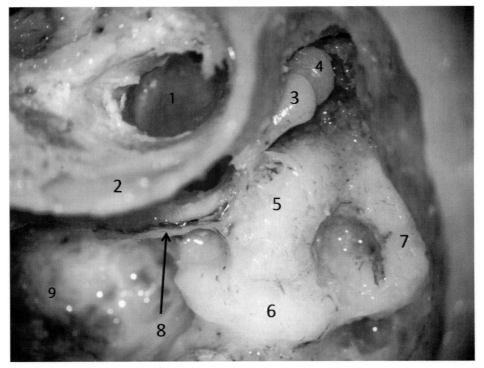

Figure 18 General view of the structures after a posterior labyrinth exposure. 1. Tympanic membrane; 2. External auditory canal; 3. Malleus; 4. Incus; 5. Horizontal semicircular canal; 6. Posterior semicircular canal; 7. Superior semicircular canal; 8. Facial nerve; 9. Area of the jugular bulb

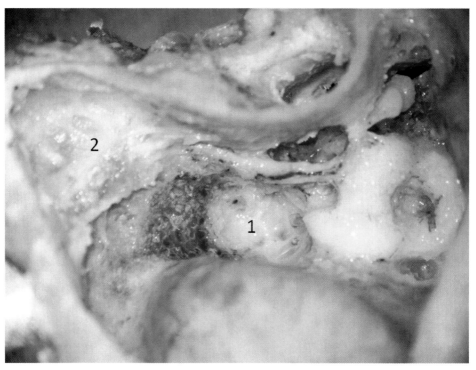

Figure 19 The jugular bulb is partially exposed in its superior portion which projects to the retrofacial region (1), medial to the digastric ridge (2) and digastric muscle

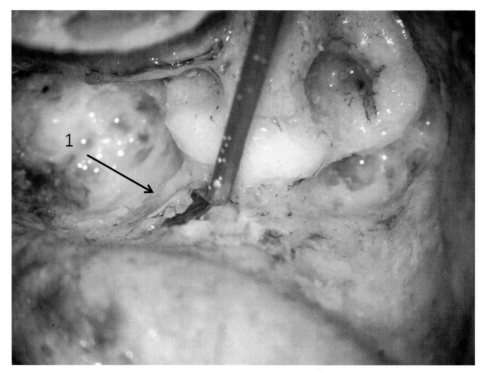

Figure 20 The endolymphatic sac (1) is dissected and appears as a fold of the posterior fossa dura in the retrolabyrinthine and presigmoid areas. The direction of the instrument shows Donaldson´s line that follows the horizontal semicircular canal and is perpendicular to the posterior semicircular canal

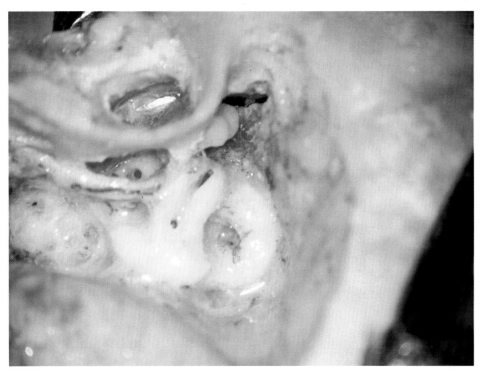

Figure 21 Progessive opening of the horizontal semicircular canal

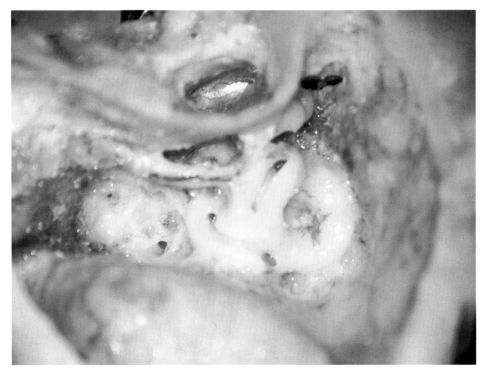

Figure 22 Progressive opening of the posterior semicircular canal

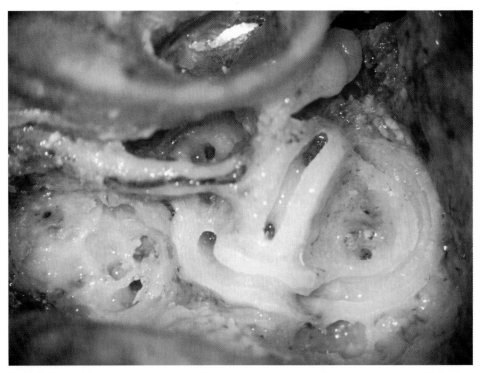

Figure 23 The semicircular canals are shown. They are open and the three-dimensional trajectory of their axis is shown

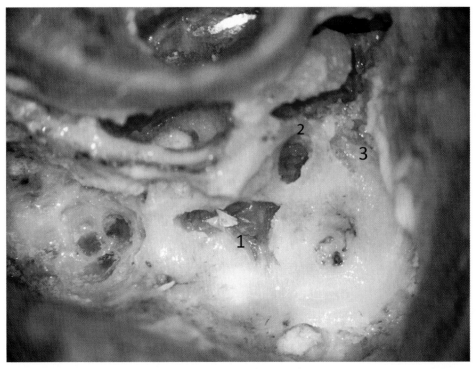

Figure 24 The labyrinthectomy is done from superior to inferior and from posterior to anterior in order not to harm the facial nerve by staying at a deeper (medial) level in relationship to the nerve. 1. Membranous structures of the vestibule; 2. Ampulla with the ampullary crest of the horizontal semicircular canal; 3. Ampulla of the superior semicircular canal

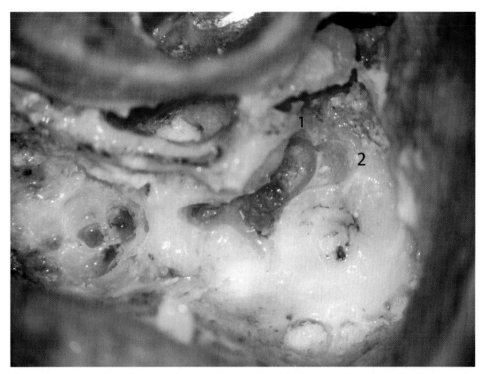

Figure 25 There is a close relationship between the ampullas of the horizontal (1) and superior (2) semicircular canals. This anatomic relationship is important because medial to them (especially medial to the superior semicircular canal) we will find the labyrinthine portion of the facial nerve

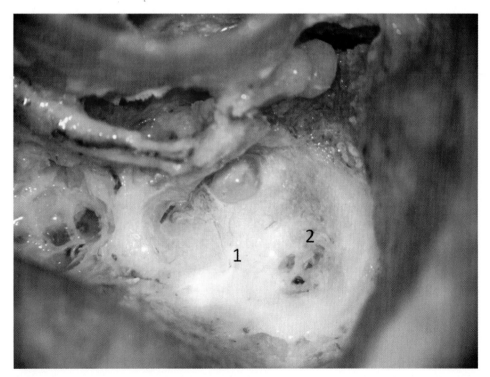

Figure 26 At this level of the dissection, the internal auditory canal (1) and the supralabyrinthine air cells (2) start to appear

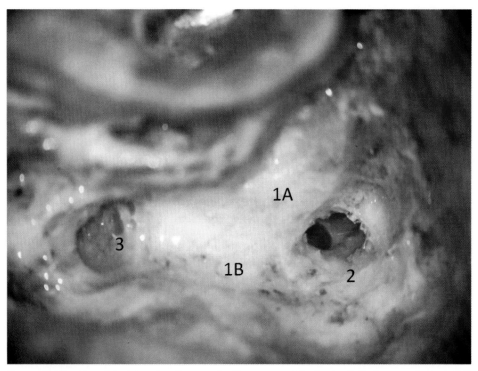

Figure 27 Dissection of the internal auditory canal with exposure of the fundus (1 A), the acoustic porus (1 B) which is much deeper, the supra (2) and infra (3) labyrinthine air cells, very close to the jugular bulb which (if it is high) has to be dissected in order to obtain access to the inferior pole of the internal auditory canal

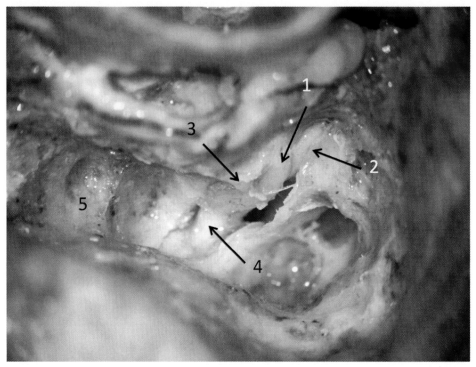

Figure 28 The internal auditory canal is open. The superior vestibular nerve can be seen (1), and anterior to it the facial nerve (2) in its initial part of its labyrinthine portion in the internal auditory canal. The transverse crest (3) divides the internal auditory canal in a superior compartment with the superior and inferior vestibular as well as the cochlear nerve (4). The proximity to the jugular bulb can be observed (5)

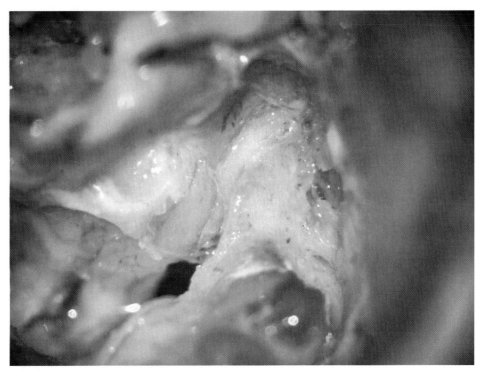

Figure 29 Higher magnification of the internal auditory canal. The inferior vestibular nerve has been removed. The transverse crest can be observed as well as the superior vestibular nerve, Bill´s bar which divides the superior compartment from the internal auditory canal into anterior and posterior. The labyrinthine portion of the facial nerve is dissected and it is approaching the geniculate ganglion

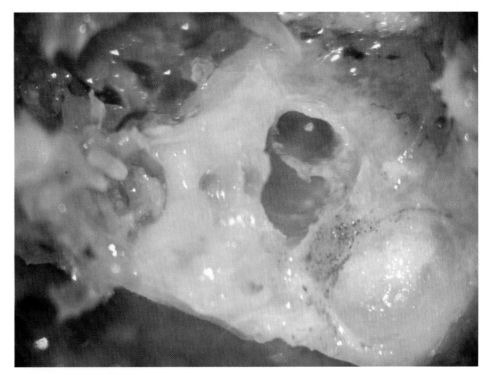

Figure 30A Dissection of the basal turn of the cochlea showing scala tympani and vestibule as well as the spiral ligament

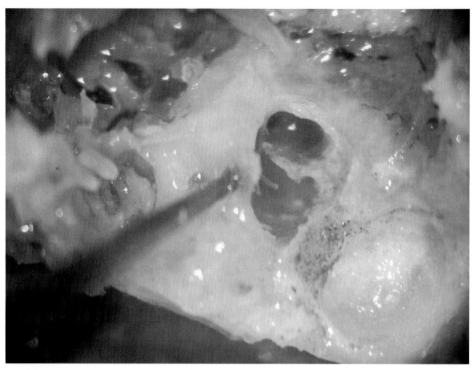

Figure 30B The instrument is placed in the anterior portion of the round window towards the scala tympani

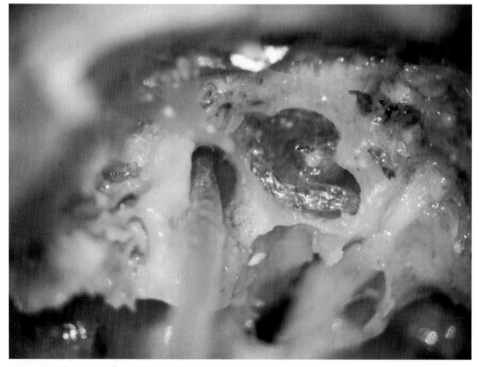

Figure 31A Placement of a cochlear implant electrode through a cochleostomy and its progression towards the second turn

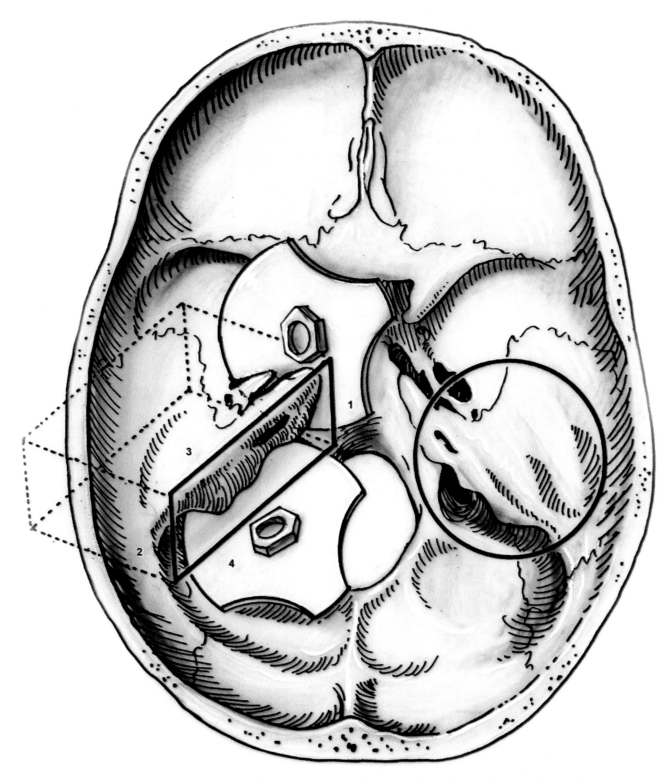

Figure 2 Stryker saw (rocker-type oscillating saw) cuts: the first cut (1) is made at a right angle, as close to the apex of the petrous bone as the regional anatomy will allow; the second cut (2) is made parallel to the first, through the mastoid process and as close to the lateral wall as possible; the third cut (3) is made approximately 2.5 cm anterior and parallel to the petrous ridge in the floor of the middle cranial fossa. It includes the bony external ear canal; the fourth cut (4) is made in the horizontal plane, close to the floor of the posterior cranial fossa

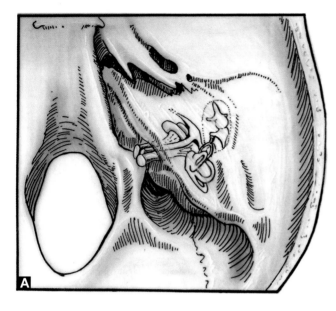

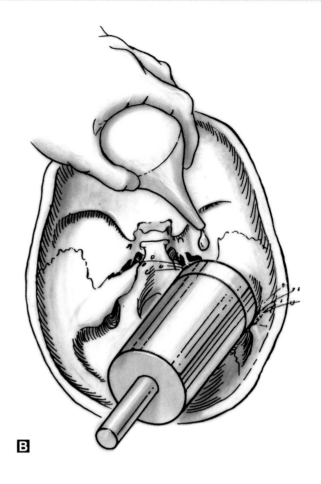

Figures 3A to C

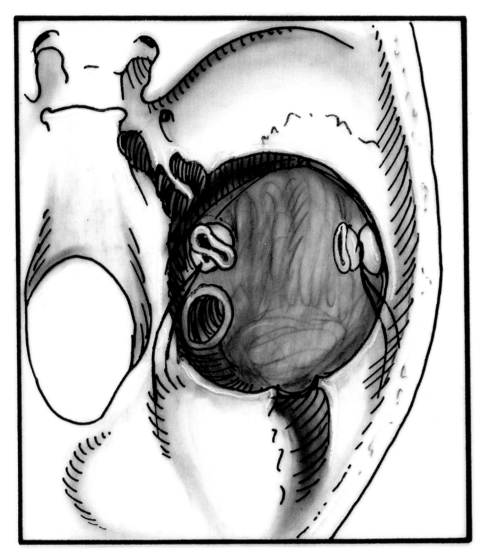

Figure 3D

Figures 3A to D Bone plug method (Schuknecht's): (A) The saw is centered over the arcuate eminence (superior semicircular canal prominence or the superior surface) and directed to the floor of the middle cranial fossa; (B) The skull is held by an assistant and a stream of water is directed at the blade for lubrication; (C) The plug is then grasped with the "lion-jawed" forceps and the bone is rotated, permitting visualization of the internal carotid artery on its inferior surface. The artery is ligated and additional attachments are sectioned with a knife, scissors or osteotome; (D) Fresh temporal bones can be wrapped in water-sealed cotton or placed in Teflon bags; the air is expelled and the bones are frozen

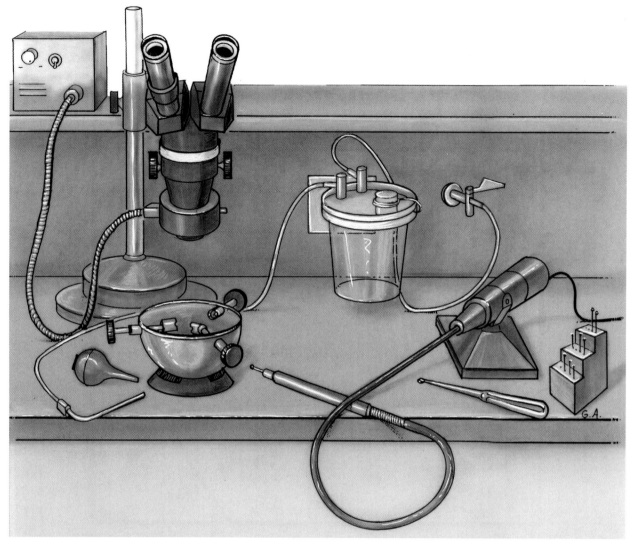

Figure 4 A temporal bone dissection station

List of Instruments and Materials

Operating microscope	Whirlybird
Drill with a set of cutting burrs	Small alligator forceps
Bulb syringe	Fenestrometer
Suction	Scalpel
Suction tips no. 1 and no. 5	4–0 silk (mounted on curved needle)
Stapes curets	0.05-mm stainless steel wire
Straight canal knife	Silastic sheeting
Sickle knife	Gelfoam
Joint knife	TORP, PORP, PE tube
Straight pick	Scissors (small plastic)
Stapes bending die	Ossicle holder
Hough hoe	Measuring rod

Residents with imagination can obviate many of these instruments and materials by adapting broken instruments and selecting similar, cheaper materials than those suggested.

SURGICAL PROCEDURES

The Guidelines in this chapter have been designed for the practical purpose of being read and followed as dissection proceeds. They are intended to serve as a dialogue between the instructor and the surgeon dissecting the temporal bone. Aims, highlights, pitfalls, pertinent anatomy and surgical steps are discussed during the dissection in an attempt to simulate a rational procedure. We encourage dissection of temporal bones as an essential prerequisite for otologic training in residency programs or for the otolaryngologists who wish to practice specific techniques. This practice, plus a knowledge of anatomy and histopathology, is essential for developing rational and not merely imitative means of surgical treatment. The succession of procedures has been organized for the fullest utilization of the bones. Four "wet" temporal bones are needed for full completion of these guidelines.

When describing or discussing a temporal bone dissection procedure, "superior" means toward the temporal line (cephalad); "inferior" is toward the mastoid tip (caudad); "anterior" is toward the external auditory canal (ventral); "posterior" is away from the external auditory canal (dorsal); "lateral" is toward the mastoid cortex (superficial) and "medial" is away from the mastoid cortex (deep).

Simple Mastoidectomy

Aim

Exenteration (removal) of all mastoid air cells while maintaining the integrity of the posterior canal.

Highlights

- Use the microscope at all times
- Drill under direct vision, avoiding "holes" (drill evenly)
- When in doubt, identify landmarks and use a mastoid curet
- Develop a gradual, step-by-step procedure
- Think anatomically and three-dimensionally. Look for structures; do not "find them"
- Keep anatomic aberrations in mind (high sigmoid sinus, anterior sigmoid sinus, Körner's septum, etc.).

Pitfalls

- Failing to identify the antrum
  - Körner's septum
  - Insufficient thinning of the tegmen and/or posterior osseous canal
- Injuring a high sigmoid sinus
- Injuring the facial nerve by going:
  - Deep to the horizontal semicircular canal
  - Too far anterior in the digastric ridge
- Dislocating the incus by drilling blindly into the antrum area.

Surgical Steps

Assess external anatomy: Place the temporal bone in surgical position (simulating its normal anatomic location for surgery). Visualize and study the lateral surface (cortex) in its entirety from the temporal line (linea temporalis) superiorly, to the mastoid tip inferiorly. Identify the posterior aspect of the osseous canal

anteriorly. Note the presence of the suprameatal spine (spine of Henle) immediately posterior to the osseous canal. Review the imaginary lines that overlie the mastoid antrum, that is, between the temporal line and spine of Henle (fossa mastoidea or Macewen's triangle). Imagine the inner structures of the mastoid cavity in a three-dimensional fashion and trace your surgical plan (Figure 5).

Initiate drilling (use large burrs, saucerize): Employing the microscope, use a large burr and start saucerizing in an even fashion, beginning at the fossa mastoidea until air cells appear (Figure 6). Make a wide cortical removal, including thinning of the posterior canal. As one goes deeper, keep thinking of one's future landmarks to orient oneself toward the antrum. One's superior limit is the tegmen mastoideum (level of temporal line), superior to which lies the dura of the middle cranial fossa. Thin the tegmen down, being careful to keep it intact; this is important if adequate access to the antrum is intended. The posterior canal wall should be thinned down as well for the same purpose. Again, drilling should remain even at all times, not straight but oriented anteriorly toward the nose of our imaginary patient. Our anterosuperior limit is the root of the zygomatic process. This should be opened without opening the epitympanum.

Identify the lateral sinus (sigmoid sinus): In drilling posteriorly one will encounter the sigmoid sinus (lateral sinus) (Figures 7A and B). It is identified in surgery by its bluish color and smooth bony plate (in this dissection we are looking for the smooth bony plate). These characteristics are the best guide to the sigmoid sinus. A change in the sound of the burrs is a helpful hint, but does not suffice as a guide; visualization far outweighs sensation in temporal bone surgery.

It must be remembered that the sigmoid sinus does not have a uniform anatomy; it can be high (lateral) or low (medial/deep). The surgeon should be cautious with the use of the drill. Inferiorly, toward the mastoid tip, the air cells are to be drilled evenly with the level of drilling superiorly. Little by little, a typical kidney-shaped mastoid cavity becomes evident.

Identify Körner's septum and antrum: In proceeding medially (deeper down), occasionally one may encounter a thick plate of bone that may give the impression of having reached the antrum. This is Körner's septum, a solid plate that represents the fusion of the squamous and petrous portions of the temporal bone. When in doubt, go back to the previously identified landmarks and structures, verify location,

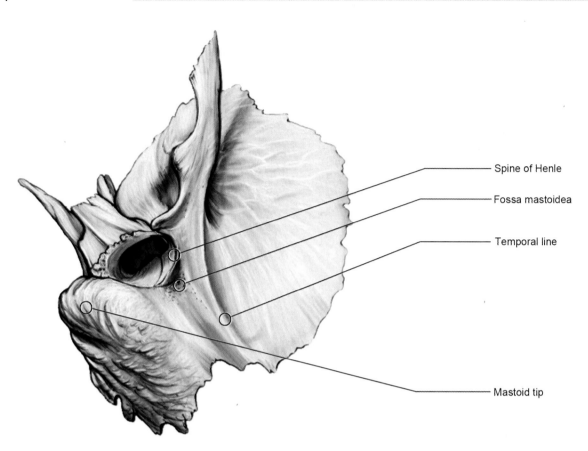

Spine of Henle

Fossa mastoidea

Temporal line

Mastoid tip

Figure 5 External anatomy of temporal bone

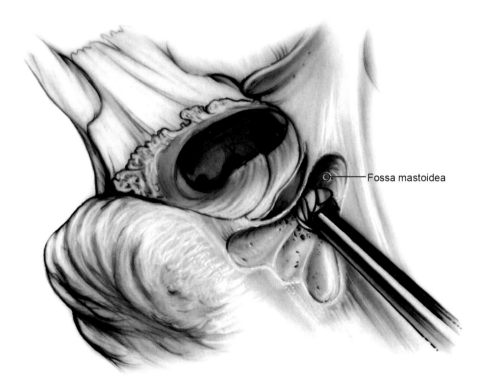

Fossa mastoidea

Figure 6 Drilling by using large burrs and start saucerizing in an even fashion, beginning at the fossa mastoidea until air cells appear

identify the chorda tympani (which is to be preserved), as it leaves the facial nerve in an anterosuperior direction; it then takes a lateral direction toward the annulus (Figure 12C). On occasion, the facial recess is quite small and the procedure is difficult. Rather than insisting on taking unnecessary risks, use a combined transcanal transmastoid approach.

Once the recess is opened, the landmarks are reidentified: the external genu of the facial nerve is medial; the fossa incudis is superior; the chorda tympani is inferolateral and posterior; and the tympanic membrane is anterolateral.

Now observe the following structures (Figure 12D): the horizontal portion of the facial nerve, the lenticular process of the incus, the incudostapedial joint, the capitulum of the stapes and the stapedial tendon. Next identify the promontory and inferomedially the round window niche.

Cochlear Implant (Facial Recess Approach)

Aim

To place an electrode into the cochlea by sliding it through the round window (we will deal only with intracochlear electrode placement and with electrodes that are placed far into the interior of the cochlea).

Highlights

- Ensure good visualization via an adequate facial recess approach
- Clearly identify the round window niche and round window membrane.

Pitfalls

- Those of the facial recess approach itself
- Inadequate visualization of the round window, with the electrode unable to be passed beyond the hook.

Surgical Steps

- Those of a simple mastoidectomy and facial recess approach
- Prepare a seat for the internal receiver
- Insert the intracochlear electrode.

Procedure

At this point in the dissection, the main drilling for the procedure has been done. You are left with inserting the electrode through the round window and drilling a seat for the internal receiver posterosuperior to the mastoid cavity. Locate a position for the internal receiver; it should be immediately posterior to the posterior limit of the drilled mastoid cavity, with its anterior border (toward the ear canal) no further than where the border of the imaginary pinna (auricle) would be if it were pushed posterior (that is, immediately posterior to the posterior border of the pinna). Superiorly, the border should not be above the superior border of the pinna. Drill a seat, using as a guideline the circumference of the internal receiver of your practice electrode (Figures 13A and B). If a practice electrode is not available, drill a seat into which a nickel-sized coin would fit. Drilling can be done carefully with a regular burr, or it can be done with either a butterfly burr or a burr specially designed by one of the cochlear implant manufacturers. If a screw type of internal receiver is to be used, drill four holes in the corresponding openings of the base of the pedestal to a maximum depth of 2 mm.

Regardless of the type of internal receiver, with a small burr drill two small holes immediately superior and inferior to the location of your already drilled seat, that is, two holes superiorly and two holes inferiorly (Figure 14A). Bring the small holes together very carefully. Then pass 2–0 silk through these openings (Figure 14B); this will be used to cross over the internal receiver and seat it in place. Do not place your internal receiver yet. Our attention is now turned back to the active electrode. Again, visualize the round window niche.

If visualization is not adequate, a transcanal approach can be made. Verify the opening of the round window niche. On occasion, it is necessary or useful to gently drill the anterior border of the niche (Figures 14C and D). This will provide a slightly larger opening with better visualization, and at the same time will present a "straight shot" at the cochlea, skipping the hook portion that sometimes is difficult to bypass. Position the electrode in the opening of the window and then gently push it in, using a blunt pick or wire guide or one of the special electrode guides provided by the implant manufacturers (Figures 15A and B). If there is some resistance, it is likely that the electrode is caught-up in the hook. Retract the electrode gently and try to rotate it, while imagining the direction of the cochlea. On the left, for example, turn gently towards the right (clockwise);

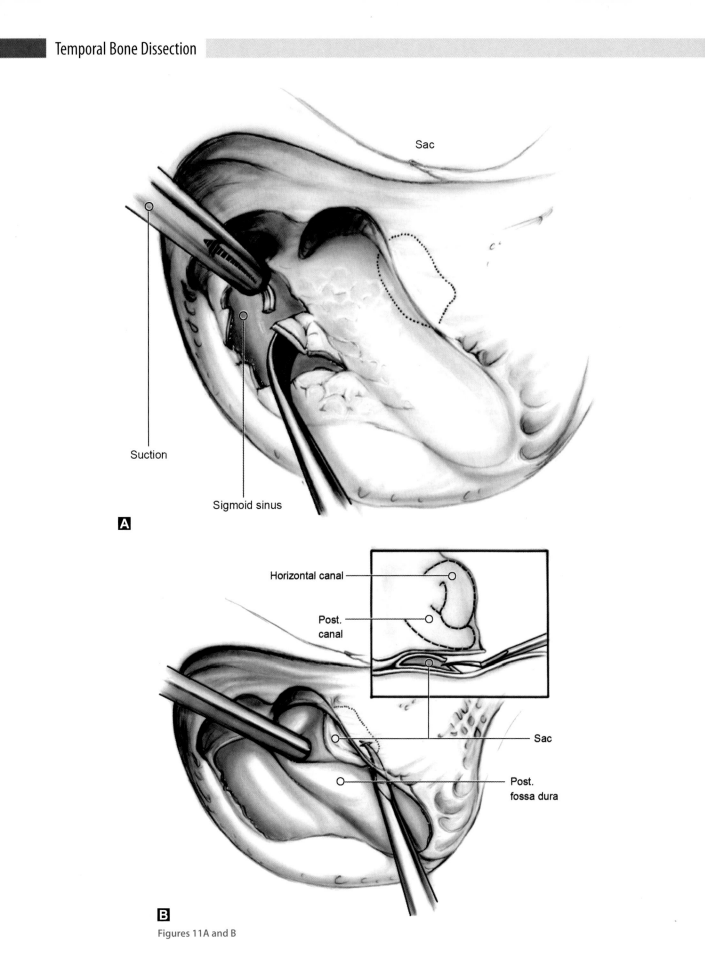

Sac

Suction

Sigmoid sinus

A

Horizontal canal

Post.
canal

Sac

Post.
fossa dura

B

Figures 11A and B

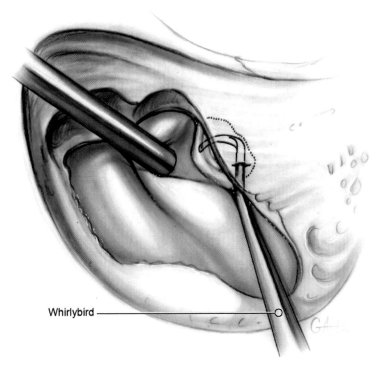

Whirlybird

Figure 11C

Figures 11A to C (A) The plate is thinned down to eggshell thickness, then gently elevated and separated from the underlying dura with a duckbill elevator; (B) The sac is identifiable as a thickened white area of the dura over the thin surrounding dura; (C) The sac is incised gently with a sickle knife and the lumen probed with a Whirlybird

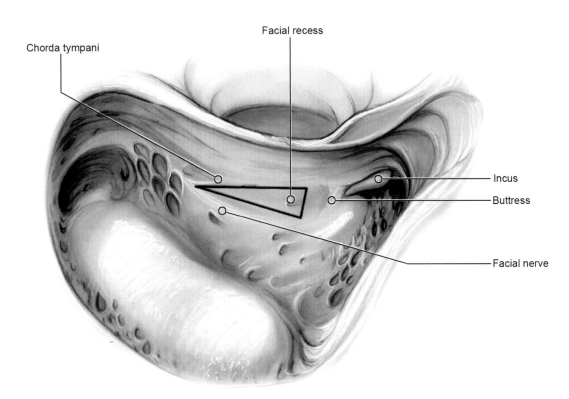

Chorda tympani

Facial recess

Incus

Buttress

Facial nerve

Figure 12A

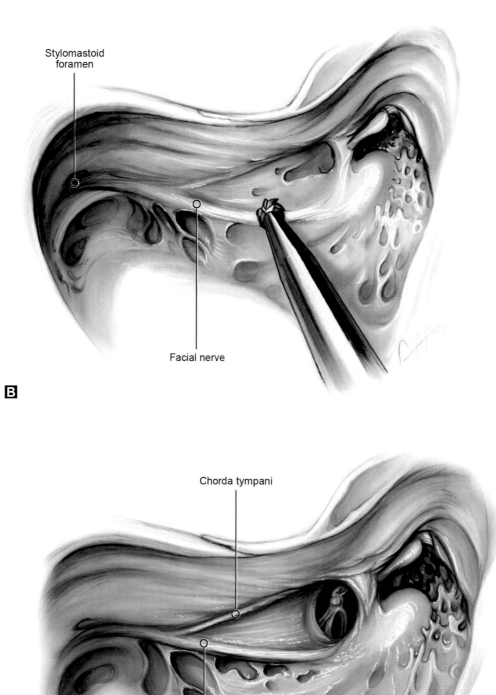

Stylomastoid foramen

Facial nerve

B

Chorda tympani

Facial nerve genu

C

Figures 12B and C

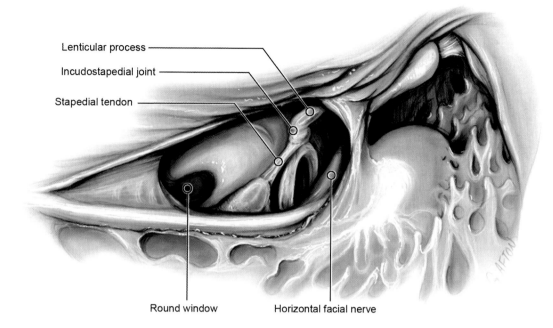

Lenticular process

Incudostapedial joint

Stapedial tendon

Round window   Horizontal facial nerve

Figure 12D

Figures 12A to D Facial recess approach, posterior tympanotomy: (A) Defining landmarks; (B) Bone is thinned down carefully by drilling parallel to the direction of the facial nerve fibers; (C) As cutting burs leaves the facial nerve in an anterosuperior direction; it then takes a lateral direction toward the annulus; (D) Once the recess is opened, the landmarks are reidentified; the horizontal portion of the facial nerve, the lenticular process of the incus, the incudostapedial joint, the capitulum of the stapes, the stapedial tendon, identify the promontory and inferomedially the round window niche

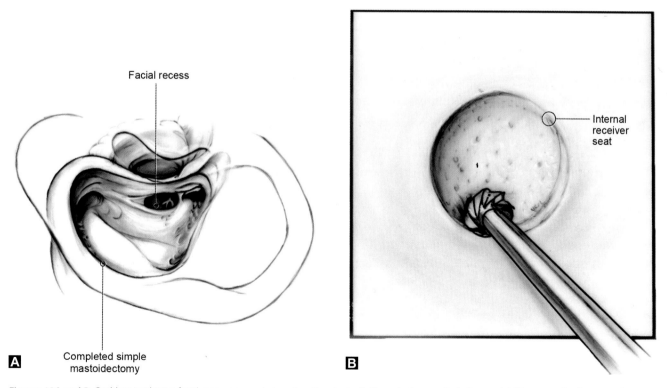

Facial recess

Internal receiver seat

A Completed simple mastoidectomy   **B**

Figures 13A and B Cochlear implant–a facial recess approach: inserting the electrode through the round window and drilling a seat for the internal receiver posterosuperior to the mastoid cavity

on the right, turn gently towards the left (counterclockwise). Place the electrode and then secure the internal receiver with either screws or sutures (Figures 16A and B).

Transmastoid Facial Nerve Decompression

Highlights and pitfalls are discussed in the text.

Surgical Steps

- Those of a simple mastoidectomy
- Identify the different segments of the facial nerve and skeletonize the fallopian canal
- Fracture and remove any bony covering
- Open the sheath of the facial canal.

Procedure

In the course of the complete simple mastoidectomy, the vertical portion and external genu of the facial nerve were fairly well delineated. For practical surgical purposes the facial nerve can be divided into three segments: (1) that within the internal auditory canal; (2) the tympanic segment (horizontal/middle ear) and (3) the vertical segment (mastoid). We will now deal with the vertical and horizontal segments, in that order.

From the external genu, the nerve proceeds vertically to the stylomastoid foramen at the level of the anterior edge of the digastric ridge (Figures 17A to C). It is important to visualize its anatomy and, if possible, compare it with other bones, since there is considerable variation. The nerve is lateral to the horizontal canal; however, it may have a posterior projection at the genu, lending itself to potential damage. It is useful to visualize the nerve anterior to the digastric ridge and to appreciate how lateral it becomes as it reaches the mastoid tip. Its tympanic or middle ear segment appears in the region of the cochleariform process at the geniculate ganglion, then runs posteriorly towards the oval window (stapes) to a point just inferior and usually medial (deep) to the horizontal semicircular canal. The vertical segment can be dissected from the level of the fossa incudis or from the digastric ridge. From the ridge it can be followed superiorly to the external genu; however, this is not a reliable landmark. Although this approach is perfectly acceptable, the authors tend to follow nerves peripherally rather than centrally, which seems both safer and simpler.

After visualization of the genu, the canal is skeletonized all the way down to the stylomastoid foramen. Drilling is done in strokes parallel to the direction of the nerve (superior to inferior or *vice versa*). Exposure of the tympanic segment is

helped by enlarging the *aditus ad antrum*. This dissection, plus enlargement of the facial recess approach, allows visualization anteriorly toward the cochleariform process. Visualize the segment at the level of the oval window and the pyramidal eminence. This is a very useful image to keep in mind. If necessary, adequate visualization can be obtained by a combined approach. Visualize the tympanic segment through the canal. It is also possible to obtain adequate visualization by removing the incus (Figure 18A). Before disarticulating the incus, try to drill under it without damaging or dislocating it, using the smallest possible burrs. Now try to remove and replace the incus. If drilling toward the geniculate ganglion was incomplete, drill now without the incus in place (the incus should be left in place for use in the next procedure; however, practice placing and replacing the incus to become familiar with its normal anatomic position). Once the entire facial canal has been thinned to eggshell consistency, fracture it with a pick and lift the bone fragments gently with a Whirlybird without using the facial nerve as a fulcrum (Figure 18B). The sheath is then opened with a sharp sickle knife (Figure 18C).

Canalplasty

Aim

Enlargement of the bony canal and visualization of the entire fibrous and bony annulus.

Pitfalls

Excessive drilling of the anterior wall and entrance into the temporomandibular joint space.

Procedure

Using a large burr, drill the canal wall evenly until visualization of the entire fibrous annulus is achieved (Figure 19). Do not drill in one spot, but "sweep" the burr gently with even pressure and go one step at a time (skin procedures will not be dealt with, since the skin is thick, tight and difficult to elevate adequately for these purposes in harvested temporal bones).

Underlay Graft of the Tympanic Membrane

Aim

Placement of a graft under the tympanic membrane, covering all edges of the perforation.

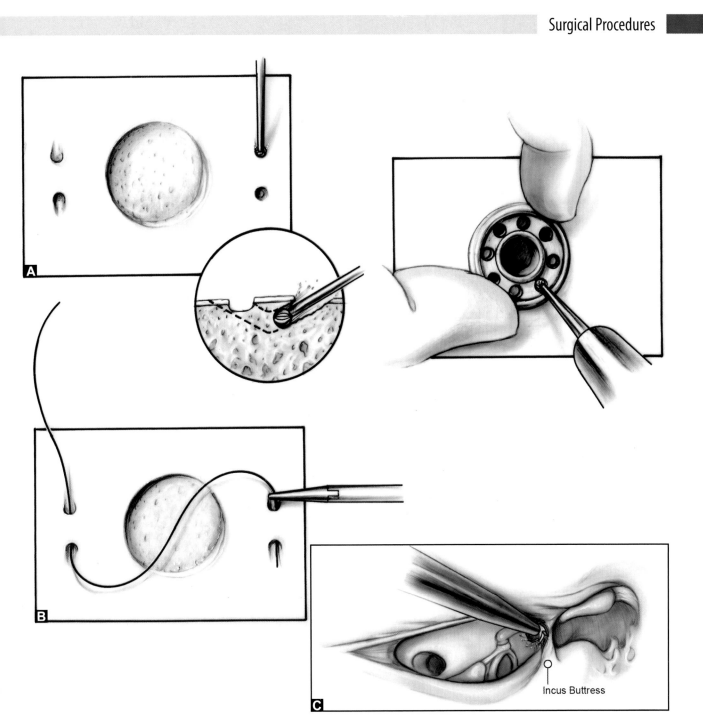

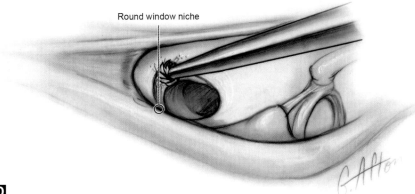

Figures 14A to D Cochlear implant—a facial recess approach; (A) Two small holes are drilled using a small bur superior and inferior to the location of already drilled seat; (B) To help cross over the internal receiver and seat it in place, 2-0 silk is passed through these openings; (C) and (D) Visualize the round window niche by gently drilling the anterior border of the niche. This will provide a slightly larger opening with better visualization

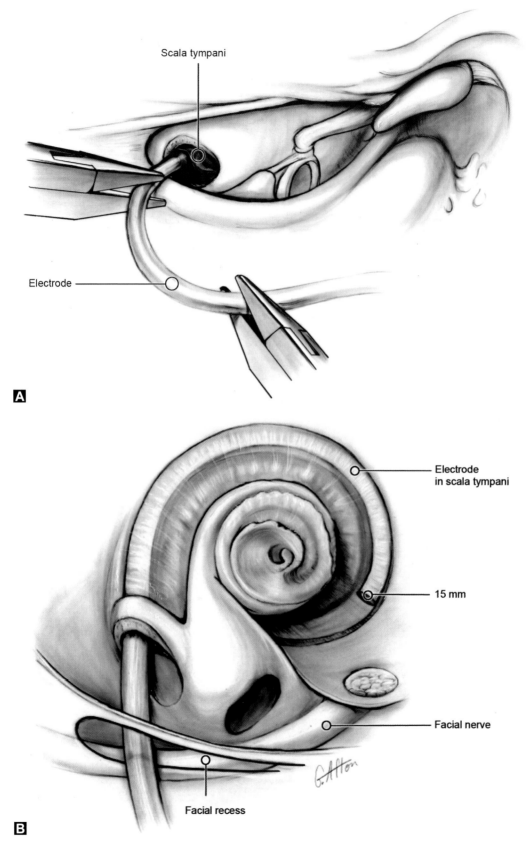

Figures 15A and B Position the electrode in the opening of the round window and then gently push it in, using a blunt pick or wire guide or one of the special electrode guides provided by the implant manufacturers

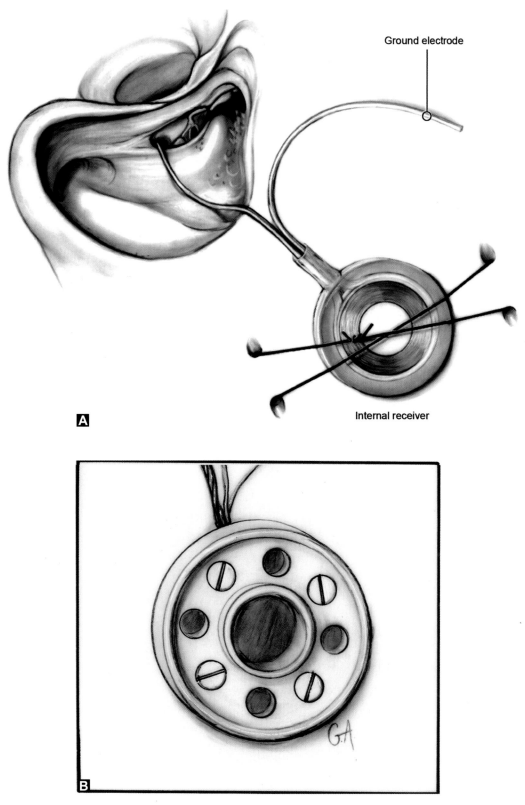

Ground electrode

Internal receiver

A

B

Figures 16A and B Placing the electrode and then secure the internal receiver with either screws or sutures

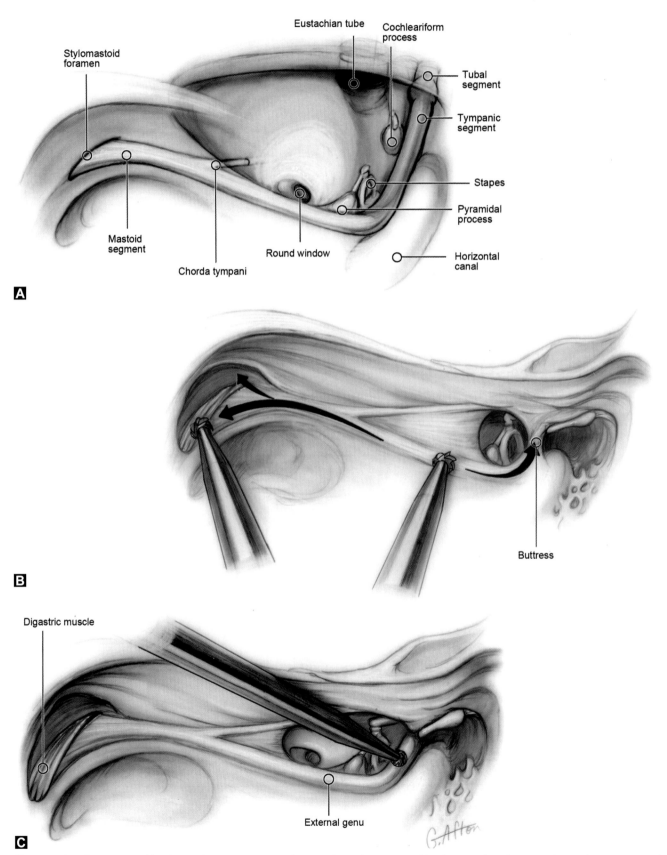

Eustachian tube

Cochleariform process

Stylomastoid foramen

Tubal segment

Tympanic segment

Stapes

Pyramidal process

Horizontal canal

Mastoid segment

Round window

Chorda tympani

A

Buttress

B

Digastric muscle

External genu

C

Figures 17A to C Transmastoid facial nerve decompression procedure: visualizing the anatomy of facial nerve—from the external genu, the nerve proceeds vertically to the stylomastoid foramen at the level of the anterior edge of the digastric ridge

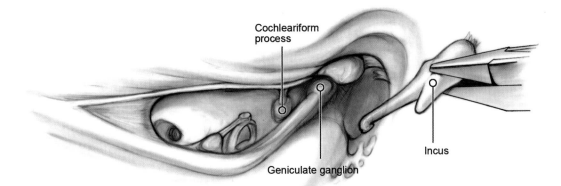

A

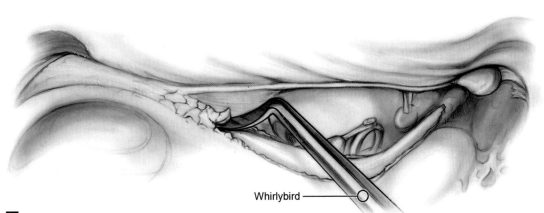

B

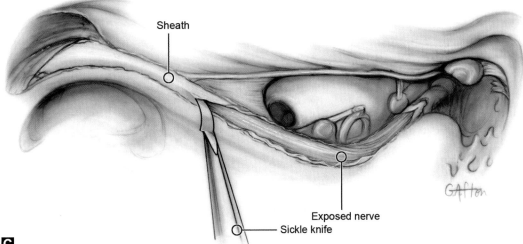

C

Figures 18A to C After visualization drilling is done in strokes parallel to the direction of the nerve: (A) Removing the incus to obtain adequate visualization; (B) After facial canal gets thinned to eggshell consistency, fracture it with a pick and lift the bone fragments gently with a Whirlybird without using the facial nerve as a fulcrum; (C) The sheath is then opened with a sharp sickle knife

223

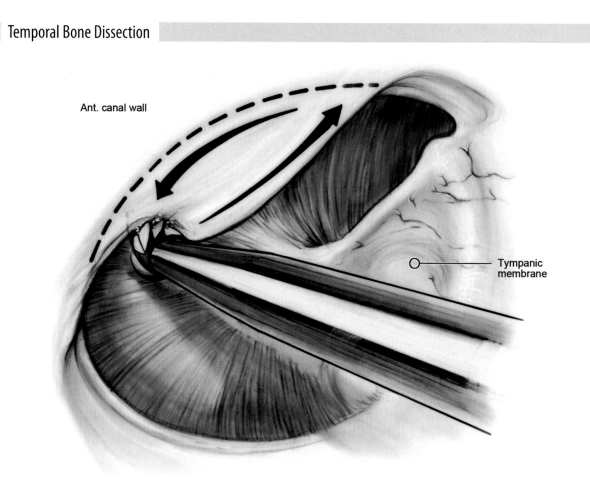

Ant. canal wall

Tympanic membrane

Figure 19 Canalplasty by using a large burr, drill the canal wall evenly until visualization of the entire fibrous annulus is achieved

Procedure

Visualize the tympanic membrane. Imagine it in four quadrants (Figure 20A). Using a straight pick and a sickle knife, make a central perforation (Figure 20B). Fill the middle ear space with gelfoam (Figure 20C). Obtain a piece of fascia (or paper) that exceeds the size of the perforation by at least 30%. Scarify the undersurface of the tympanic membrane around the perforation, using a Hough hoe. Now place the graft over the perforation and position it medially by using the Hough hoe (Figures 20C and D).

Ossiculoplasty (Incus Procedures)

Aim

Restoration of ossicular chain continuity (in this case, where incus problems are the cause of the loss).

Procedure

Remove the "graft," the entire tympanic membrane, and the gelfoam filling the cavity. Now visualize the cavity and what is found beneath the different quadrants (see Figure 20A). Familiarize yourself with the anatomy. Mobilize the temporal bone and learn what areas can be seen best at different angles. Palpate the ossicles with a blunt pick, and observe the round window niche area, the opening of the Eustachian tube, the stapedial tendon and other features. Compare the views of the middle ear cavity with the transcanal and posterior tympanotomy approaches. The incus is already loose.

Clip the distalmost portion of the long process of the incus ("necrosis of the lenticular process") (Figure 21A). Since the mastoidectomy has been done already, remove a piece of "cortical bone" posterior to the mastoid cavity opening (Figure 21B). Using a small burr, delineate a square of bone and remove it.

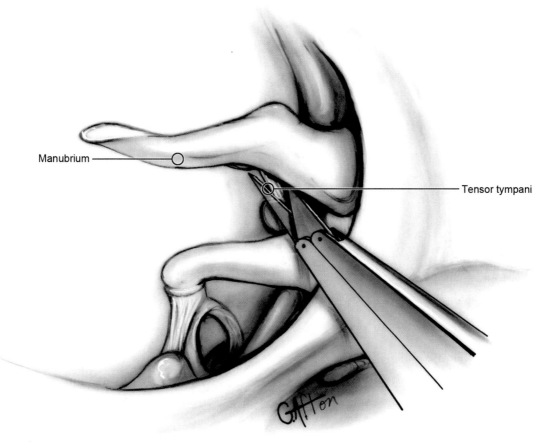

Manubrium

Tensor tympani

Figure 23C

Figures 23A to C Intact bridge mastoidectomy: (A) Drill the anterior canal wall, enlarging it until clearly visualizing the entire fibrous and bony annulus but without entering the temporomandibular joint space; (B) Lower the posterior canal wall, leaving the bridge intact; (C) Visualize and section the tensor tympanic tendon (this maneuver lateralizes the manubrium)

to the semicircular canal, leading into the supracochlear air cells; visualize this tract and its relationship to the facial nerve. The third tract is posterior to the superior canal, and runs between the tegmen mastoideum and common crus of the membranous labyrinth toward the internal auditory canal. Do not expose the common crus, this is to be done later. The intention here is to obtain a better visualization of this anatomic relationship.

The fourth or retrolabyrinthine cell tract is inferior to the posterior semicircular canal, medial to the vertical segment of the facial nerve and superior to the jugular bulb.

Anterior Cell Tract

A radical mastoidectomy has already been done. The tegmen should be skeletonized and the anterior wall thinned; both of these procedures have already been performed. The cells of the anterior tract are found in the "peritubal" and carotid areas in the bony wall just medial to the Eustachian tube orifice anterior to the promontory. These cells are closely associated with the tegmen mastoideum; therefore, dissection must be done very carefully. The authors prefer to use small curets at this level.

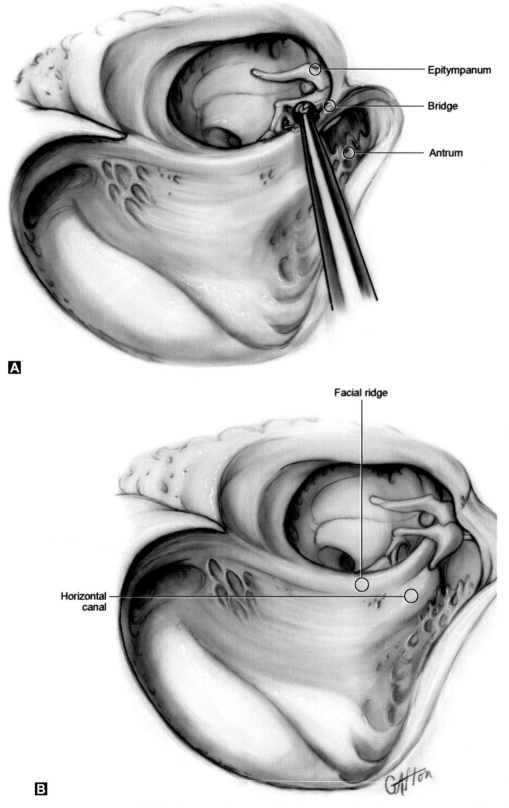

Epitympanum

Bridge

Antrum

A

Facial ridge

Horizontal canal

B

Figures 24A and B Modified radical mastoidectomy: (A) Drilling is started in the epitympanum and followed posteriorly into the antrum. The bridge is removed. The antrum and the horizontal canal are identified; (B) Mastoidectomy is performed and the posterior bony wall is lowered to the level of the facial ridge

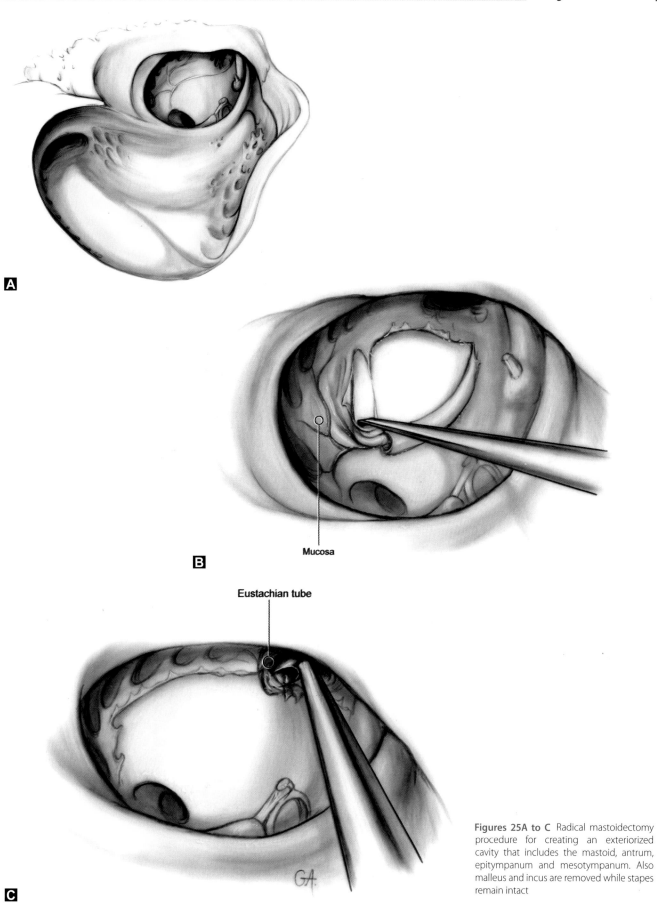

A

B

Mucosa

Eustachian tube

C

Figures 25A to C Radical mastoidectomy procedure for creating an exteriorized cavity that includes the mastoid, antrum, epitympanum and mesotympanum. Also malleus and incus are removed while stapes remain intact

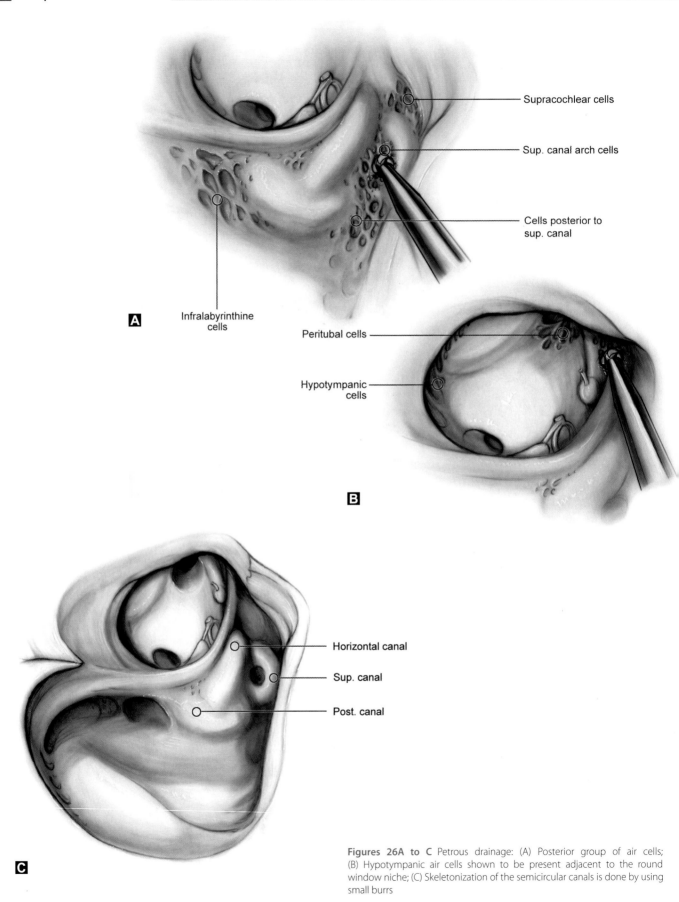

A

Supracochlear cells

Sup. canal arch cells

Cells posterior to
sup. canal

Infralabyrinthine
cells

B

Peritubal cells

Hypotympanic
cells

C

Horizontal canal

Sup. canal

Post. canal

Figures 26A to C Petrous drainage: (A) Posterior group of air cells;
(B) Hypotympanic air cells shown to be present adjacent to the round
window niche; (C) Skeletonization of the semicircular canals is done by using
small burrs

Labyrinthectomy (Transmastoid Labyrinthine Dissection)

Aim

Complete removal of the semicircular canals and soft tissues of the vestibule.

Highlights

- The sinodural angle must be completely thinned for adequate exposure of the vestibule
- The tegmen must be thinned for adequate visualization of the superior aspect of the semicircular canals.

Procedure

The three semicircular canals are skeletonized until the membranous labyrinth is visible through the bone as a thin blue line (Figure 27A). Note the relationship of the facial nerve to the horizontal semicircular canal (Figure 27B). Fenestrate the horizontal canal. Unroof the posterior and anterior portions of the superior semicircular canal. Follow the superior semicircular canal until it reaches its common crus with the posterior semicircular canal. The arcuate artery penetrates the hard labyrinth in the center of the arch of the superior semicircular canal. Go back to the superior semicircular canal, identify the superior vestibular nerve and follow it into the internal auditory meatus (Figure 27C). Visualize the common crus. Now identify the endolymphatic duct as it enters the posterosuperior end of the vestibule. Verify its presence and its direction toward the endolymphatic sac; this is a useful anatomic relationship to keep in mind, since this area is not visualized in endolymphatic sac enhancement procedures. Bone is now removed from the floor of the vestibule where the inferior vestibular nerve is encountered.

Follow the common crus anteriorly into the vestibule. Open it widely and try to identify the membrane of the utricle and saccule. Notice the relationships and distances between the footplate, saccule and utricle. Now skeletonize the round window, since two additional observations can be made in this area.

First, drill carefully at the inferior margin of the round window and identify the singular nerve (Figure 27D). Second, drill this area and identify the hook of the basal turn of the cochlea (Figure 27E). Cochlear electrodes may be obstructed in this area when being inserted into the cochlea. Visualize its anatomy in order to see the direction in which the electrode should be pointed and the amount of bone that should be drilled to bypass the hook.

Middle Ear Dissection

Procedure

This procedure is started with a new wet bone. Skin procedures will not be dealt with since the skin is thick, tight and difficult to elevate adequately for these purposes. Identify the walls of the ear canal. Visualize the tympanic membrane; imagine it in four quadrants (Figure 28A). Make openings in the anterosuperior, anteroinferior, posteroinferior and posterosuperior quadrants. Now gently elevate the tympanic membrane and identify the areas and structures beneath the four openings. Visualize what is found beneath the posterosuperior quadrant opening. Now bend the tympanic membrane forward; if it is too brittle, remove it. Visualize the middle ear (Figure 28B). Palpate the ossicles, Jacobson's nerve, the round window niche area and the opening of the Eustachian tube, and identify the tensor tympani. Remove the skin, leaving the annulus intact. Identify the tympanosquamous suture superiorly and the tympanomastoid suture posteriorly. Between the sutures is the vascular strip. Identify the anterior wall and carefully drill the anterior bony overhang without entering the temporomandibular joint space. Enlarge the canal until the entire tympanic membrane annulus is clearly visualized (Figures 28C and 29A).

Using a large stapes curet, curet the scutum from superior to inferior, thus avoiding injury to the ossicles (Figure 29B). Visualize the stapedial tendon. Make sure it is clearly in sight. At this point you are ready for a stapedectomy. Instead of sectioning the stapedial tendon (which can be done, as well), try to lift it along with its periosteum with the incudostapedial joint knife, leaving it attached to the periosteum of the long process of the incus (Figure 30A). This is not a simple procedure. Using the incudostapedial joint knife, separate the joint very gently. Fracture the footplate in the middle with a straight pick (Figure 30B). Mobilize the stapes, using superior-to-inferior and inferior-to-superior movements and remove it, hooking the joint knife to the area immediately inferior to the capitulum (Figure 30C). The remaining footplate portions are lifted gently with a Hough

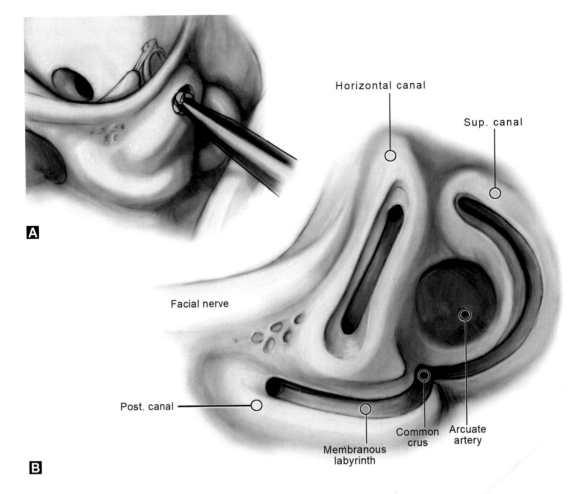

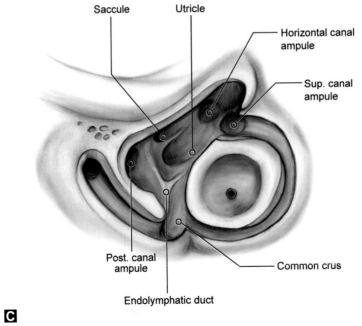

Figures 27A to C

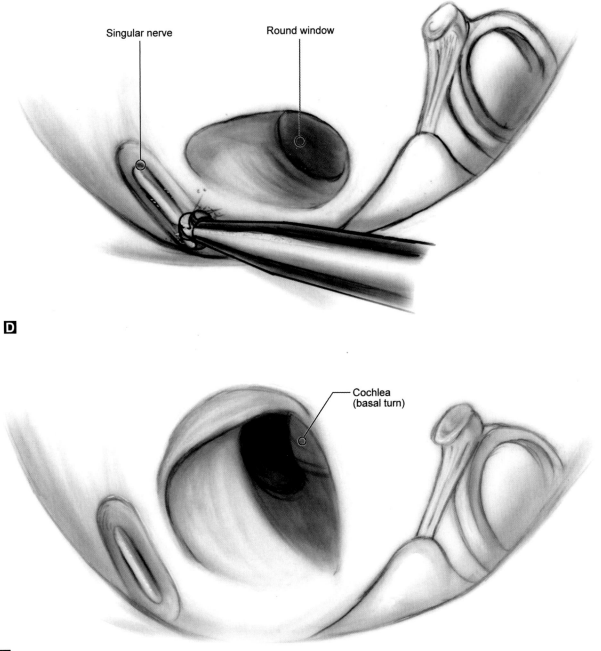

D

E

Figures 27D and E

Figures 27A to E Transmastoid labyrinthine dissection: (A) Skeletonized the three semicircular canals until the membranous labyrinth is visible through the bone as a thin blue line. (B) Relationship of the facial nerve to the horizontal semicircular canal is shown. (C) Fenestrated horizontal canal, unroofed posterior and anterior portions of the superior semicircular canal are shown. Following the superior semicircular canal till it reaches its common crus with the posterior semicircular canal. Identify the superior vestibular nerve, and follow it into the internal auditory meatus. (D) Drilling at the inferior margin of the round window one can identify the singular nerve. (E) Also drill this area and identify the hook of the basal turn of the cochlea

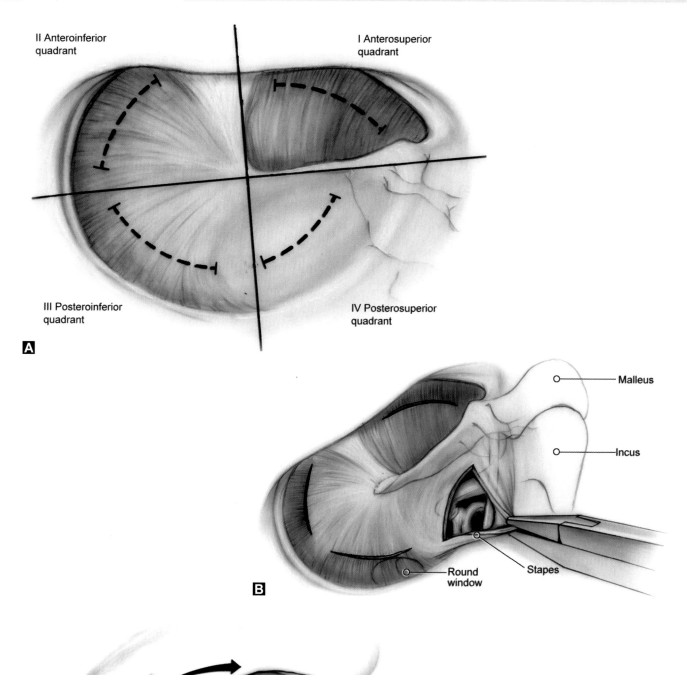

Figures 28A to C Middle ear dissection: (A) Visualizing the four quadrants of tympanic membrane and openings in the anterosuperior, anteroinferior, posteroinferior and posterosuperior quadrants are made; (B) Beneath the posterosuperior quadrant opening, middle ear, ossicles and other structures are visualized; (C) Enlarging canal for better visualization of entire tympanic membrane annulus

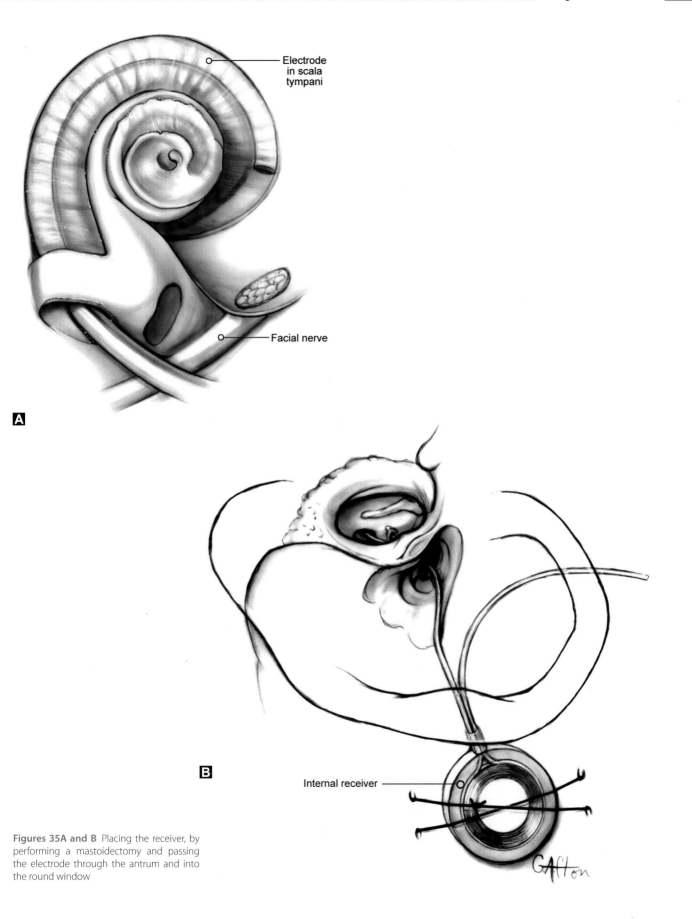

Electrode
in scala
tympani

Facial nerve

A

B

Internal receiver

Figures 35A and B Placing the receiver, by performing a mastoidectomy and passing the electrode through the antrum and into the round window

the antrum by visualizing the attic area directly through the middle ear. In order to ascertain the location of the antrum, a Whirlybird can be used for direct probing. Even if a mastoidectomy is not precisely a cortical mastoidectomy, the opening should be large enough; a blind, small opening is dangerous. The mastoidectomy itself is a useful exploratory tool for the antrum when blockage is suspected or improved aeration of the middle ear is desired. Insertion of the electrode through the round window is the same as in the posterior tympanotomy approach; the electrode is passed through the opening into the cochlea.

Transcanal Labyrinthectomy

Procedure

Visualize the middle ear cavity (Figures 36A to D). Identify the oval and round windows and promontory, as well as the facial nerve. The purpose of this procedure is to destroy the labyrinth.

The stapes footplate has been removed, and the vestibule containing the saccule and utricle is exposed. By the use of a hook or Hough hoe, the saccule can be destroyed (Figure 36B). Using this same route, the ampule of the superior semicircular canal can be reached above and in front of the facial nerve, that of the posterior canal below and behind the nerve and the ampule of the horizontal canal inferiorly beneath the nerve (Figure 36C). In this process, the utricle is destroyed as well. It is important to stay within the bony confines and to destroy only the "membranous labyrinth". Immediately inferior to the vestibule is the internal auditory canal, where the bony plate is quite thin. The facial nerve also can be injured. To complete the procedure, drill the promontory and join the oval and round windows, exposing the beginning of the basal turn of the cochlea (Figure 36D). Additional drilling can be done at this point for purposes of orientation to the cochlear anatomy. Placing an electrode via the basal turn can give the surgeon a clearer grasp of this procedure and its anatomic location.

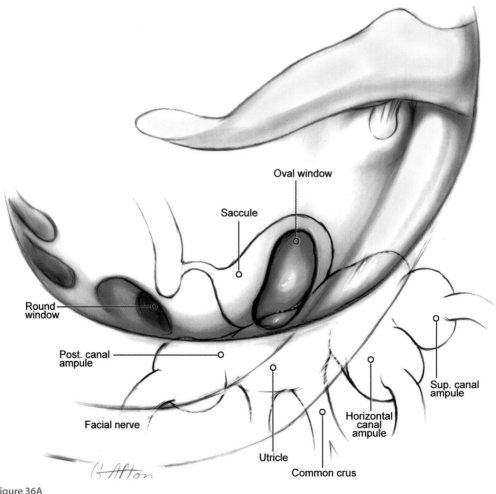

Oval window

Saccule

Round window

Post. canal ampule

Facial nerve

Utricle

Common crus

Horizontal canal ampule

Sup. canal ampule

Figure 36A

labyrinthectomy, as described earlier. The internal auditory canal is then outlined and the facial nerve is identified as it enters the labyrinthine segment of the fallopian canal. This is found by using the ampulla of the superior semicircular canal as a landmark for the superior vestibular nerve. With a small diamond burr, the tegmen is followed medially in this area to develop the superior aspect of the internal auditory canal. The facial nerve will be blue-lined as it leaves the internal auditory canal and begins its course in the labyrinthine segment of the fallopian canal (Figure 39A).

The next step is to completely skeletonize the facial nerve from the stylomastoid foramen to the internal auditory canal. An extended facial recess opening is made (Figure 39B). After adequate thinning of the posterior external auditory canal, a cutting or diamond burr is used to enlarge an area immediately inferior to the fossa incudis and lateral to the facial nerve at the beginning of its mastoid segment. It is important to use as large a drill as possible to prevent tunneling and poor visualization. In a true facial recess, care must be taken not to disrupt the chorda tympani (lateral limit) and the tympanic membrane. These structures will be removed in this approach so that dissection may be accomplished more swiftly. After the opening is made into the middle ear, the incudostapedial joint is visualized and separated. The incus is removed through the attic. The facial recess is then enlarged superiorly through to the fossa incudus and inferiorly to the level of the floor of the tympanum.

The external auditory canal is then removed with a rongeur to improve visualization of the facial nerve. The anterior buttress is drilled to the level of the middle fossa tegmen and inferiorly as a smooth transition to the floor of the tympanum is accomplished. With the diamond drill, the facial nerve is then skeletonized completely within the temporal bone. The chorda tympani has already been sacrificed. When the bone has been completely removed, the greater superficial petrosal nerve is cut at its origin from the geniculate ganglion (Figure 39C).

This frees the facial nerve from all attachments in the temporal bone. It is then carefully reflected posteriorly out of its bony bed. Any remaining tympanic membrane is now removed, as well as any skin remaining on the anterior part of the external auditory canal. The anterior external auditory canal and any bony overhang are drilled to the level of the temporomandibular joint. The stapes is also removed at this point. Starting with the basal coil, the cochlea is completely drilled out, as well as the remnant of the fallopian canal (Figures 39D and E) (it is a good practice to follow the cochlea's coils to gain a better understanding of its anatomy). Bone removal is carried forward to the septum that lies between the internal carotid artery and anterior wall of the basal coil. The internal carotid artery can be blue-lined with the diamond drill, much as the jugular bulb is bluelined in the translabyrinthine approach. Inferiorly, bone removal extends to the inferior petrosal sinus and jugular bulb. Superiorly, the superior petrosal sinus and tegmen are followed medially to Meckel's cave (Figure 39F). Medially, removal of bone continues to the lateral clivus. When bone removal has been completed, a large window covered by dura (bounded superiorly by the superior petrosal sinus, and inferiorly by the jugular bulb and inferior petrosal sinus, with its apex just below Meckel's cave and the internal carotid artery located anteriorly) is created into the skull bone. If the dura is still intact, this window can be opened posterior to the internal auditory canal and extended as far forward as needed for exposure. Cuts may run medially, anteriorly, and parallel to the superior petrosal sinus and jugular bulb. In an actual procedure, the dural defect is packed with abdominal fat and the external ear canal is sewn shut to prevent postoperative leakage of cerebrospinal fluid.

Middle Fossa Approach to the Internal Auditory Canal

Aim

To expose the floor of the middle cranial fossa and identify the structures contained within, including the cochlea, arcuate eminence and contents of the internal auditory canal.

Highlights

- To decompress the labyrinthine segment of the facial nerve or remove facial nerve lesions
- To remove small intracanalicular acoustic tumors in an attempt to preserve residual hearing
- To repair large defects of the tegmen and dura that have resulted in cerebrospinal fluid leaks
- To section the superior and inferior vestibular nerves, and retain hearing.

Procedure

When practicing this approach in the laboratory, placement of the bone within the bone cup is important. Imagine a patient

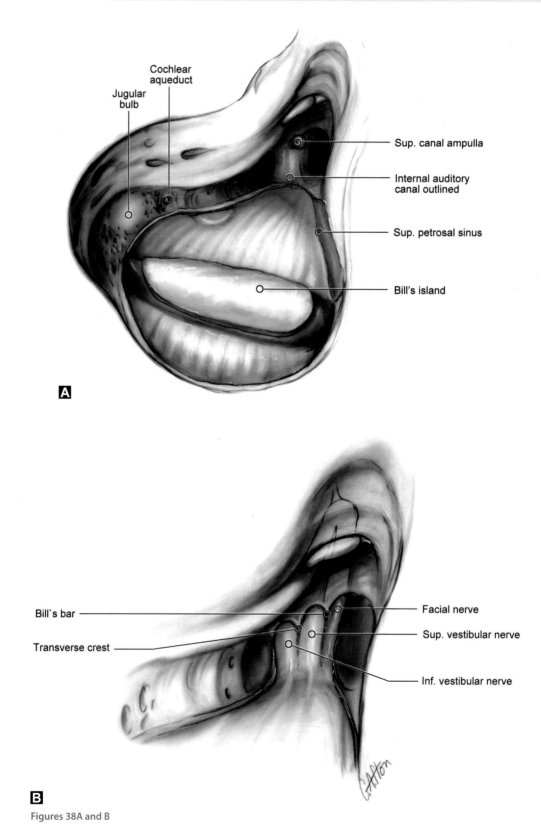

Figures 38A and B

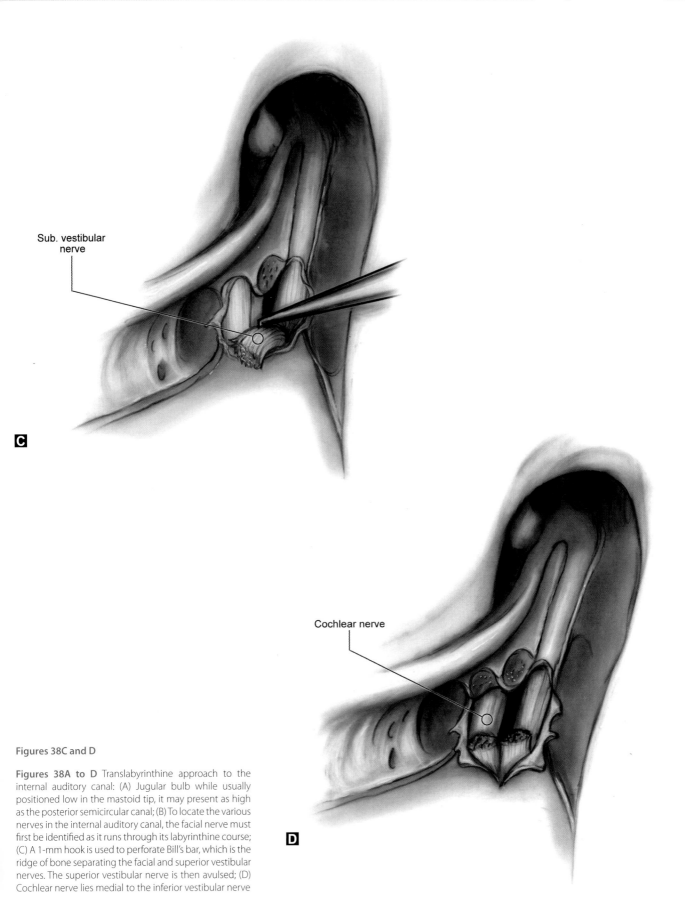

Figures 38C and D

Figures 38A to D Translabyrinthine approach to the internal auditory canal: (A) Jugular bulb while usually positioned low in the mastoid tip, it may present as high as the posterior semicircular canal; (B) To locate the various nerves in the internal auditory canal, the facial nerve must first be identified as it runs through its labyrinthine course; (C) A 1-mm hook is used to perforate Bill's bar, which is the ridge of bone separating the facial and superior vestibular nerves. The superior vestibular nerve is then avulsed; (D) Cochlear nerve lies medial to the inferior vestibular nerve

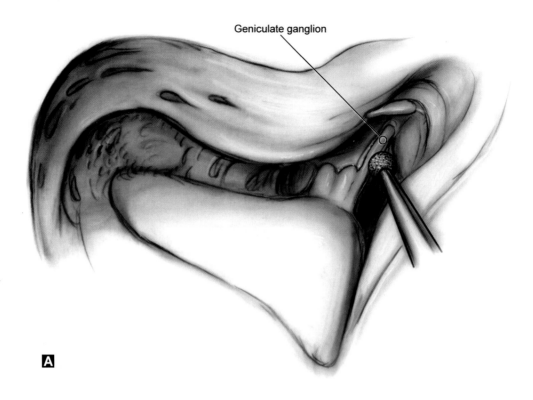

Geniculate ganglion

A

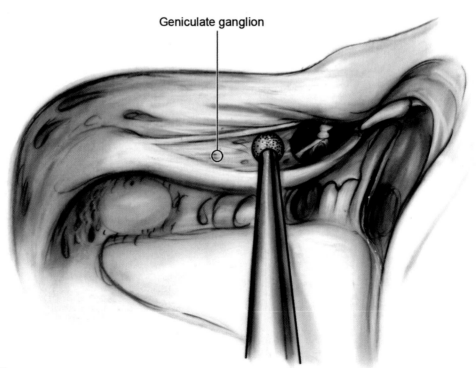

Geniculate ganglion

B

Figures 39A and B

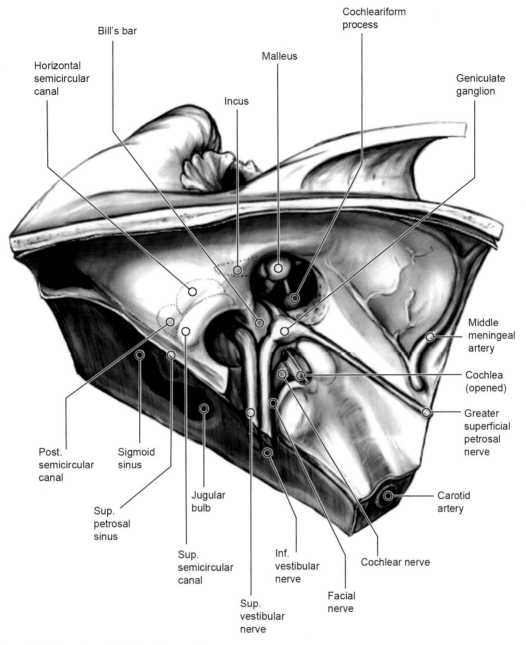

Figure 41 A three-dimensional view of temporal bone anatomy

facial nerve lies the cochlear nerve and the inferior vestibular nerve lies beneath the superior vestibular nerve. These represent the anteroinferior and posteroinferior compartments respectively. For the sake of completeness, the following structures should be found and followed in their courses. This will help to further the understanding of temporal bone anatomy in a three-dimensional view (Figure 41). Slightly lateral to the greater superior petrosal, the Eustachian tube runs medially from the middle ear cavity to the nasopharynx. Upon dissection of the Eustachian tube, the carotid artery may be found on the inferomedial floor of the tube; it courses horizontally from the middle ear to the cavernous sinus. The semicircular canal and cochlea should be entered and followed to gain a clear understanding of their positions within the temporal bone.

Section III

General Principles and Approaches in the Operating Room

Francisco Soto, Hortensia Guzmán, Josefina Ernst, Marcos Goycoolea, Pedro Cubillos, Raquel Levy, Verónica Briones, Viviana Orellana

3.1

General Principles

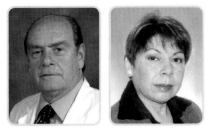

Marcos Goycoolea, Verónica Briones

EVALUATION

All patients should have a complete history obtained and be given a physical examination. Although, proper surgical indications and adequate laboratory studies are essential, their discussion is beyond the scope of this chapter. A complete assessment of the patient's general condition as well as of the otologic problem itself, is to be made. It should be remembered that the ear is not an isolated organ; it interrelates anatomically and functionally with other organs and systems for example, the nasopharynx and nasal cavity that must be evaluated in detail. The local condition of the ear, including the skin of the pinna, the ear canal, middle ear mucosa and so forth, must be improved as much as possible before surgery.

An otologic evaluation includes a number of basic tests in addition to the history and physical examination. A recent complete audiogram that includes pure tones and speech discrimination is essential. Equally important is confirmation of the results by the surgeon, utilizing tuning forks at 512 Hz.

Radiologic studies include computed tomographic scans, magnetic resonance, and other imaging modalities depending on the specific needs. Specific indications of such studies will not be discussed here except to mention that tomographic studies should provide (in addition to the specific disease being treated) information on mastoid aeration, the position of the sigmoid sinus, facial canal, etc.

X-rays must be available in the operating room. A number of additional tests are used, such as, brainstem auditory evoked responses (BAER), electrocochleography, promontory stimulation and others; the indications for which are outside the scope of this atlas. The essential concept in this section is that the patient must be evaluated from a general as well as a local standpoint and that the tests serve the purpose of screening, ruling out or confirming specific questions in the mind of the surgeon. They are not a "routine blanket ordered according to trends", nor are they intended to replace common sense and clinical acuity.

PATIENT CONSENT

As important as informed consent is from a legal standpoint, it is much more important in that it provides the patient with

information and improves patient safety. It is essential that the patient (or his or her parents) be aware of the rationale for and purpose of the surgical procedure. Is the aim, reconstruction of the ossicular chain? Is it eradication of disease? What are the chances of success and the risks involved?

A well-informed patient is the best guarantee of success. Information on the postoperative course and care is also essential and should be provided by the surgeon. If printed instructions are to be provided, commercially printed instructions are very helpful. However, they do not approach the usefulness of instructions given by the surgeon. The purpose is to provide information so that the patient is well-informed and not to provide it in order to avoid legal suits.

In the operating room, we have an additional so-called "security pause" in which the surgical team must describe the surgical procedure to be performed and the side (ear) in which it will be performed.

ANESTHESIA

Most otologic procedures can be performed under local anesthesia with or without sedation. The decision will depend on the specific case and the surgeon's judgment and common sense. General anesthesia has significantly improved the safety and currently, in most (but not all) cases, it carries a small risk at times comparable or even less than that of local procedures under sedation. If a local anesthetic is to be used, it is important to know the innervation of the area to be anesthetized (See the anatomy and anesthesia sections). Different agents are utilized and these are described in the anesthesia section. In cases of myringotomies and tubes, the topical use of phenol or iontophoretic anesthesia is a useful method in the office. Iontophoresis is based on a battery-operated unit (iontophoretic applicator) that generates a constant direct current allowing ion transfer of a local anesthetic (placed in the ear canal) into the ear canal and tympanic membranes. Because it does not require an injection, it is very well-accepted by some patients. However, it takes some time to take effect and topical use of phenol is much faster. Topical use of phenol is just wonderful, however, it should be used cautiously since excessive amounts and repeated use on the same site (e.g. for injection of local steroids or gentamicin) can result in a tympanic membrane perforation. In these cases, the injection site should be changed or a ventilation tube should be placed.

ANTIBIOTICS

The use of antibiotics is a controversial subject that will not be dwelled upon here. The authors use them prophylactically when there is a risk that infection will extend into the inner ear or intracranially or there is a potential compromise of a graft or a reconstructive procedure or potential local spread (e.g. to the auricular cartilage). When a prophylactic antibiotic is used, it is immediately before, during and after the operation.

Use of antibiotics does not mean that strict aseptic techniques are disregarded; they are used only when there are additional risks in spite of a flawless technique that includes asepsis, meticulous hemostasis and gentleness with tissues.

OPERATING TABLE

The operating table must be comfortable but hard enough to allow for resuscitation procedures, if needed. It should be easily adjustable so that it can be raised or lowered or the patient can be placed in a Trendelenburg's or reverse Trendelenburg's position (Figures 1A and B). The headpiece should be separable in order to change the position of the patient's head independently from the rest of the table (Figure 2).

At times, a simple small "donut" will suffice, since currently most operating tables can be moved in different directions and heights quite easily with automatic controls. A Juers head

holder is also useful as it allows adjustments in angulation of the head as needed (Figures 3A and B). The patient's head should be taped to the head holder (which in turn is taped to the head of the table) and moved with the holder as a unit (Figure 4).

The patient lies supine with the head turned and lowered in order to bring the external auditory canal, which has a bony orientation that is downward and forward, into a nearly vertical position. Another useful feature, especially in cochlear implant cases, is the use of a table that allows intraoperative radiologic evaluations.

PREPARATION OF THE SKIN

At our institution (as in most others) skin preparation is done according to a protocol based norms of hospital infection control.

The skin is prepared after shaving the hair. Shaving of the hair is done with a dry razor blade at the time of surgery avoiding any lacerations of the skin. Enough hair is shaved to provide a clean operative field (generally a very little shaving will suffice). For a postauricular approach, the authors shave an area of approximately 2.5 cm. If a large flap is to be raised, more hair is shaved. For an endaural approach, 0.5 cm of hair superiorly along the superior helix will suffice. A germicidal soap and solution, such as povidone iodine is used.

The operative field is isolated with sterile drapes avoiding excessive bulk that would compromise mobility. The "hanging drapes" are clamped together in order to allow the surgeon's legs to fit comfortably under the head of the table without interference.

FOREIGN BODY REACTION

Particles contained in gloves (powder), prosthesis or surgical instruments can cause inflammatory reactions that are potentially harmful. It is a good habit to keep a sterile solution and moist gauze to rinse and clean the surgical gloves before initiating the surgery. The scrub nurse should have on his or her table a container with saline in order to clean the instruments and prosthesis prior to use. In the past, we used to recommend that instruments should be rinsed meticulously after the use of sterilizing chemicals, since these can be very damaging to tissues. We do not use sterilizing chemicals any more.

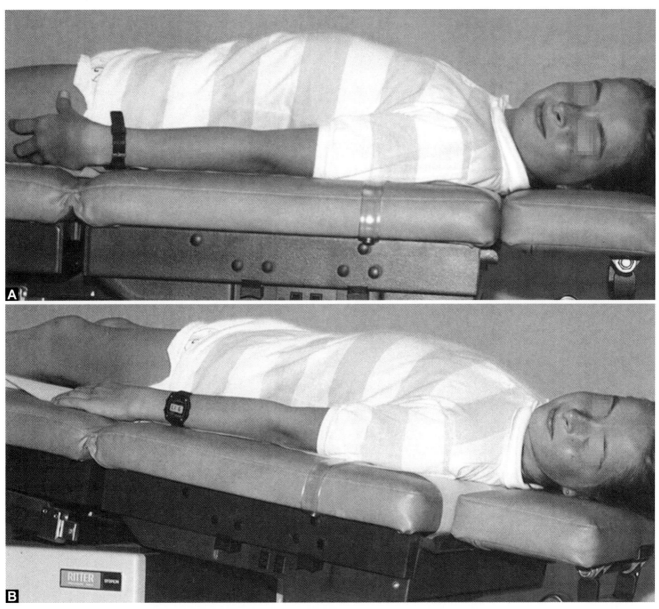

Figures 1A and B Different position of the patient on operating table

POSITIONING OF THE SURGICAL TEAM

Like any surgical event, the general organization and distribution in the room must be efficient and its organization must be done according to the particular need of each surgical procedure.

The surgeon must be in a comfortable and stable position with both the feet on the floor and with the back supported by a chair that can be moved easily (by the surgeon), while retaining its position. The patient must be placed such that the surgeon is not bent or forced into uncomfortable positions. This is usually achieved by positioning the head of the operating table virtually over the surgeon's lap with the surgeon capable of "comfortably writing on a desk", while looking through the microscope.

The surgical team is of the utmost importance. A successful surgical procedure represents the combined efforts of a team of surgeons, anesthesiologists and, scrub and circulating nurses. No matter how skilled the surgeon, his or her work is not possible without a safely and adequately anesthetized or sedated patient; no matter how skilled the anesthesiologist, adequate anesthesia will not be possible if the surgeon does not inform him or her of the moment of injection of epinephrine, mobiliza-

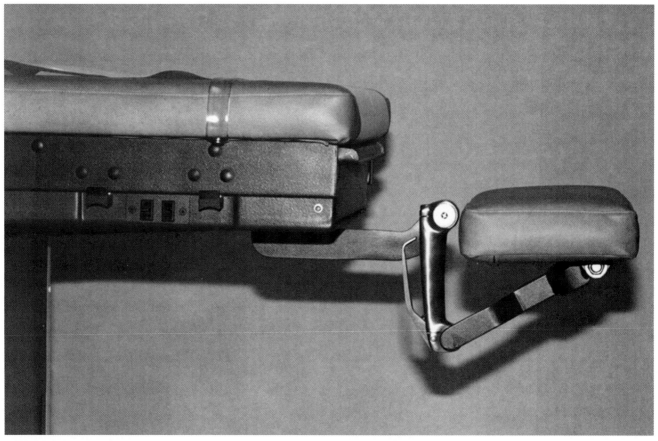

Figure 2 The headpiece should be separable in order to change the position of the patient's head

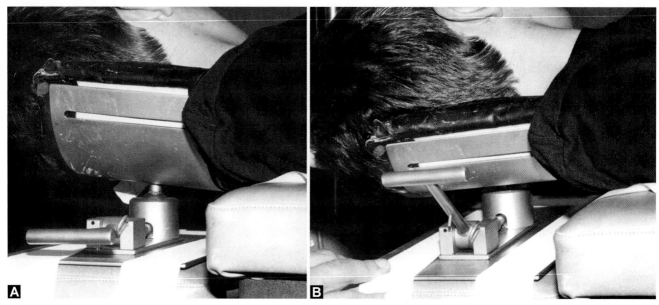

Figures 3A and B Juers' head holder for adjustable angulation of head

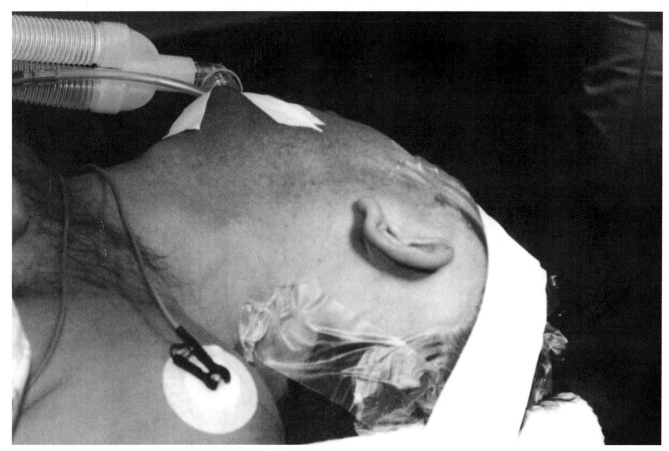

Figure 4 The patient's head is taped to the head holder

tion of the head of the patient, elevation of the operative table or other procedures. The same rules apply, in principle, for the circulating and scrub nurses. The precept of this chapter is that in surgery teamwork yields better results than "wonder man" or "wonder woman" alone.

The author's positioning of the team and the instruments in the operating room is shown in Figures 5A and B. The scrub nurse is to the right of the surgeon and the assistant is to the left. Other surgeons prefer different setups. The best position is one that provides the most comfort and efficiency to a particular team (Figure 6).

The scrub nurse and the operating room nurse and assistants are shown in Figure 7.

Technological advances in medicine and in particular in surgical equipment, have caused significant changes in the operating room. Current devices (microscopes, drills, lasers, video equipment, etc.) have become sophisticated and complex,

requiring special training and permanent updating of the operating room team. The operating room nurse and scrub nurse must be capable of operating these devices efficiently (assisted by our electronic, technical and maintenance departments).

More importantly, and especially, since we are dedicated to people's needs, we require adequate human profile and attitudes. Our scrub nurse team requires the following professional profile for their members:

1. Interest and empathy
2. Respect for others
3. Emotional self-control
4. Honesty and ethical conduct
5. Manual ability
6. Organizational abilities
7. Concentration
8. Capability to solve problems
9. Sense of humor.

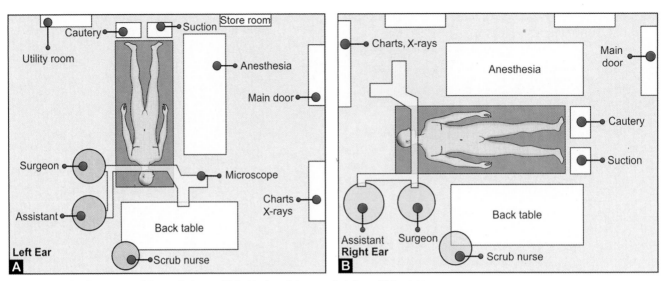

Figures 5A and B Positioning of the surgical team: (A) Positioning of the team for left ear; (B) For right ear

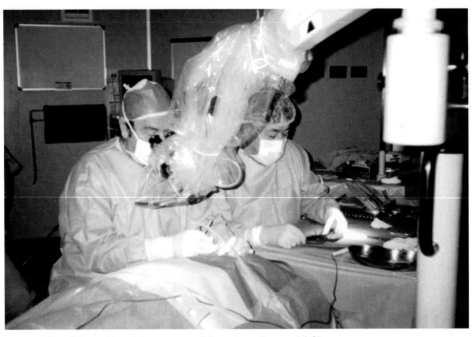

Figure 6 One of the position of the surgeon and the assistant (surgeon's left)

INSTRUMENTS

The operating microscope obviously must be binocular with a focal length of at least 20 cm. The authors prefer to use the 25 cm length as it provides a range of magnification from 6x to 40x, with 6x, 10x and 16x the most commonly used. Along with good light, it requires good handling ability. Current microscopes with Xenon light and with easy regulations of zoom and focus have resulted in greater ease. Both the surgeon and the scrub nurse must be familiar with the different knobs that provide maneuverability. Authors prefer to use an angled eyepiece that provides an angle of 45° and allows a more comfortable head position for the surgeon (Figures 8A and B).

The arm of the microscope should be at a 90° angle, which permits a full range of motion (Figure 9). In the case of the classical OPMI-1, the "longer leg" of the pedestal should point toward the patient's shoulder on the operated side. In the newer models, this does not make that much difference (Figure 10). The side viewer (teaching lens) is placed at the opposite side of the ear to be operated upon (left side; for right ear and vice versa) and a video camera is attached (Figure 11). This allows the operating team to be aware of the procedure, anticipate the use of instruments and even maintain a permanent record of the operation. A suitable sterile drape of either cloth or disposable plastic must be used (Figure 12). For insertion of pressure equalizer tubes, rubber handles for focusing and magnification are useful. If they are not available, a sterile towel will suffice. The microscope should be checked preoperatively (Figure 13) and when the procedure is over, it must be cleaned and carefully covered (Figure 14). Skipping these steps in the past has resulted in unpleasant surprises related to microscope damage or malfunctioning.

A variety of drills are commercially available. A high-speed drill should suffice, provided that it is a durable instrument capable of withstanding continuous use. At least two drills should be available in the operating room. The drill handles should be light and easy to manipulate; the instrument should have several speeds, including reverse and forward. Control by a foot pedal is preferable since handle-controlled drills tend to have more vibration. The reverse speed is useful for saucerizing small bleeding points in the mastoid and bony ear canal. Different metal burrs, usually made out of tungsten or steel are available (Figures 15A and B). Rounded burrs work best

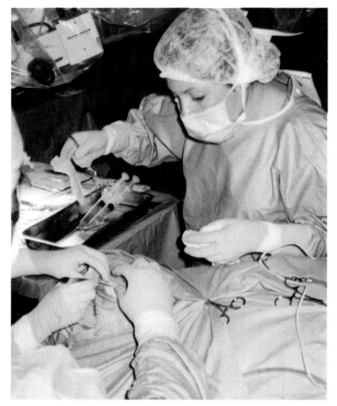

Figure 7 Showing position of the scrub nurse (right to the surgeon)

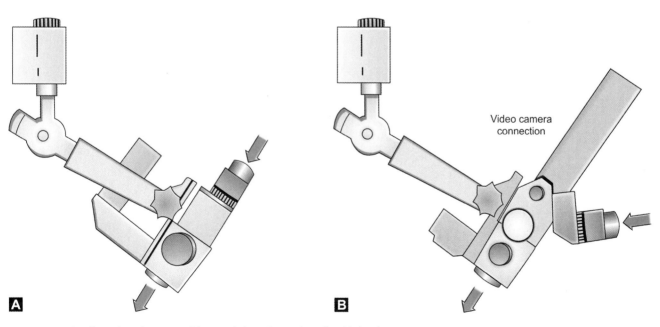

A　　　**B**

Figures 8A and B Operating microscope with an angled eyepiece and comfortable head position

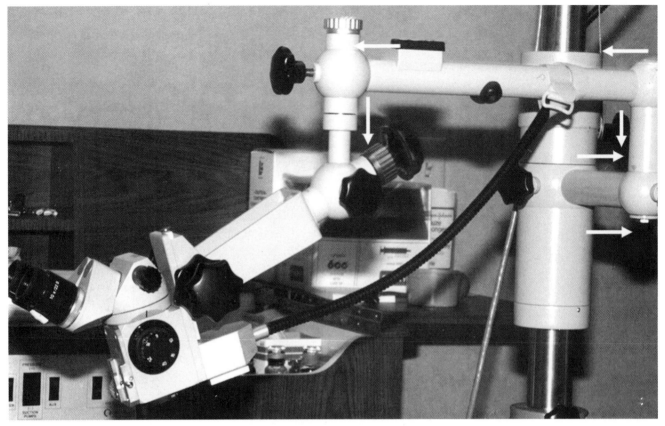

Figure 9 The arm of the microscope at a 90° angle which provide full range of motion

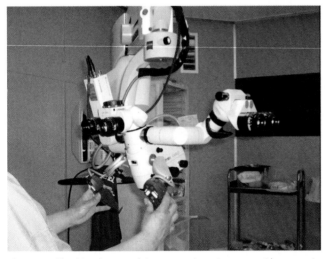

Figure 10 Checking the controls in an operating microscope with automatic focus and zoom controls

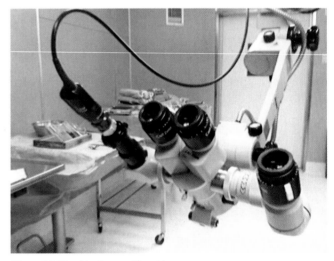

Figure 11 The side viewer with a video camera

for otology; they can be of six or eight teeth. In general, burrs with more teeth accumulate more debris and are less effective. However, a burr full of debris is useful in areas requiring gentle work and is similar in this regard to a diamond burr (a metal burr coated with diamond powder). Burrs must be sharp; dulling

leads to overheating. Sizes of burrs vary according to the needs (discussed in specific chapters) as shown in Figure 16.

The "suction irrigation" feature is commonly used today. Drills with continuous irrigation (variable flow) are available and are useful in avoiding drilling over "dry bone," which promotes

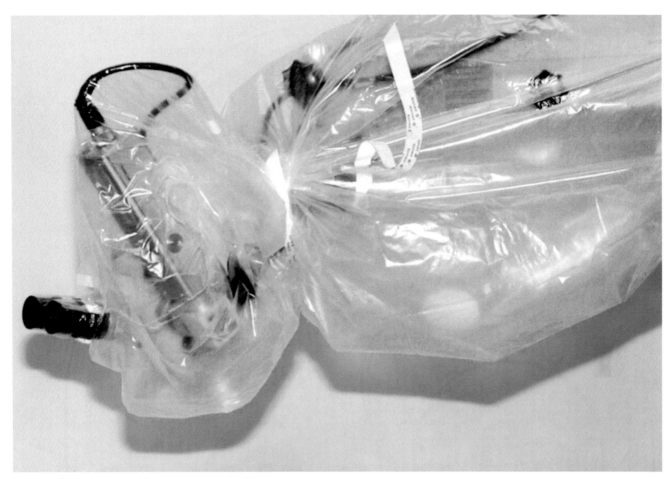

Figure 12 Sterile drape is used for covering operating microscope

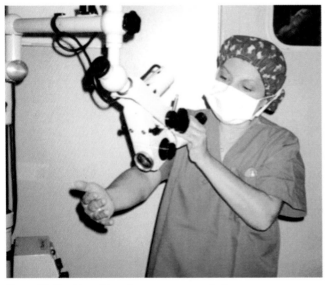

Figure 13 Checking of the microscope preoperatively

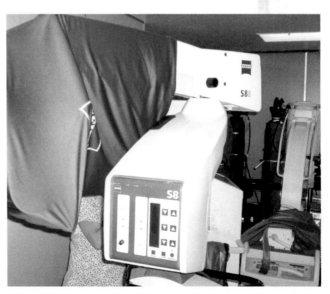

Figure 14 Microscope is carefully cleaned and covered after operating procedure gets over

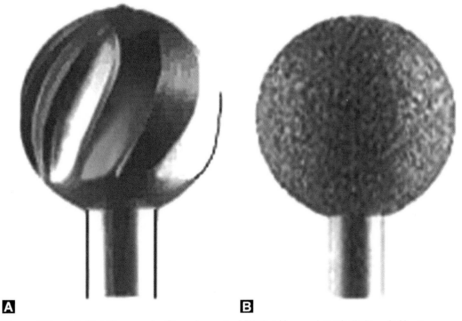

Figures 15A and B Metal burrs made of tungsten or steel: (A) Metal burr with teeth; (B) Rounded burr

0.5	1	1.5	2	2.3	2.5	3	3.2	3.5	4	4.5	4.8	5	5.5	6	6.5	7

Figure 16 Metal burrs of different sizes

overheating and necrosis. Some surgeons prefer to use intermittent suction irrigation, with moments of a bulb syringe use, to provide moisture as needed and thus, avoiding the visual distortion that occurs at times with "underwater drilling." Again, the purpose is to avoid heating and necrosis of bone that is best achieved in a manner that is efficient for the surgeon.

Good suction is essential. The tubing should be flexible, soft but not collapsible and not too rigid, so that it is easy to handle. A number 5 suction tip is used for cleansing the ear canal, a number 20 for raising flaps and for middle ear work, and a number 24 for work in the oval window.

Fenestrated handles are preferable, since they allow control of the degree of suction. Some surgeons prefer to control the degree of suction with a foot control. For drilling, larger suction tips are used (number 7–9 French). A syringe for forced irrigation as well as a wire to clean the suction tip should be available. Small sponges or cotton balls should be used at the suction tip, when working over grafts or prostheses that can be loosened or dislodged by the suction (Cotton must not be left in the ear since it is a guarantee of infection). The author's usual instrument set-up is shown in Figures 17A and B.

Standard cautery units will not be described. It is suffice to mention that the authors routinely use a bipolar unit. Monopolar cautery is faster but healing is more compromised. Both the suction and cautery units should be adequately positioned and clipped to the drapes with sufficient length to allow easy

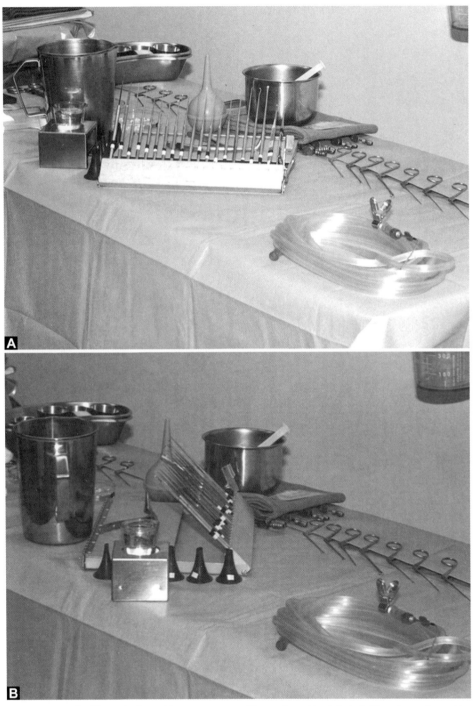

Figures 17A and B The author's usual instrument set-up. The suction tubing is included in order to give an idea of the size and type used

handling, but short enough to prevent contamination if the units are dropped (Figure 18).

A variety of instrument sets are commercially available. Since, the purpose of this atlas is descriptive and not promotional, the author's specific preferences are not listed; they will be sent upon request. It is important to acquire quality instruments, particularly for work inside the ear. Apparent savings from buying cheaper but poorly made instruments can be illusory. Instruments are designed for specific purposes and should be purchased with this in mind.

Instruments bearing the endorsement of a particular surgeon provide a sense of security and should be considered for acquisition. However, they represent the preference of that surgeon and may not necessarily meet your needs.

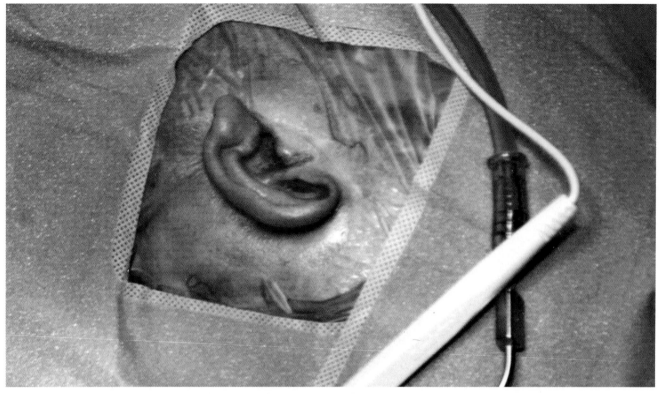

Figure 18 Suction tip and cautery "hanging" in the operating field. They are not left in this position during surgery; this figure simply shows that if clipped correctly, the suction tip and cautery will not become contaminated if they fall

Instruments should be positioned in such a manner that they are accessible to the scrub nurse and in a position that is efficient in order to be handled to a surgeon that is looking through a microscope.

Finally, otology instruments are extremely delicate and have been developed to work in microsurgery. Cleansing and handling should be done carefully and preferably by the scrub nurse or under her direct supervision.

Operating room cards describing the instruments and materials required for different surgical procedures should be available. They make the nurses' jobs easier and more effective. Ear instruments preferably are placed in a rack and numbered in the order in which they are used for example, number 1 straight canal knife, number 2 curved canal knife, number 3 duckbill elevator and so on. If the scrub and circulating nurses rotate or the operating room "committee" believes that nurses can be "jacks of all trades", it is useful to print the names of the instruments (beside their numbers) and to place on the table a plasticized, "sterilizable" card listing the names and positions of instruments and materials. In addition, cards describing the

position of the team in the operating room should be taped to the wall in a clearly visible place. Otologic surgery has become too specialized. As in other surgical specialties, currently there are many (too many) sophisticated and very expensive instruments. Therefore, in our surgical team, the scrub nurses do not rotate in other specialties and are an exclusive and integral part of the team.

RECORD OF OPERATION

As important as describing what was done is describing what was found, preferably with CD documentation. Problem areas should be noted. Such records are useful in evaluating prospective causes and factors in both failures and successful results. Packing techniques are described in specific sections and will not be discussed here. Illustrations of how to apply an oval eye pad (Figures 19A to C) and a mastoid dressing (Figures 20A to M) are included as well as a photograph showing the application of ointment with a rubber-tipped syringe (Figure 21).

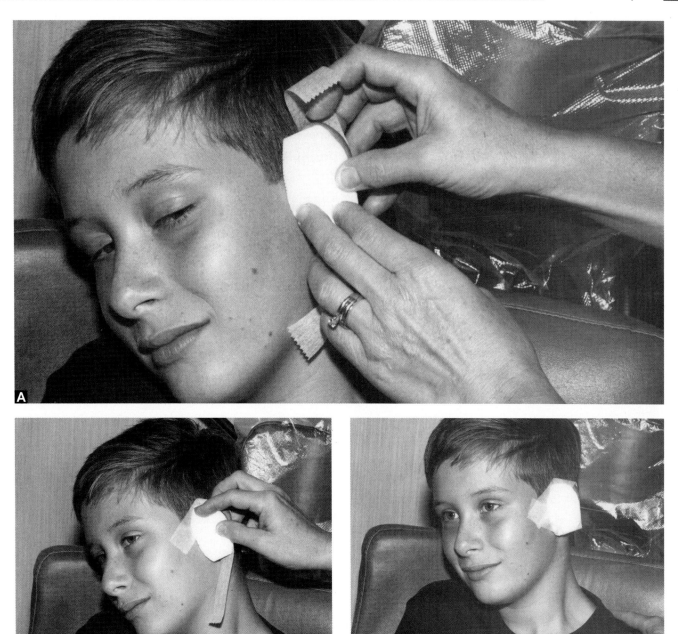

Figures 19A to C Placement of an oval eye pad

SURGICAL TIME

It is important to develop surgical techniques and habits that allow a systematic and efficient use of time, but completeness and thoroughness are equally essential. As mentioned in previous sections, hours of temporal bone drilling and practice (using the head as well as the hands) allow the acquisition of a functional three-dimensional mental view of the ear. This acquisition that becomes natural overtime, allows anticipation and coordination, just as a golfer or a violinist or a chess player of excellence, acquire with time.

This is something that the surgeons notice when it occurs, but is difficult to describe in words and reflects established neuronal circuits. In measuring success, results have more

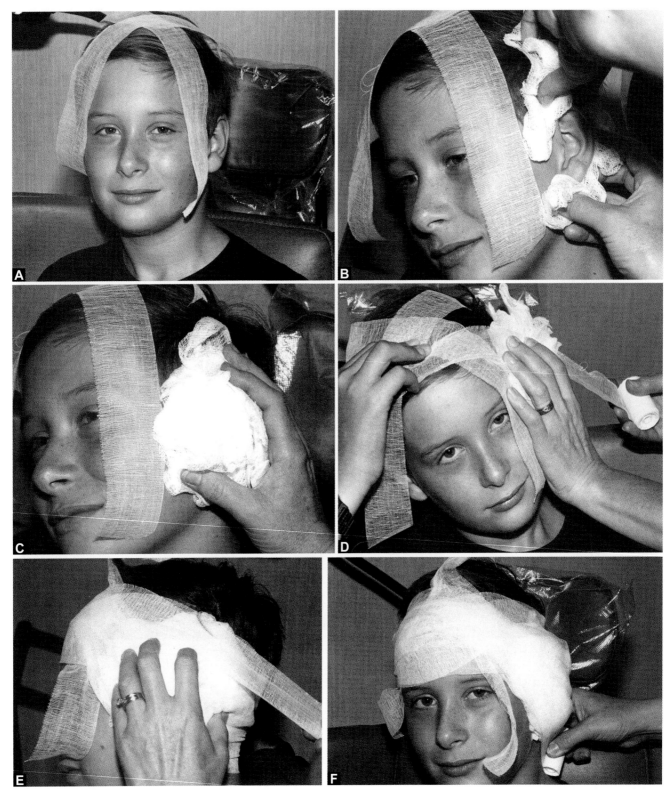

Figures 20A to F

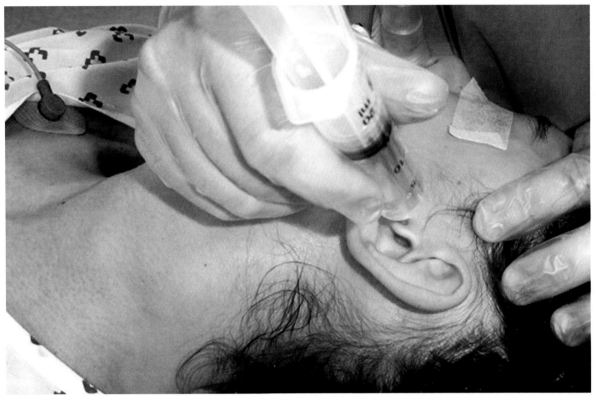

Figure 2 Auriculotemporal nerve block
Photo courtesy: Dr P Canepa, Clinica Las Condes

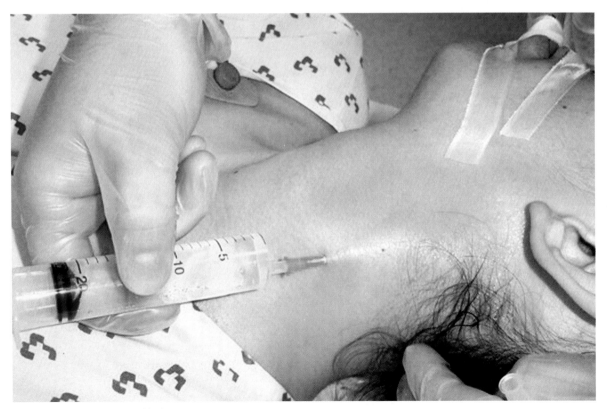

Figure 3 Great auricular nerve block
Photo courtesy: Dr P Canepa, Clinica Las Condes

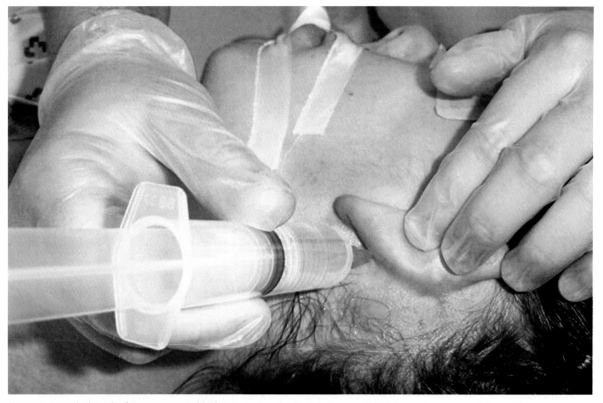

Figure 4 Auricular branch of the vagus nerve block
Photo courtesy: Dr P Canepa, Clinica Las Condes

REFERENCES

1. Miller RH (Ed). Miller's Anesthesia Textbook, 6th edition. Elsevier Inc; p. 5657.

2. Bernard JM, Péréon Y, Fayet G, et al. Effects of isoflurane and desflurane on neurogenic motor and somatosensory evoked potential monitoring for scoliosis surgery. Anesthesiology. 1996;85:1013-9.

3. Duff B. Use of LMA in otologic surgery. Laryngoscope. 1999;109:1033-6.

4. Fujii Y, Toyooka H, Tanaka H. Prophylactic antiemetic therapy with a combination of granisetron and dexamethasone in patients undergoing middle ear surgery. Br J Anesth. 1998;81(5):754-6.

5. Vega R, Cabrera C. Dexmedetomidine: a new alfa-2 agonist anesthetic agent in infusion for sedation in middle ear surgery with awake patient. Anesthesiology. 2005;(A623).

6. Heard C, Houck C, Johnson K, et al. A comparison of dexmedetomidine and propofol for pediatric MRI sedation. Anesthesiology. 2007;107:A13.

3.3

Basic Audiology

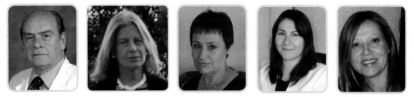

Marcos Goycoolea, Hortensia Guzmán, Raquel Levy, Viviana Orellana, Josefina Ernst

BASIC HEARING EVALUATION

Hearing testing is done using a number of tests that are oriented toward identifying the type of hearing loss, the degree and the location of the problem within the auditory pathway. A detailed history and clinical examination (including the use of tuning forks) are essential, and contribute to have a good general idea of the situation prior to doing the tests that will be described. These tests are done using electronic devices.

Tests to be described are as follows:
- Classic pure tone audiometry
- Special tests:
  - High frequency audiometry
  - Special and suprathreshold tests
  - Play audiometry and visual reinforcement audiometry
- Speech audiometry
- Sound field audiometry
  - Play audiometry and visual reinforcement audiometry
  - With and without hearing aids
- Evoked response audiometry
- Otoacoustic emissions
- Acoustic immittance evaluation.

Classic Pure Tone Audiometry

This is the basic test for measuring hearing. The aim is to establish the threshold (the stimulus of lowest intensity that can be perceived) for each of the frequencies. The pure tones that are electronically generated by the audiometer are delivered by ear phones (air conduction) or by bone vibrators (bone conduction). Testing is done in a soundproof room. Thresholds are expressed in decibels (intensity measure). The frequencies that are used in conventional audiometry for air conduction are 250–500–1000 Hz, up to 8000 Hz (cycles per second; a high frequency audiometer can give higher frequencies) and 250–500–1000 Hz, up to 4000 Hertz for bone conduction. The written record of a person´s hearing

level measured with pure tones is termed as an audiogram. There are different forms; the most common being the one described in Figure 1.

There are number of conventional forms of writing an audiogram, for the sake of uniform reporting and comparison purposes which are:
- Tone frequencies (Hz) are placed from left to right
- Tone intensities (dB) are placed up and down
- The left ear is marked with the color blue (crosses) and the right ear with red (circles)
- Air conduction is written with a full line and bone conduction with an interrupted line
- The symbols that are used are described in the audiogram.
- In case masking is required for air conduction, the right ear thresholds are triangles and the left ear are cubes. For bone conduction, masking the staples is red or blue according to the side (right or left) and come together with an interrupted line.
- Audiograms are calibrated to a standard reference level that has to be described in the audiogram (e.g. ANSI, 1969). The zero of the audiometer is an average and not a mathematical zero. Therefore, normal hearing is between –5 and 20 dB.

Recapitulating Some Basic Concepts

Sound is produced by a vibrating object and is transmitted as waves. Sound waves travel in straight lines in all directions away from the source. They travel through a medium, being faster in solids but do not travel in a vacuum. A pure tone is a simple type of wave. It has two main characteristics: (i) frequency; and (ii)

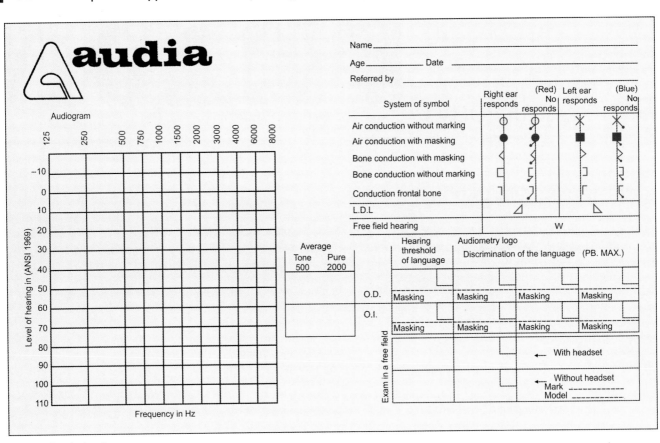

Figure 1 Standard audiogram

intensity. Frequency is the number of times per second that a complete vibration occurs. It is expressed in cycles per second; the unit is Hertz and is abbreviated Hz. One thousand Hertz is also expressed as 1 Kilo Hertz and is abbreviated KHz. The human ear can pick up frequencies from 20 Hz to 20 kHz. Speech sounds range between 250 Hz and 4000 Hz. Frequency gives the sensation of pitch, which is what the person hears.

Intensity is the sound energy or pressure. It is represented in pure tones by the height of the wave from the baseline. Intensity is expressed in decibels, abbreviated as dB. Intensity gives the sensation of loudness.

Frequency and intensity are the expressions of a stimulus. Pitch and loudness are the experiences perceived. The study of perceived experiences is termed as psychoacoustics.

In daily life one hears complex sounds, rarely just pure tones. Noise is composed of unrelated random frequencies. Musical tones are composed of frequencies related to one another. Background noise is composed of unrelated random frequencies that convey competing messages to the listener.

Decibels: Sound is a form of energy and the ear responds to pressure fluctuations. The units of pressure are the microbars (or dynes/cm²). The weakest detectable is 0.0002 microbars and the strongest is 20000 microbars. Since this range is too wide, it is very difficult to tabulate for practical clinical purposes. Therefore, a unit was developed that is termed decibel (dB).

A decibel is a logarithmic ratio. One decibel refers to the smallest change in the intensity between two sounds that a human ear can distinguish. A decibel is therefore, a unit of intensity; a unit of comparison between two sound pressures. For example, 40 decibels is a sound that is 40 dB above a standard or reference level. Just the term 40 dB alone has no meaning. The following are the reference levels used:

1. Acoustic zero or SPL (sound pressure level) is based on the sound pressure of 0.0002 microbars.
2. The zero of hearing loss of average normal hearing or HL (hearing level) refers to the average normal hearing of young healthy adults. The most common average used is American National Standards Institute (ANSI), 1969 (set down in 1969 by the ANSI). It is very important that the records (or audiogram) describe the reference (for example ANSI 1969) because the references for average normal hearing used can be different.

3. Sensation level (SL) is in relation to the threshold. Therefore, decibel values vary according to the reference that is used.

What do we Measure?

The threshold of hearing at different frequencies is what is measured. The threshold is the minimal intensity that can be heard by bone or by air conduction.

Curves are obtained for air conduction, using ear phones in each ear and then for bone conduction using a bone vibrator on the mastoid in each ear. Normally, air conduction and bone conduction should be the same and should be superimposed on top of each other. In reality, one hears better by air conduction but the audiometer is regulated so that they are at the same level (Figures 2A to D).

In conductive losses, air conduction thresholds are increased and bone conduction is normal (Figure 2B). This difference, gap or space in the audiometric curves is termed as an air-bone gap (for example, a 30 dB air-bone gap) and gives the degree of conductive loss. This degree can give an idea of the type of problem. For example, fluid in the ear gives rise to a small gap whereas ossicular disruption or fixation gives a larger gap.

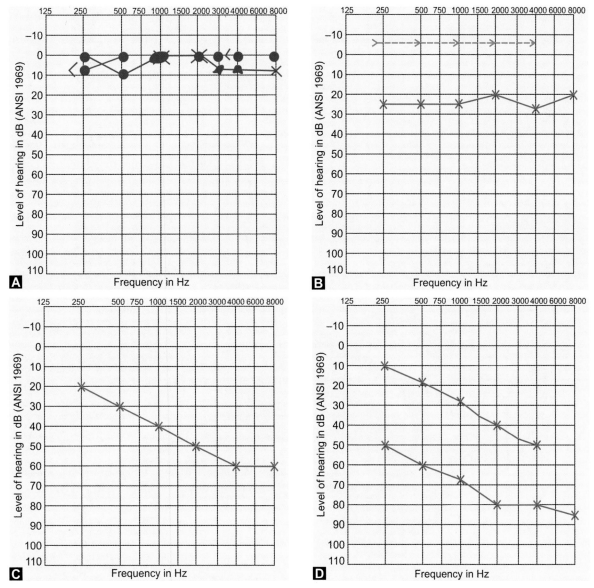

Figures 2A to D Audiograms: (A) Normal audiogram; (B) Conductive hearing loss; (C) Sensorineural hearing loss; (D) Mixed hearing loss

In sensorineural losses, the thresholds of both curves are increased and the curves (air and bone) are superimposed (Figure 2C). If one ear has a profound sensorineural hearing loss and a tone of 50 dB is applied to it, which is intense enough to be carried by bone conduction to the other ear giving a false audiogram. This curve that is obtained is termed as a shadow curve. Therefore, it is necessary to use sound in the other ear to 'mask' this effect, when the ear that is being tested has a threshold of 40 dB or more. It is important to use the 'masking' noise adequately (both the type of noise and its intensity) in order to fulfill the purpose and prevent this sound in turn from reaching the tested ear (over the 'masking' sound) and give false results in the tested ear. When there is an air-bone gap also, 'masking' should be used.

In mixed losses, the thresholds of both curves are increased but air conduction thresholds are higher than those of the bone (Figure 2D).

Degrees and Percentages of Hearing Loss

There are two questions that keep coming up:
1. What is my percentage of hearing loss?
2. Is my hearing loss severe or profound?

The percentage of hearing loss is obtained by averaging pure tone responses according to a mathematical formula. It is used for calculation of percentages for compensation because of acquired hearing loss. The formula does not represent real (clinical) percentages of hearing losses (Table 1).

Table 1 Division of hearing loss

-5-20 dB	Normal hearing
20-40 dB	Mild hearing loss
40-70 dB	Moderate hearing loss
70-90 dB	Severe hearing loss
90 dB and more	Profound hearing loss

Special Evaluations

High Frequency Audiometry

For this test, the frequencies tested are 8000 Hz and above, until 12000 to 16000 Hz. It is useful for early detection of hearing loss in patients treated with ototoxins, however, currently otoacoustic emissions are commonly used (to be described).

Special and Suprathreshold Tests

Pure tone audiometry evaluates hearing thresholds. Speech audiometry evaluates hearing and understanding of speech. Special tests evaluate what is heard by the patient and help to localize the site of lesions. As mentioned earlier, frequency gives the sensation of pitch and intensity, and the sensation of loudness. Distortion in the sensation of pitch is termed as diplacusis and in the sensation of loudness is termed as recruitment. Recruitment occurs when the intensity of sound in the diseased ear is perceived louder than it should be in relation to the threshold of hearing. If the intensity is perceived softer than it should be, it is termed reverse recruitment.

Alternate binaural loudness balance: Both the ears are tested by increasing the intensity of the tones comparing both ears in terms of sensation of loudness. In patients with problems within the cochlea, an uncomfortable loudness is reached quite early due to an abnormally rapid growth of loudness. This is called abnormal loudness recruitment. Another test that is used to evaluate cochlear losses is the short increment sensitivity index test.

Tone decay: In this test, a pure tone is given at 5 dB above the threshold. So, we know that the patient hears it and the tone is maintained. The patient must be able to hear it for 60 seconds. If this does not occur, the intensity is increased by 5 dB, step-by-step. When 30 dB SL or more is required to hear the tone for 60 seconds this is an indication of a positive tone decay, suggestive of a retrocochlear lesion (for example, an acoustic nerve tumor). Tests that are conducted above the threshold level (such as word recognition and special tests) are also termed suprathreshold tests.

There are also special tests that can measure tinnitus by determining the tone that is most similar as well as the intensity and the capability of having residual inhibition (capacity to mask the tinnitus).

Play Audiometry and Visual Reinforcement Audiometry

Visual reinforcement audiometry is a technique used for children between the ages of six months and two years. Turning the head toward a sound is conditioned by visually reinforcing the response with the appearance of a lighted toy, such as a bunny that plays a drum.

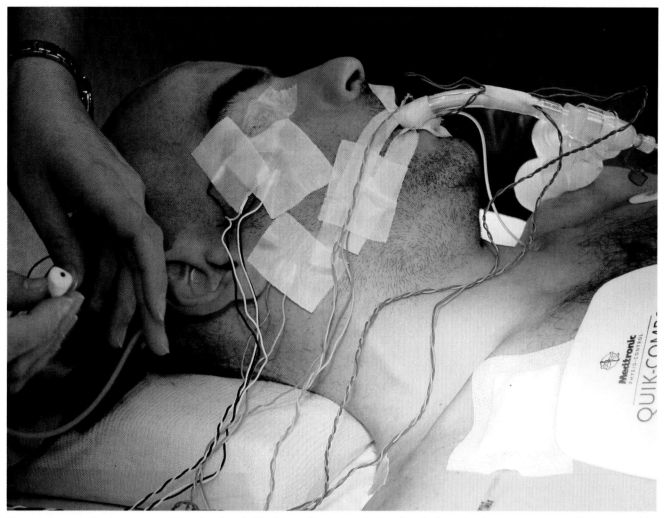

Figure 1 Electrodes for electromyographic registration of orbicularis oculi and oris are in place. Ear olive for registration of acoustic nerve is in the hands of the examiner

I must warn the you that the acoustic nerve is extremely sensitive and the waves can be altered by traction, temperature and even vibration of an adjacent tumor caused by an ultrasonic suction. Therefore, we must be alert and in a multimodal and simultaneous fashion we must look out for the facial and acoustic nerves giving pauses or rests if there are alterations in order to decrease the risk of lesions.

I also suggest—especially, in larger tumors or tumors that descend in the cerebellopontine angle—to monitor the adjacent nerves with needles. In the trapezius muscle for the XI cranial

nerve or accessory, in the masseter, for localization of the motor component of V cranial nerve (trigeminal). Recording needles in the orotracheal tube will allow us to localize cranial nerves IX and X (glossopharyngeal and vagus nerves). Last, needles in the ipsilateral "hemitongue" orient about the hypoglossal or XII cranial nerve (Figure 3).

Not all the facial discharges are ominous. Some only tell us that we are close, without harm and this is also useful. The ones that are described as dangerous and are associated with postoperative deficits are the sequential prolonged discharges

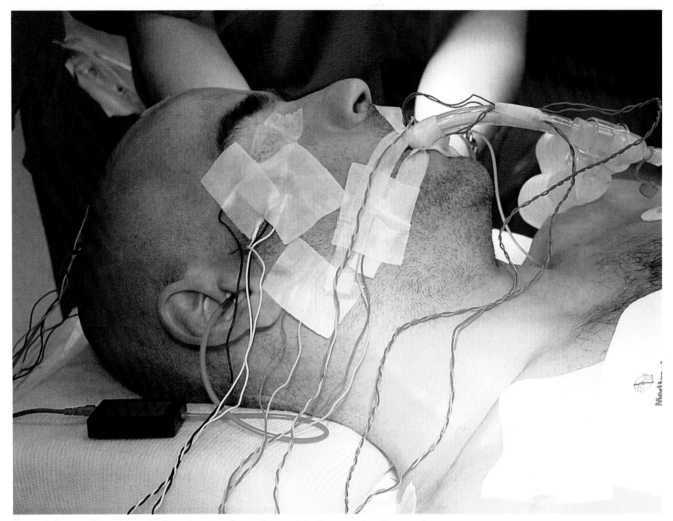

Figure 2 Same as Figure 1 but olive for registration of acoustic nerve is in the external auditory canal

that have a tail in which the electromyographic activity remains after the surgical manipulation has ended. This is also the case for discharges that repeat themselves again and again. There are reports that describe that intraoperatively discharges of more than 10 continuous seconds have more risk of having postoperative harm.

The suggested anesthetic agents are balanced halogenated agents or intravenous with the use of short acting muscle relaxants only at the beginning of the procedure.

PITFALLS

The main causes of failure are failures in communication. If the anesthesiologist administers muscle relaxants, monitoring is impaired until such effects cease. Hypotension and hypothermia can also alter the recordings.

Communication and mutual understanding with the surgeon are crucial. Some surgeons are perturbed by alarms and become tense with them. On the other hand, the neurophysiologist cannot be insecure in moments in which he must tell the surgeon to stop. For this to work, the neurophysiologist must have authority and most of all, credibility, and for that, experience and "flying hours" are essential. Just like in surgical teams, it is important for a young specialist to acquire proper practice working at the side of an experienced neurophysiologist.

Other causes of error are technical difficulties. It is useful to have a system that measures impedance of recording electrodes in the facial musculature, because this will allow the surgeons to know if one of them is loose and needs to be repositioned. In the same manner, in order to check that the stimulator is working properly, the surgeon should test it over a muscular tissue exposed in the surgical field and visualize its

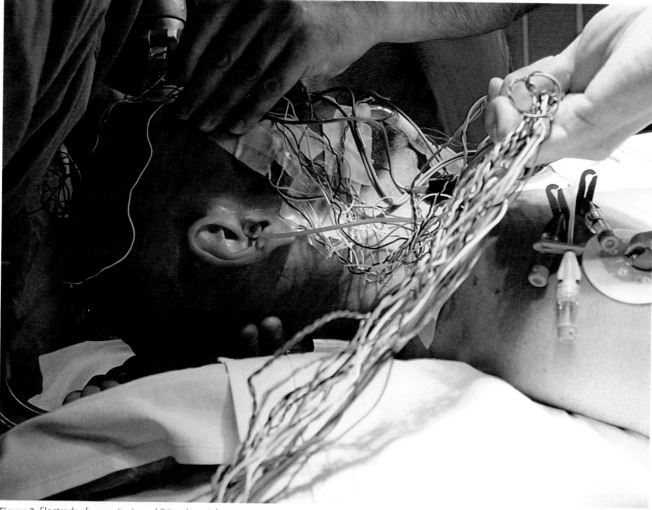

Figure 3 Electrodes for monitoring additional cranial nerves

contraction, thus, confirming that the function is adequate. This is harder to do in the case of auditory stimulation. The olives that are placed in the external ear canal can become displaced. If they are not stable they can be fixed with a fine suture. Giving small taps to the facial electrodes can help to test this system.

COMPLICATIONS

From a safety standpoint; there are no risks to the patient if things are done the right way. This is especially true for facial nerve monitoring. In past years there was concern about neuro-endocrinological effects in children, however, in the last 20 years no adverse effect of this type or others have been described.

One important aspect is that the system always has to have a ground. There are reports in the literature about burns related to the lack of ground.

When the parameters of the facial nerve stimulator are to be established, I suggest determining a superior limit of stimulation of 10 milliamperes. In this manner, it is impossible to stimulate with too much intensity by error and to cause neural damage by direct stimulation.

In practical terms, the most common complication is losing one of the facial recording electrodes. This can be avoided by fixing them adequately, as is described in methods, and to keep the surgeon informed of what is going on in case an electrode has to be reinstalled. As mentioned earlier, it is best not to have monitoring if monitoring is not going to be reliable.

CONCLUSION

The advent of intraoperative monitoring has allowed us to recognize the anatomical structures in a safe and trustworthy

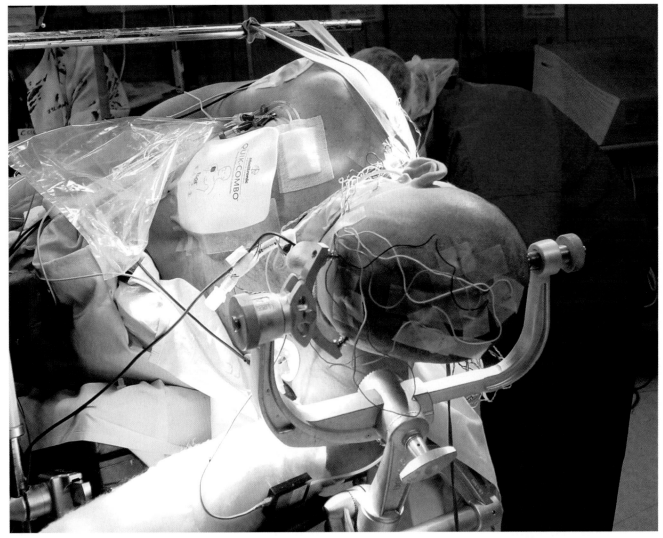

Figure 4 Patient with monitoring electrodes in place and in position for the surgical procedure

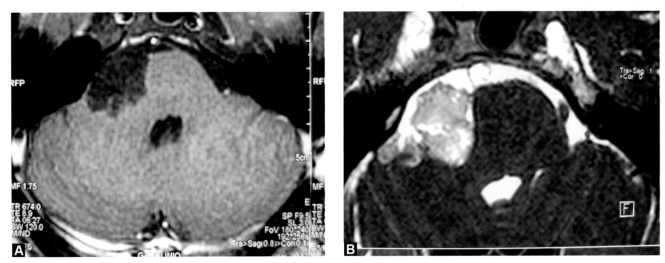

Figures 5A and B Magnetic resonance images showing cerebellopontine angle tumors; the most common lesions requiring surgical monitoring during their removal

and the dissection is started from this point (beware of the tensor tympani area, where the facial nerve is dehiscent in 11.6% of temporal bones). The chorda tympani can also serve as a guide to follow. Whatever is the choice, thickened tissue should not be removed blindly.

Exposure of the Middle Ear

The middle ear is visualized and the mucosa as well as the different anatomical structures are identified before any planned procedure is begun (Figure 3C). Methodical evaluation of the cavity is a good practice. This includes evaluation of ossicular mobility, which is done by mobilizing the long process of the malleus with a drumhead elevator or joint knife (Figure 3D) followed by palpation of the incus and stapes (Figure 3E). Testing the mobility of the stapes includes the footplate, not the head alone. If more complete exposure of the oval window is needed, the posterior canal wall should be curetted. The tip of the curet should always be in view. A sharp curet that is as large as possible should be utilized. An angled curet is used to remove the bone of the posterior canal, including the area of the scutum. In general, it is better to curette from 12 o'clock to 6 o'clock position in order to avoid accidental dislocation of the ossicles. The curet should not be used in a perpendicular fashion. Special time should be dedicated to completely remove bone fragments, which if left in the middle ear stimulate localized tissue reaction and make the cavity prone to infection. Again, for good visualization it is important to position the patient appropriately with the surgeon and microscope in the correct position as well.

Closure

Upon completion of middle ear work (procedures are described in later chapters), the flaps are repositioned. At the same time, they are carefully cleansed, freed of debris with thin suction tips, a joint knife or both, and examined for tears. The tympanic membrane is also examined for small punctures or lacerations; if any are present, their edges are closely approximated and small pieces of Gelfoam® are used to cover them. The paramount consideration, requiring great care, is the anatomic position. The fact that flaps shrink initially must be taken into account.

Revisions

Ideally, previous reports should be available, but only as a general reference of what was done. Revisions should be approached as a "box of surprises" from beginning to end. The main points to keep in mind are that flaps are quite thin

and tear easily and the bony defects of the ear canal are to be expected. Careful incisions and elevation are used. Adhesions are common and should be sectioned carefully and sharply in order to avoid tears. Repositioning of the flaps should be carefully done and anatomically adequate; adequate packing is of the utmost importance as well.

Packing

Alternatives to packing exist, depending upon the particular case and the surgeon's preference. They are all satisfactory and will work if done correctly. Different materials can be utilized; if used properly, most of them suffice. Excessive pressure must be avoided. Antibiotic or steroid ointments or solutions, or both, are useful in preventing localized inflammation and infection. Only the most common packing techniques will be mentioned.

1. A basket is fashioned from surgical rayon or Owen's silk strips moistened with antibiotic or steroid ointment. Cotton soaked in antibiotic solution fills the space and the silk is used as a rosebud packing. A 1/2 inch gauze pack with antibiotic ointment is placed in the lateral third of the canal (Figures 4A to C). This type of packing provides adequate pressure to keep the flaps flat, but not enough to damage them. It should be removed at intervals of 1 week for the gauze and 2 weeks for the rosebud; if left for a longer period, granulation tissue invades the silk making it difficult, if not impossible, to remove it by simply pulling.

2. The canal is filled with Gelfoam® soaked in antibiotic solution. It is placed initially in layers with Gelfoam® strips covering all areas of incision. The lateral aspect of the canal can be filled with ointment or a piece of sterile cotton can be placed (Figure 4D). The disadvantage of this method is that it takes a long time for the Gelfoam® to come out spontaneously. Thus, removal must be done very carefully in order to avoid flap disruption. Gelfoam® promotes granulation. This type of packing may require the use of otic drops or ointments.

3. The canal is filled with an antibiotic ointment as the sole packing and a piece of cotton is placed in the meatus (Figure 4E). This method of packing requires perfect approximation of the intact flaps.

4. The incisions are completely covered with compressed, dry Gelfoam® strips and a flat, round piece of Gelfoam® is placed over the tympanic membrane. In order to do this, the Gelfoam® is compressed with the press that is used for the fascia in cases of tympanoplasty and the round pieces are obtained by using a paper punch (US $ 1.5 dollars) that can be bought in any office store.

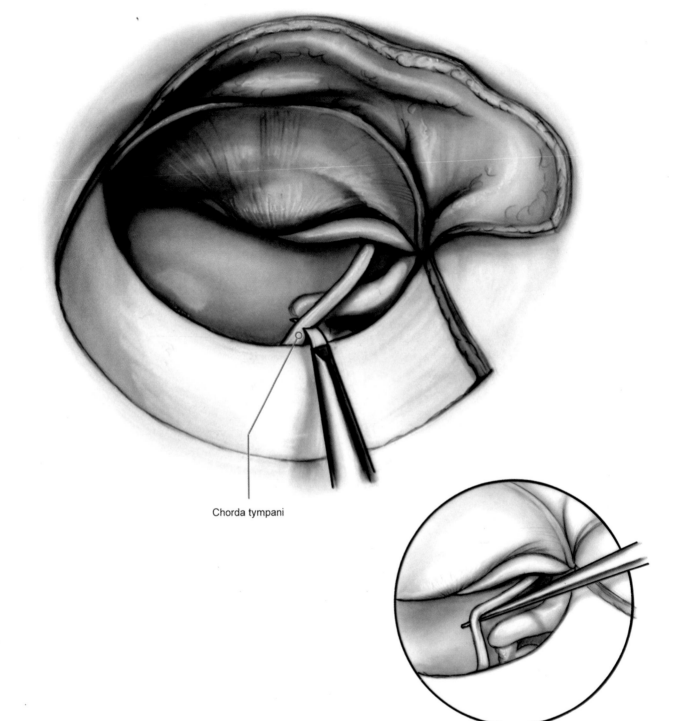

Chorda tympani

Figure 3A

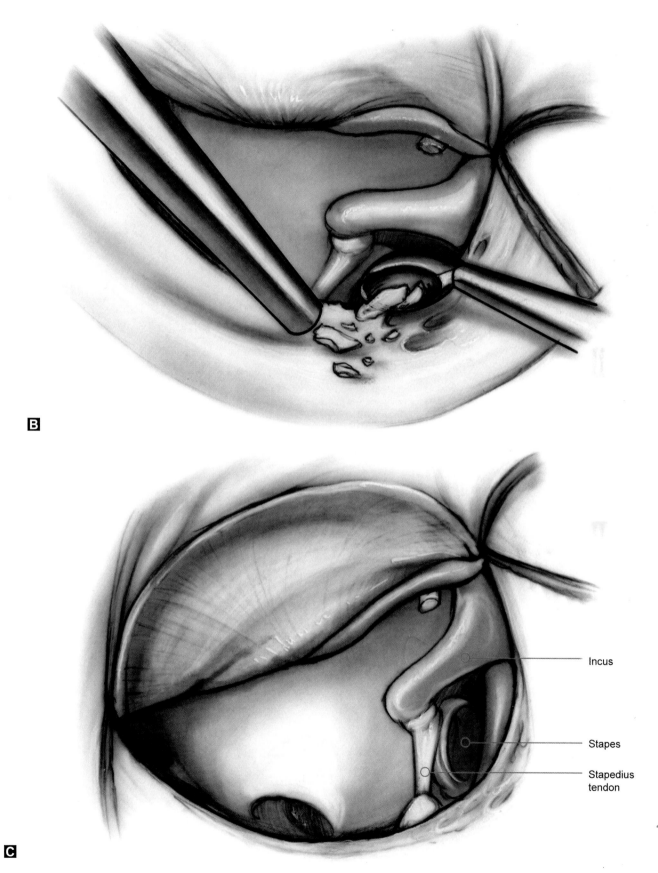

B

C

Incus

Stapes

Stapedius
tendon

Figures 3B and C

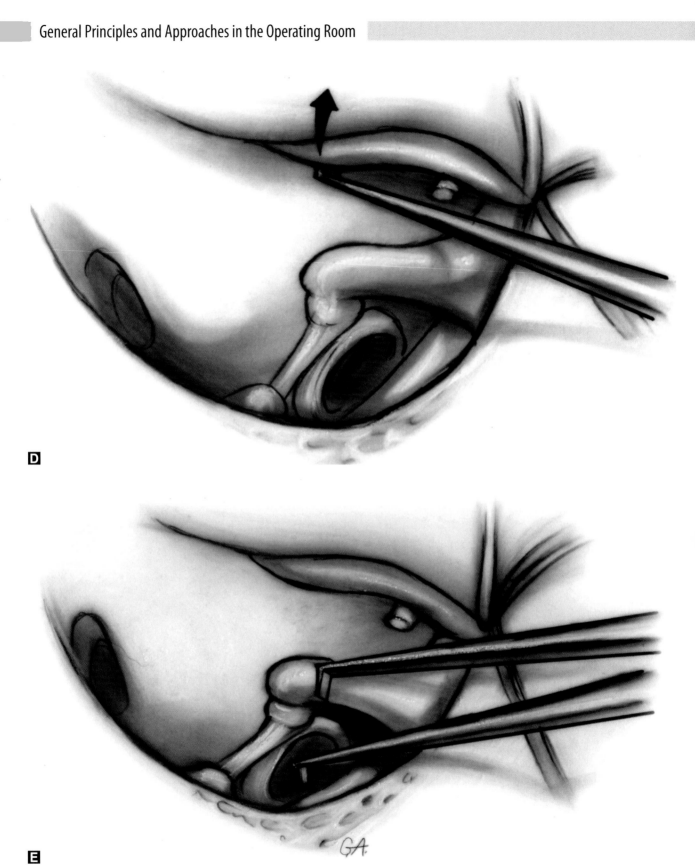

Figures 3D and E

Figures 3A to E (A and B) Moving chorda tympani out of the field of vision; (C) Visualizing the middle ear and the mucosa as well as different anatomical structures; (D) Methodical evaluation of ossicular mobility by mobilizing the long process of the malleus with a drumhead elevator or joint knife; (E) This is followed by palpation of the incus and stapes

between the tragus and helix (at the incisura) and immediately anterior to the helix (Figure 6A). The endaural approach avoids the use of an ear speculum and provides a direct view of the middle ear.

Incisions

For purposes of exposure, it is best to use a curved nasal speculum. Incisions are made with a scalpel. The first incision (Lempert I) is made semicircumferentially between 6 o'clock and 12 o'clock position on the posterior wall at the bony cartilaginous junction (Figure 6B). This incision must extend down to the bone. The second incision (Lempert II) runs between the tragus and helix and incisura; care must be taken not to expose or cut the helix. The extension of this incision depends upon the degree of exposure needed, varying from a few millimeters (for an exploratory tympanotomy) to a full 3/4 cm (for a mastoidectomy). This incision is made in the ear. Caution must be exercised not to deepen it immediately after going through the subcutaneous tissue, since branches of the superficial temporal artery and vein are present in this area; too deep a cut may also section the temporal fascia, which might be needed for grafting purposes. It is important to completely section the connective tissue and to expose the bony canal at the level of the incisura, allowing more space. Small bleeding vessels are cauterized. The remaining posterior canal skin (cartilaginous portion) is preserved and gently elevated with a small periosteal elevator, leaving the whole posterior bony canal clearly exposed

(Figure 6C). On occasions, a small free skin graft can be taken safely from this area. Two two-prong retractors (two) are used for exposure. It is useful to position them at right angles to each other, one pointing cephalad (superiorly) and the other pointing caudad (posteriorly); this provides better exposure and stability, and is less inconvenient for the surgeon. Temporal fascia is harvested at this point (discussed in a different section) and all bleeding vessels are controlled. With the scalpel, incisions can be made at 6 o'clock and 1 o'clock or 2 o'clock position (Figure 6D). These incisions allow for easier development of the flap; however, the flap can be elevated without the incisions. The flap is elevated in the same manner as in a transcanal incision. The same principles and technique also apply for a canalplasty.

Closure

The flap is repositioned anatomically; particular attention is paid to repositioning the skin, which must cover the cartilaginous canal. Subcutaneous tissues are approximated with interrupted absorbable sutures (for example, 3-0 chromic catgut). Approximation does not need to be very tight at the incisura. Skin is approximated with absorbable 4-0 sutures or 4-0 silk or nylon sutures. The first skin suture should be at the incisura; as in other ear incisions, there is remarkably good healing in this area. Packing is done as in transcanal procedures for the bony canal; however, it is best to use 1/2 inch gauze impregnated with antibiotic or steroid ointment in the lateral third (cartilaginous canal), followed by a mastoid

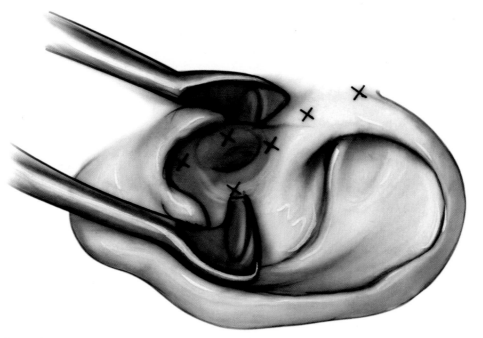

Figure 6A

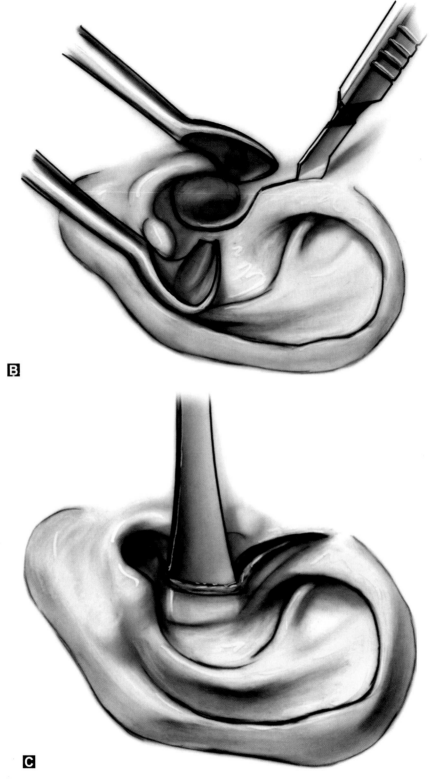

Figures 6B and C

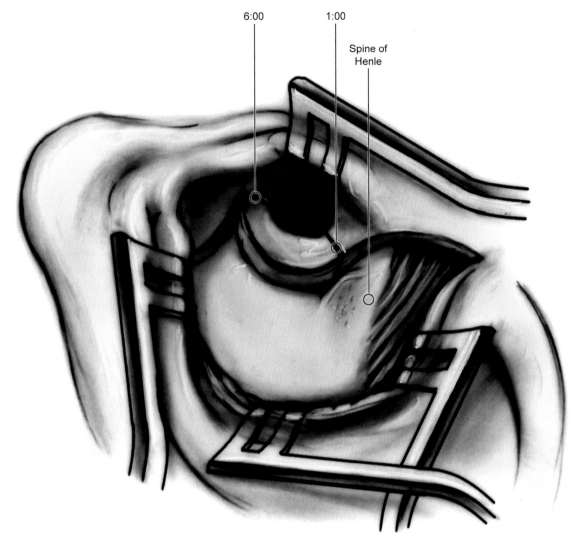

Figure 6D

Figures 6A to D Endaural approach. (A) Additional injections are made between the tragus and helix (at the incisura) and immediately anterior to the helix; (B) The first incision (Lempert I) is made semicircumferentially between 6 o'clock and 12 o'clock position on the posterior wall at the bony cartilaginous junction; (C) The remaining posterior canal skin (cartilaginous portion) is preserved and gently elevated with a small periosteal elevator, leaving the whole posterior bony canal clearly exposed; (D) With the scalpel, incisions can be made at 6 o'clock and 1 o'clock or 2 o'clock position

dressing. The gauze and the skin sutures are removed one week after the procedure. At this time, the authors usually fill the space with antibiotic ointment for one additional week.

POSTAURICULAR APPROACH

Highlights

- Same as for transcanal and endaural approaches
- The postauricular incision should be made plane-by-plane

- The canal should be reached in the "avascular" plane
- Cleansing of all debris should be done carefully.

Pitfalls

- Tearing of the canal with three-prong retractors
- Inadequate cleansing of debris leads to wound infection.

The postauricular approach can be used for an exploratory tympanotomy, a tympanoplasty and a mastoidectomy. It provides a good view of the anterior rim of the annulus, unless there is a prominent bony overhang or a "tight" canal;

however, it is useful for dealing with these two problems as well.

Positioning, inspecting, and cleansing are done in transcanal and endaural procedures; however, shaving of some hair might be needed. Injection of a local anesthetic is similar to the transcanal procedure, as far as the canal is concerned; however, a postauricular injection is necessary in the whole area where the incision is to be made, as well as in the posterior aspect of the canal from behind. It is useful to lift the auricle, pull it forward and inject posteriorly, while feeling the tip of the needle and the flow of anesthetic and vasoconstrictors with the index finger placed in the meatus of the canal. This maneuver ensures adequate injection.

Incisions

The classic incision is made 3/4 cm behind the posterior sulcus, with the inferior end deviating posteriorly (see Figure 1A). In children, the incision is high and posterior with the inferior limb far posterior, since the facial nerve can be very superficial in its exit at the stylomastoid foramen (because of lack of development of the mastoid tip) (see Figure 1B). For cosmetic purposes, the incision can be made in the crease itself, but the cosmetic advantage is relative; this location lends itself to minor healing problems, small epidermal cysts and so on. An additional incision that can be made is the posterosuperior (Portmann) (see Figure 1C), which is a compromise between the posterior incision and the anterosuperior (Hermann) incision. In spite of its good exposure, the latter is not used because it may lead to necrosis of the helix. The posterosuperior incision provides excellent exposure.

Procedure

The incision is made with a scalpel and deepened perpendicularly through subcutaneous tissues without advancing too far. The purpose is to reach the musculoaponeurotic or "avascular" plane. Cautery can be used for bleeding vessels; however, even if it takes a little longer it is preferable to use bipolar cautery. Healing is definitely better than with monopolar cautery. If the planes are developed carefully, large branches of the posterior auricular artery usually will not be sectioned. If this does occur, it is best to tie them with a nonabsorbable suture. Many surgeons use cutting cautery in the skin, which is effective in terms of surgical time and dryness of the field. However, this must be weighed against the disadvantage of skin healing secondary to a cutting cautery burn.

If the right plane is reached, the auricle is pulled anteriorly (forward) and the cartilaginous canal is identified, as well as the spine of Henle (at this point the temporal fascia can be harvested). Once this is done, the connective tissue plane behind the cartilaginous canal can be developed sharply and safely. All bleeding vessels, if there are any, should be controlled. Elevating the plane toward the zygomatic root, gains room to mobilize the auricle forward (anteriorly) easily (Figure 7A). A circumferential incision is made at the bony cartilaginous junction posteriorly, as in the endaural procedure (here exploratory approaches alone are discussed; other types of flaps for other purposes, for example, Korner's will be dealt later). A piece of twill tape passed gently through the incision ensures that the skin of the meatus posteriorly is not torn when using a retractor, and at the same time serves to keep this flap out of the field of vision (Figure 7B). With the use of a three-prong Wullstein retractor, the auricle (pinna) is gently pulled anteriorly with the posterior cartilaginous canal, protected by the twill tape (Figure 7C). Care must be taken not to tear the skin and cartilage. If a Wullstein retractor is not large enough, a modified Schuknecht three-prong retractor is used (This is usually necessary in a mastoidectomy but uncommon in exploratory procedures).

From this point on, the same procedure is followed as in endaural or transcanal incisions. Closure is preceded by careful removal of debris. The packing of the bony canal is similar to that in other approaches; the lateral aspect of the canal (cartilaginous) is packed as in the endaural approach. Postauricular closure is done with interrupted absorbable sutures for subcutaneous tissues (for example, 3-0 chromic catgut). This layer should be approximated carefully; otherwise, the pinna may lack adequate subcutaneous support and show a tendency to project anteriorly. Skin is approximated with interrupted, nonabsorbable silk or nylon suture. Some surgeons close the skin with 4-0 catgut sutures; although this method may be adequate, the authors do not use it. Instead, and especially in children we use a "subdermal" absorbable running suture with opsite R coverage (collodion spray) and steristrips. A mastoid dressing is applied. Removal of sutures and packing is done as in the endaural approach.

SIMPLE MASTOIDECTOMY AS A SURGICAL APPROACH

A simple mastoidectomy is described here as a general surgical approach for different procedures. It is discussed as a specific procedure in other sections of the atlas.

Aim

Exenteration (removal) of all mastoid air cells while maintaining the integrity of the posterior canal.

Highlights

- Skin incision is performed with the scalpel perpendicular to the skin.
- Incision should be deepened in layers
- Careful elevation of intact periosteum should be done
- Retractors must be adequately positioned
- Complete exposure of landmarks is important
- Carefully close in layers.

Pitfalls

- Tearing of the skin of the posterior ear canal
- Inadequate exposure
- Injuring a high sigmoid sinus
- Injuring the facial nerve by going:
  - Deep to the horizontal semicircular canal
  - Too far anterior in the digastric ridge
- Dislocating the incus by drilling blindly into the antrum area
- Exposing the dura mater
- Drilling the semicircular canals.

Positioning, patient preparation and draping, and injection have already been discussed. As described in previous sections, a classic postauricular incision will be used, starting at the level of the linea temporalis and following the contour of the external meatus to turn posteroinferiorly at the level of the mastoid tip.

Incision and Exposure

Before initiating postauricular work, it is a good idea to place a piece of sterile cotton in the canal in order to avoid accumulation of debris and bone dust.

The incision is made in layers with a scalpel held perpendicularly to the skin. Subcutaneous vessels are cauterized. A plane between the musculoaponeurotic layer and connective tissue is reached by sharp dissection and developed. It is possible in this plane to avoid damaging branches of the posterior auricular artery; if damage does occur, it is better to ligate than to cauterize them.

The periosteum is identified and sectioned, following the contour of the external ear canal. Vertical incisions at 45° angles are made at 6 o'clock and 12 o'clock position (toward the linea temporalis and toward the mastoid tip) (Figure 8A). The intact periosteum is elevated carefully using periosteal elevators (Figure 8B). This is important for closure, since re-establishing the periosteum in position will avoid a marked postauricular depression. As soon as the periosteum is elevated, the landmarks become apparent. It is useful to expose the root of the zygoma; this provides better mobility when positioning the retractors. Two three-prong retractors are positioned at right angles to one another (Figure 8C).

Specific surgical steps are described in surgical procedures under the section on Temporal bone dissection. The discussion here will focus on closure and treatment of intraoperative complications.

Closure

Careful washing and thorough removal of all debris and bone dust are of the utmost importance in order to prevent postoperative inflammation and infection. The retractors are removed and the periosteal flap is repositioned and secured to the posterior canal by nonabsorbable sutures. If the flap is intact and the approximation is adequate, marked postauricular depression will be avoided. Subcutaneous tissues are approximated with layers of interrupted absorbable sutures (for example, 3-0 or 2-0 chromic catgut) and skin with interrupted nonabsorbable sutures (for example, 4-0 silk or nylon), making sure that the skin and subcutaneous sutures do not overlap. A mastoid dressing is then applied.

Intraoperative Complications or Problems

- Facial nerve trauma
- Exposure of the dura mater
- Drilling of the semicircular canals
- Damage to the sigmoid sinus
- Dislocation of the incus.

Facial Nerve Trauma

Inadvertent exposure of the facial nerve sheath does not necessarily imply injury to the nerve and requires no treatment. However, if the nerve itself is injured in its course through the Fallopian canal, it should be opened for several millimeters to ensure continuity. The nerve sheath should not be opened unless discontinuity of nerve fibers is suspected. Opening of the sheath might allow ingrowth of fibrous tissue, which can compromise nerve regeneration. If discontinuity of fibers exists, they should be apposed cleanly to each other. If the injury is

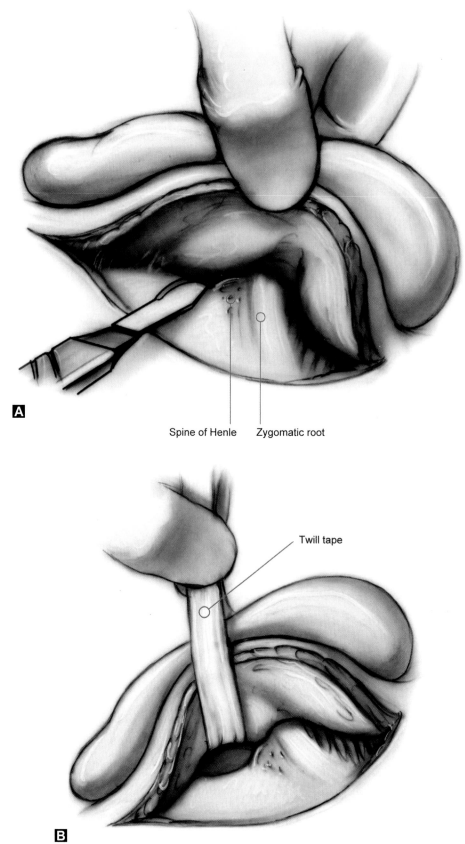

Spine of Henle   Zygomatic root

Twill tape

Figures 7A and B

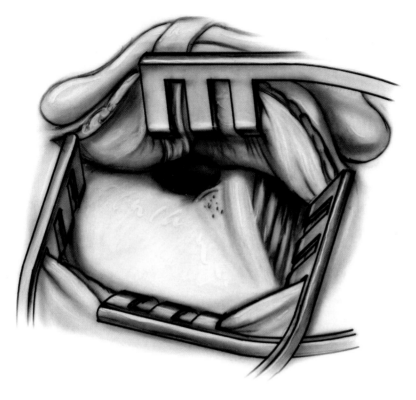

Figure 7C

Figures 7A to C Postauricular approach. (A) Elevating the plane toward the zygomatic root to mobilize the auricle forward (anteriorly); (B) A piece of twill tape is passed gently through the incision ensures that the skin of the meatus posteriorly is not torn when using a retractor, and at the same time serves to keep this flap out of the field of vision; (C) With the use of a three-prong Wullstein retractor, the auricle (pinna) is gently pulled anteriorly with the posterior cartilaginous canal, protected by the twill tape

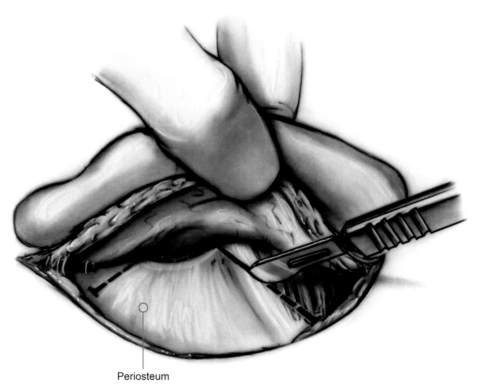

Periosteum

Figure 8A

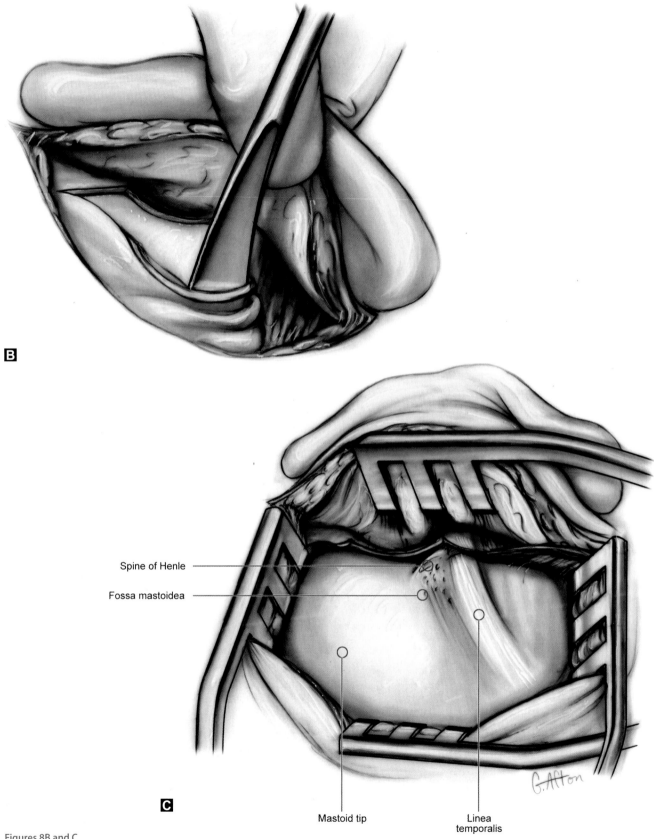

Figures 8B and C

Figures 8A to C Simple mastoidectomy. (A) The periosteum is identified and sectioned. Vertical incisions at 45° angles are made at 6 o'clock and 12 o'clock position; (B) The intact periosteum is elevated carefully using periosteal elevators; (C) Exposing the root of zygoma, two three-prong retractors are shown positioned at right angles to one another

to provide adequate skin coverage for the newly created surface area. It is crucial to remember that the meatus also comprises cartilage and bone; that the flap is an important part, but only a part, of the meatoplasty. Despite a flap that is beautifully designed "on paper," an inadequate meatoplasty may result because of lack of attention to the underlying subcutaneous tissues, cartilage or bony meatus.

Meatoplasty in Closed-Cavity Tympanomastoidectomy

An endaural Lempert I incision is made at a level approximately 7 mm below the mastoid cortex level. A Lempert II incision is made that is large enough to admit the surgeon's forefinger freely. The bony canal, especially the posterior bony canal, is enlarged; conchal cartilage is then removed by carefully everting the conchal skin using sharp scissors or a scalpel (Figures 10A and B). Packing, suturing and postoperative care are identical to those for an open-cavity tympanomastoidectomy.

Management of Pitfalls and Complications

A torn skin flap or a flap with poor vascularity due to a thin base may not survive; however, a thin flap may behave for all practical purposes as a skin graft. Lack of flap survival necessitates surgical debridement and a Thiersch graft. Excessive bleeding may lead to infection or appearance of granulation tissue, or both; if bleeding occurs underneath the flap, the flap may become medially displaced. An "organized clot" often leads to fibrosis, calling for careful elevation of the flap, meticulous hemostasis, debridement, and tight packing. Fibrosis can also occur when using a tight packing, but there will be no secondary problems, provided that the packing is removed at the proper time (no longer than 2 weeks afterward). Management of open areas with granulation tissue has already been described. On occasions, especially when an infected mastoid has been dealt with, a perichondritis might occur, characterized by edema, induration and pain over the entire pinna. In early stages, the possibility of allergy to the antibiotic ointment or solution must be considered. These signs (misnamed "cellulitis") require change of antibiotic solution, systemic antibiotics, daily (at least twice) soaks with Burow's solution or any astringent solution, and application of packing saturated with antibiotic steroid solution. If the symptoms progress (which they rarely do) debridement, drainage and placement of drains may be needed. Cultures should be obtained, if possible.

If general principles including adequate follow-up, are not observed, meatal stenosis requiring a revision may occur. The meatal skin is carefully elevated, the underlying bone (which usually displays new bone formation, bony spicules, ridges and so on) is widely drilled or curetted, and a large meatus is developed. Remember that for practical purposes a meatus cannot be made too large or too small.

THIERSCH GRAFT

Granulation tissue may develop in the mastoid cavity after canal wall down mastoidectomy. Drainage may persist from granulation tissue until the entire mastoid cavity is epithelialized. A Thiersch graft is a thin skin graft that helps to epithelialize and eliminate drainage from the mastoid cavity.

Aim

Placing a thin skin graft in the mastoid cavity, in order to achieve complete epithelialization.

Highlights

- Remove infected granulation tissue
- Harvest thin skin from the upper medial arm
- Cut the skin into proper sizes on Owen's silk
- Cover the entire nonepithelialized mastoid cavity surface with the skin graft.

Pitfalls

- Inadequately removing infected granulation tissue
- Harvesting too thick skin.

Operative Procedure

The procedure is usually carried out under local anesthesia. Local injection of 1% lidocaine with 1:100,000 epinephrine combined with topical application of 4% cocaine solution soaked in 1/2 inch gauze strip provides adequate anesthesia.

Debridement of Granulation Tissue from Mastoid Cavity

The mastoid cavity is irrigated with warm saline to remove any debris or mucopus. Using cupped forceps, ring curets and suction tips, all infected granulation tissue and necrotic tissue is removed; any thin, clean, raw tissue over the bone is left intact (Figure 11A). Hemostasis is obtained with 1:1,000 topical epinephrine (Adrenalin) soaked in 1/2 inch gauze strip.

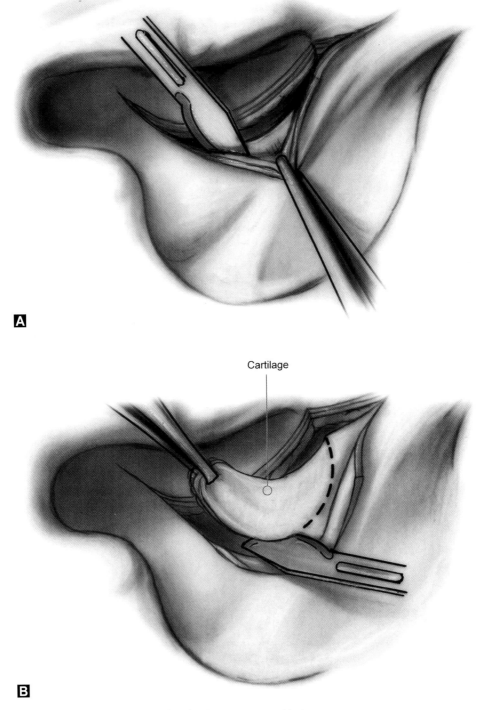

Figures 10A and B Meatoplasty in closed-cavity tympanomastoidectomy

Harvesting Thin Skin

After the mastoid cavity is cleaned out and while hemostasis is being attained, thin skin is harvested from the medial upper arm. Local anesthesia is obtained with 1% lidocaine with 1:100,000 epinephrine injection. Adequate strips of skin can be obtained using a razor blade held in a clamp (Figure 11B) or with other instruments (e.g. dermatomes). In order to obtain a thin skin graft, the razor blade is pressed down only by the weight of the instrument and a slicing motion is used. The area of the upper arm where the skin is harvested is made tight by pulling the lateral part of the arm with the surgeon's free hand. A thin coat of mineral oil over the skin helps to harvest thin pieces of skin. The area of the mastoid cavity requiring a skin graft determines the amount of skin to be harvested; the donor site is then dressed with scarlet red or Xeroform gauze dressing. The thin pieces of harvested skin are laid on a piece of Owen's silk impregnated with gentamicin sulfate (Garamycin) ointment and placed on an upside down petridish (Figure 11C). Extreme care should be taken to lay the skin on the Owen's silk with the shiny dermis side up. The skin and Owen's silk are then cut into the proper size (usually about 0.5 cm) with sharp scissors.

Skin Graft of Mastoid Cavity

The gauze strips soaked in topical epinephrine solution are removed from the mastoid cavity. The pieces of skin and Owen's silk are placed over the raw tissue in the mastoid cavity with the dermis side down (toward the bone) and the Owen's silk up (Figure 11D). The entire nonepithelialized surface of the mastoid cavity is covered carefully; slight overlap of coverage is acceptable. An eye patch dressing is then applied over the ear.

Postoperative Care

The pieces of Owen's silk are removed in two weeks. If the skin has taken well, drainage is ended and only routine care of the mastoid cavity is required.

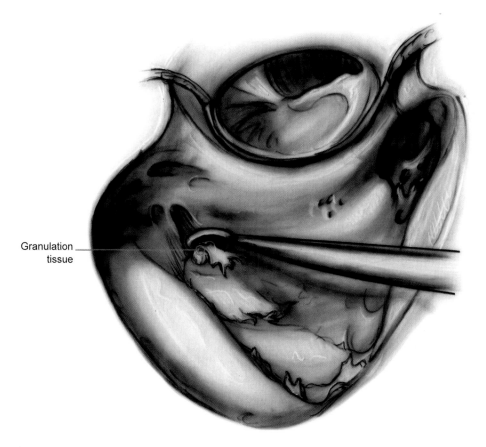

Granulation tissue

Figure 11A

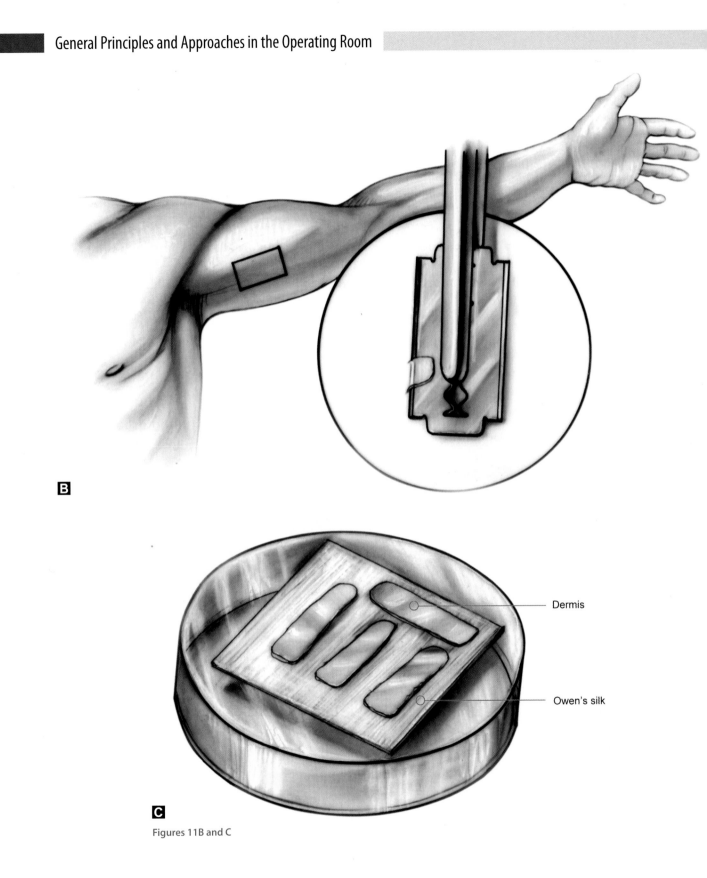

Figures 11B and C

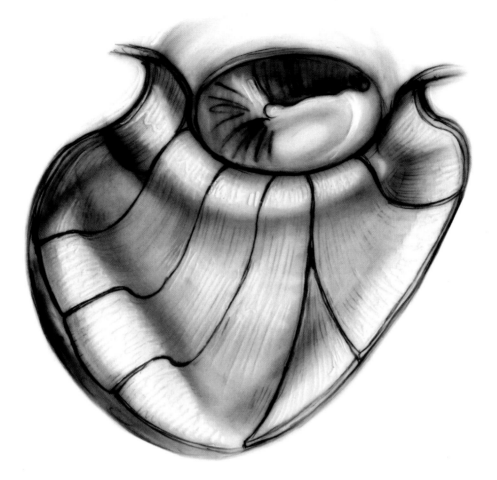

Figure 11D

Figures 11A to D (A) Debridement of granulation tissue from mastoid cavity; (B) Adequate strips of skin can be obtained using a razor blade held in a clamp; (C) The thin pieces of harvested skin is then laid on a piece of Owen's silk impregnated with gentamicin sulfate (Garamycin) ointment and placed on an upside down petridish; (D) The pieces of skin and Owen's silk are placed over the raw tissue in the mastoid cavity with the dermis side down (toward the bone) and the Owen's silk up

Section IV

Surgery of the Pinna and the External Auditory Canal

Antonio Soda Merhy, Carmen Gloria Morovic, José Javier Zepeda Rodríguez, Marcelo Hueb, Marcos Goycoolea, Mirko Tos, Peter Hilger, Raquel Levy, Timothy Jung, Viviana Orellana

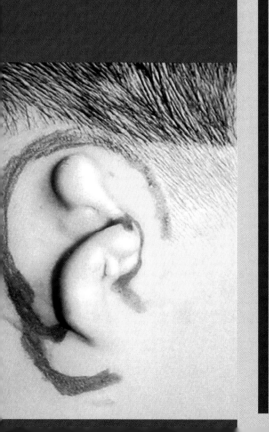

4. It is suggested that transparent nylon be used and it should not be transfixiating.
5. Before closure, abundant irrigation and suctioning is recommended.

Potential Complications and How to Manage Them

- Hematoma under tension in the antihelix—cleansing and abundant cold irrigation followed by compressive dressing
- Loss of bending because of laceration of the cartilage suture—use adequate suture and needle, thus avoiding to damage the cartilage
- Sectioning of auricular cartilage—careful tunnel dissection with adequate instruments and moderate erosion of cartilage.

Postoperative Management

Management of pain: By regional block plus oral analgesics. Elasto-Gel™ dressing is maintained for 48 hours. In the first check-up, the bandage and cotton bowl are removed from the auricular concha and the Tegaderm™ is maintained. A protective headband is used for 15 days. The patient is allowed to go back to normal exercising and sports after 1 month.

ANOMALIES BECAUSE OF ABSENCE: MICROTIA (CONCHAL OR LOBULAR)

Purpose

The anomaly because of absence or agenesia of the pinna is manifested by either absence of the upper-third [(conchal microtia) Figure 3], or by absence of the upper two-third [(lobular microtia) Figure 4], which occurs most frequently. It can be unilateral or bilateral and may or may not be associated with a syndrome.

Highlights

The surgical procedure intends to reconstruct the anomalous pinna. The aim is to construct a pinna that is similar to the normal, using existing remnants and the costal cartilage graft.

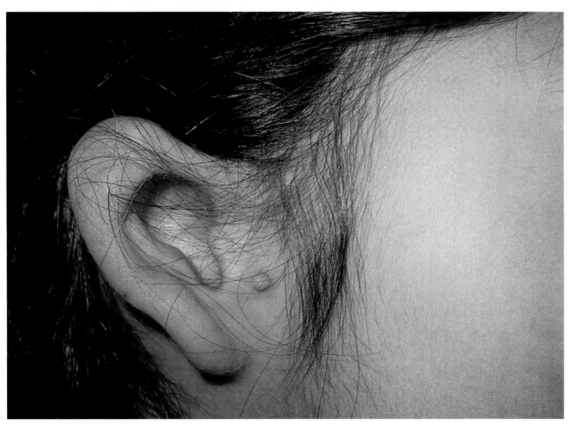

Figure 3 Conchal microtia

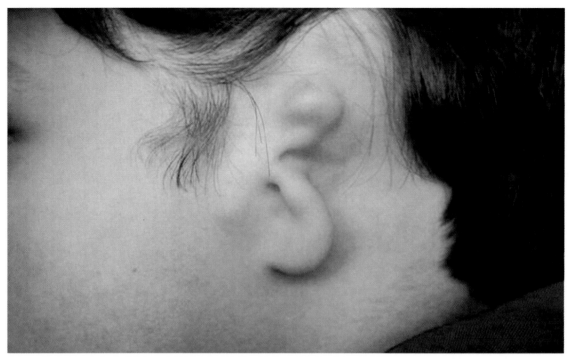

Figure 4 Lobular microtia

Surgical Steps

- Two surgical fields: pinna and costal donor site
- Infiltration of local anesthetic (bupivacaine 0.25 with epinephrine 1:100,000)
- Small incision over the rib cage exposing the cartilaginous segment and obtaining graft from C5, C6 and C7 (Figures 5A and B)
- Check hemostasis and pleural indemnity
- Closure by layers (muscle, subcutaneous tissues, skin) with 3-0 vicryl and 4-0 monocryl.

Surgical Field of the Pinna

Delineation of the absent segment to be reconstructed; considering the rotation of the remnant be it lobule or lobule and concha [(modified Nagata's technique) Figure 6].

Infiltration with local anesthetic with epinephrine.

Development of a subdermal pocket for placing the cartilage graft.

Meticulous hemostasis and placement of two drain tubes in the auricular pocket.

The cartilage (graft) is sculptured using the grafts that are brought together with wire sutures with a shape according to the healthy normal pinna (Figures 7A and B).

Placement of the sculptured pinna in the subdermal pocket and connection of the drains to a vacuum in order to accommodate the skin and closure of skin with a running 6-0 nylon suture (Figures 8A and B).

Double check the adequate functioning of the drains and vacuum; steri-strip over the sutures, moist cotton in the concha and Tegaderm™ covering the "new" pinna.

Hidden Dangers

- Loss of vacuum (less adhesion of the skin to the cartilage graft)
- Partial or total loss of vitality of the skin flap with exposure of the cartilage graft.

Practical Suggestions

1. Double check pleural indemnity.
2. Infiltration of local anesthetic with vasoconstrictor.
3. It is important to use a firm suture, such as the wire filament, in order to avoid tension in the cartilage graft, which might lead to loosening of the segments of the reconstructed pinna.
4. Make sure to place the cartilage framework in an adequate axis using other anatomical structures as reference.

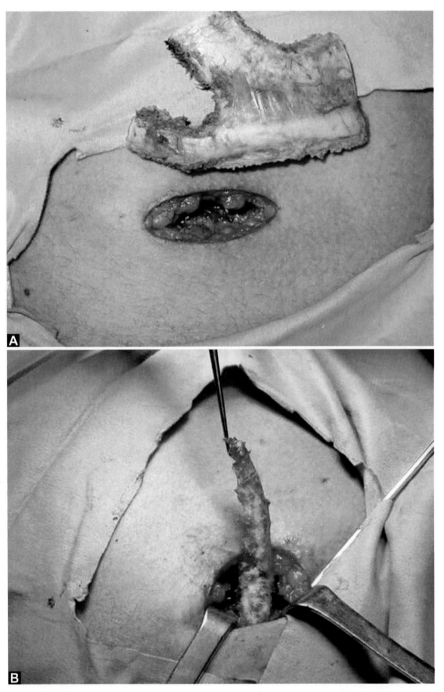

Figures 5A and B Small incision over the rib cage exposing the cartilaginous segment and obtaining graft from C5, C6 and C7

5. Make sure that the vacuum is adequate, otherwise seal the suture areas with an impermeabilizer.
6. The use of Tegaderm™ allows observing the vitality of grafts that cover the cartilage without seal loss or local manipulation.

Potential Complications and How to Avoid Them

- Hematoma of the reconstructed pinna—cleansing with abundant cold saline solution plus careful hemostasis

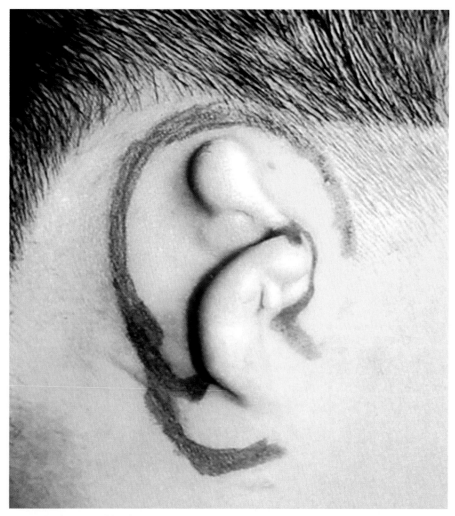

Figure 6 Delineation of the absent segment which needs to be reconstructed

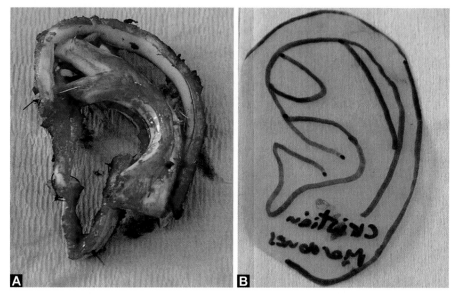

Figures 7A and B The cartilage (graft) is sculptured using the grafts that are brought together with wire sutures with a shape according to the healthy normal pinna

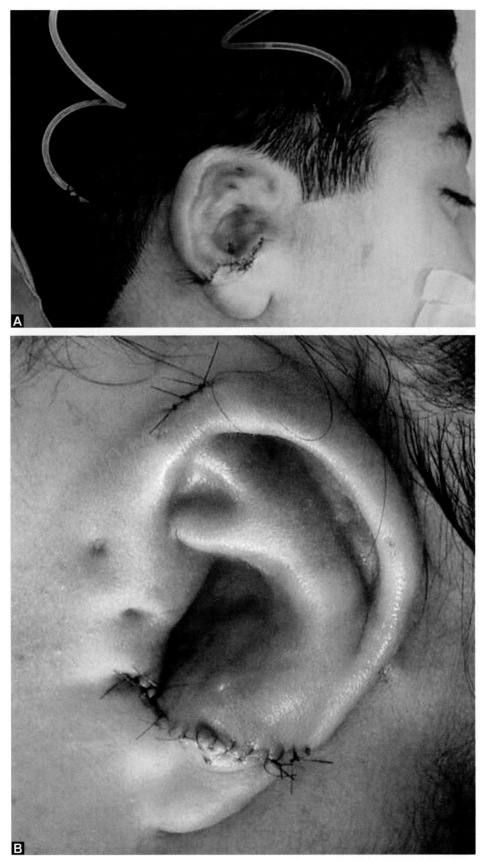

Figures 8A and B (A) Placement of the sculptured pinna in the subdermal pocket and connection of the drains to a vacuum in order to accommodate the skin; (B) Closure of skin with a running 6-0 nylon suture

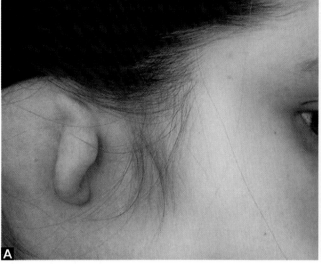
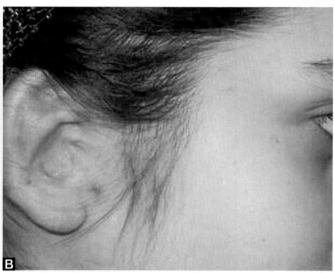

Figures 9A and B (A) Condition before treatment; (B) Postoperative result

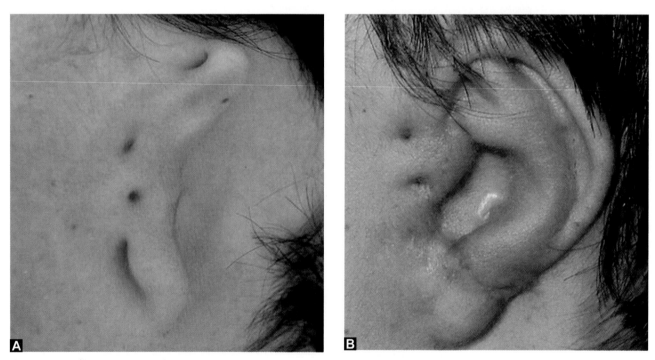

Figures 10A and B (A) Condition before treatment; (B) Postoperative result (shown in a different patient)

- Partial or total loss of skin flap—avoid large flaps and tension in flaps
- Exposure of cartilage—resection of the exposed cartilage and coverage with a vital flap.

Postoperative Management

- Appropriate analgesics that are capable of controlling pain in the donor site

- Semiseated position
- Antimicrobial prophylaxis (48 hours)
- Maintaining drains connected to a vacuum with the skin adherent to cartilage of the reconstructed pinna for 2 or 3 days
- Protection of the operated site with a cone
- Suture removal in 7–10 days
- Reinitiate usual physical activity, one month after the operation [Figures 9A and B and 10A and B].

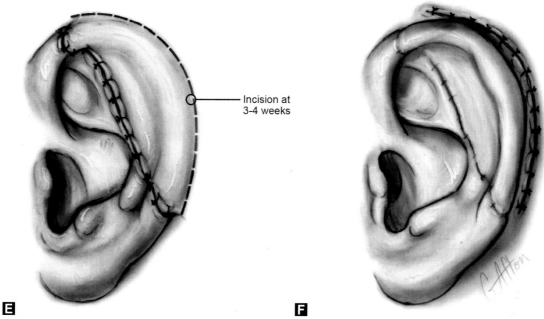

— Incision at
3-4 weeks

E

F

Figures 3E and F

Figures 3A to F Reattaching completely amputated pinna. (A and B) When microvascular repair is not available or indicated, the cartilaginous framework is salvaged by dermabrading all of the epidermis from the cartilaginous skeleton; (C) Burying the pinna in a postauricular pocket for 3–4 weeks; (D to F) The cartilaginous skeleton can then be "released" from this pocket and allowed to slowly re-epithelialize

Aim

To reconstruct the pinna after resection of a neoplasm.

Highlights

- Gentle handling of the tissues is necessary to reduce operative trauma.
- Small defects are repaired by primary closure or composite graft.
- Larger defects most often are repaired with a postauricular pedicled graft.
- The less complex the repair, the greater is the likelihood of good results.
- All margins of resection should be histologically examined.

Pitfalls

- Imprecise closure may lead to a cosmetic deformity.
- A composite graft may be lost if it is too large (greater than 1.5 cm).

- A pinna may "cup" after a wedge resection if wedges of skin and cartilage are not removed along the antihelical fold.

Instruments

The instruments listed below form the basics of a plastics tray used for most soft tissue surgeries of the head and neck. These instruments will be used for the procedures described in the rest of this chapter.

- No. 11 and No. 15 scalpel blades and handles
- Medium and fine needle holders
- 0.5 mm ophthalmic forceps
- Brown-Adson forceps
- No. 3 single or double skin hooks
- No. 2 Senn retractors
- Storz "stitch" scissors
- Curved and straight iris scissors
- Small Metzenbaum scissors
- Tenotomy scissors
- Sutures: 4-0 and 5-0 Vicryl, 4-0 and 6-0 nylon, 6-0 chromic
- Marking pen

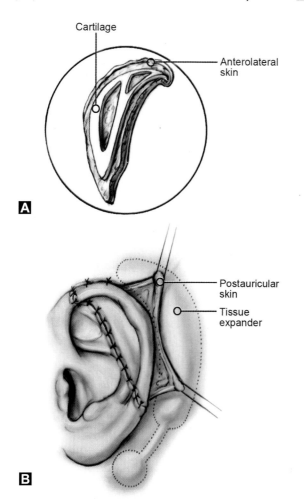

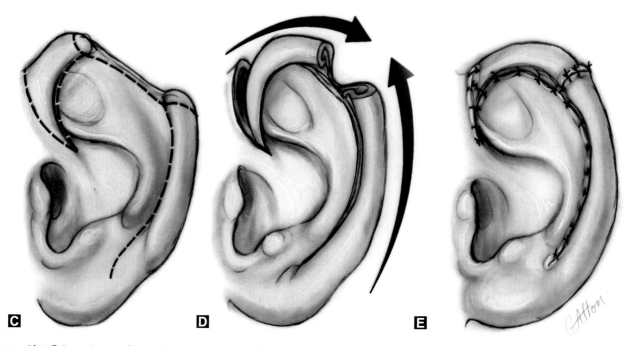

- Cotton-tipped applicators
- Dressing: Tincture of benzoin, Steristrips, 4 × 4 "Fluffs", 2" rolled bandage, cotton balls, and Betadine ointment.

Procedure

Depending on the extent of the reconstruction, either local anethesia with 1% lidocaine and 1:100,000 epinephrine or general anesthesia can be used. After the resection of a neoplasm, the pinna can be reconstructed by many methods, limited only by the surgeon's imagination and ingenuity. The following discussion, which is not intended to be encyclopedic, outlines methods that have worked well over the years and that are based on general principles of flap design.

After removing the neoplasm, all margins must be examined histologically. The pinna can be reconstructed in three ways: (1) primary closure; (2) a composite graft from the other ear, and (3) a pedicled skin/cartilage flap.

Primary closure: When less than 30% of the pinna has been excised, the defect often can be closed primarily, especially if it involves the upper and middle portions of the pinna (Figures 5A and B). When closing a defect primarily, it is usually necessary to use any of a variety of releasing incisions along the antihelical fold and conchal bowl to allow for the advancement of

Figures 4A to E Reattachment of the total amputated pinna. (A) If the postauricular area is badly injured then a soft tissue from the cartilage is removed, making a pocket under a cervical skin flap and left there until the postauricular skin has healed; (B) A crescent-shaped tissue expander can then be placed in the postauricular/mastoid region and slowly expanded over 4–6 weeks until twice as much surface area is expanded; (C) Another method of salvaging the cartilaginous skeleton of the amputated ear is to remove the skin from the medial surface of the pinna and perforate the cartilage; (D) The postauricular skin is removed; (E) Ear is reattached by suturing the helical rim to the free margin of remaining postauricular skin

adjacent tissue. The rigid cartilaginous framework of the pinna, the densely adherent skin, and the lack of subcutaneous tissue hinders the closure of even small defects. Without these incisions, closure of the defect may cause cupping of the pinna.

Often, small wedges of conchal bowl cartilage must be removed so that proper closure can be obtained. Closure is accomplished with interrupted 5-0 Vicryl suture in the cartilage and a cutaneous layer of running locked 6-0 chromic or interrupted 6-0 nylon suture.

Composite graft: Another satisfactory method of repairing small defects of the pinna (not greater than 3 cm) is to use a composite graft from the opposite ear. A through-and-through graft up to 1.5 cm in size can be harvested from the donor ear. The size of the graft is usually half the size of the defect, i.e. for a 2 cm defect a 1 cm composite graft is harvested. The donor site is closed primarily as described above. The composite graft is then sutured in place with a minimal number of sutures, securing the cartilage with 5-0 Vicryl and closing the skin with 6-0 chromic or nylon suture. Too many sutures can compromise the viability of the graft. Composite grafts often undergo epidermolysis with discoloration and blister formation, but usually re-epithelialize if infection is avoided.

Pedicled skin flap: For larger defects, a skin flap based either anteriorly or posteriorly on the postauricular skin is elevated and sutured into the defect (Figures 5C and D). If the defect has been created by resection of a neoplasm or a traumatic tissue loss, an anteriorly based flap is not feasible. The blood supply is better when the flap is based posteriorly, but anteriorly based flaps usually do not require a secondary takedown procedure. The length-to-width ratio is usually low (1:1 to 2:1) because of the close proximity of the donor site. A piece of contralateral conchal bowl cartilage or costal cartilage can be placed under the flap primarily, or secondarily when the flap is taken down (Figure 5E).

For small defects, the use of cartilage is not necessary. The postauricular sulcus can often be preserved by leaving a strip of postauricular skin intact when developing the flap. The free margin of skin on the medial surface of the pinna is sutured to the free margin of the postauricular skin. The leading edge of the elevated flap is sutured to the free margin of the lateral skin of the pinna. After 3 or 4 weeks the pedicled flap can be separated from the postauricular skin and rolled around to make a new helical rim (Figures 5F and G). If the helical fold is not well defined, small cotton bolsters can be placed on the lateral surface of the pinna and sutured in place with 4-0 nylon to help recreate this portion. Subcutaneous and cartilaginous sutures are 5-0 Vicryl, with 6-0 chromic or

nylon used for the cutaneous layer. The donor site usually can be closed primarily with extensive undermining, but a skin graft may be necessary.

Defects of the conchal bowl can be closed primarily if they are small. For a larger defect, a full-thickness postauricular skin graft works well. Large defects may also be repaired with a postauricular pedicled skin flap, which is elevated and laid through a slit made through the conchal cartilage (Figure 6A). The flap is sutured anteriorly, superiorly and inferiorly, leaving the posterior through-and-through slit (Figure 6B). After 3 or 4 weeks, the flap is released along the posterior slit and the defect is closed primarily (Figure 6C). Loss of the ear lobe can be repaired by designing a bilobed flap based anteriorly, which is lifted and folded upon itself (Figures 7A and B). The donor site is closed primarily or with a skin graft. Alternatively, an inferiorly based flap is elevated and sutured to the inferior edge of the remaining pinna. After 3 or 4 weeks, the flap is separated inferiorly and folded upon itself (Figures 7C to E).

Postoperative Care

Bacitracin ointment is applied to the incisions. A light mastoid dressing is applied to prevent the patient from disturbing the

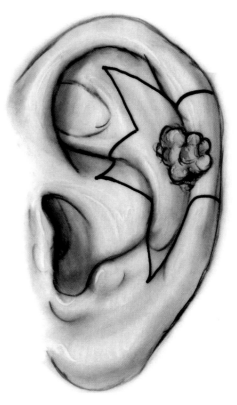

Figure 5A

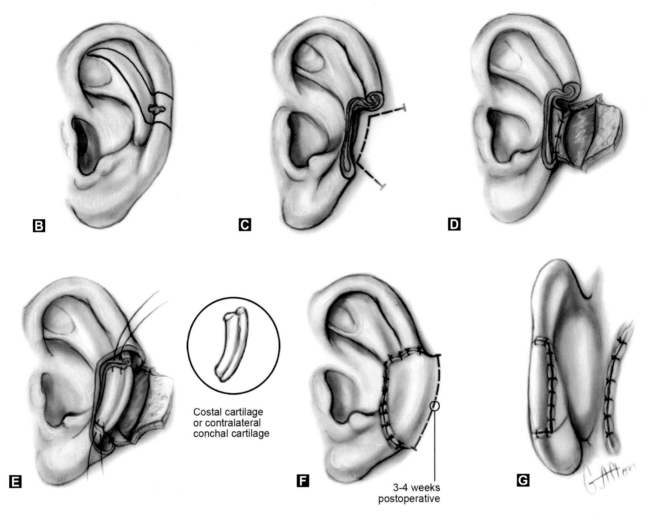

Figures 5B to G

Figures 5A to G (A and B) Primary closure of the small defects, if it involves the upper and middle portions of the pinna; (C and D) For larger defects, a skin flap based either anteriorly or posteriorly on the postauricular skin is elevated and sutured into the defect; (E) A piece of contralateral conchal bowl cartilage or costal cartilage can be placed under the flap primarily, or secondarily when the flap is taken down; (F and G) After 3–4 weeks the pedicled flap can be separated from the postauricular skin and rolled around to make a new helical rim

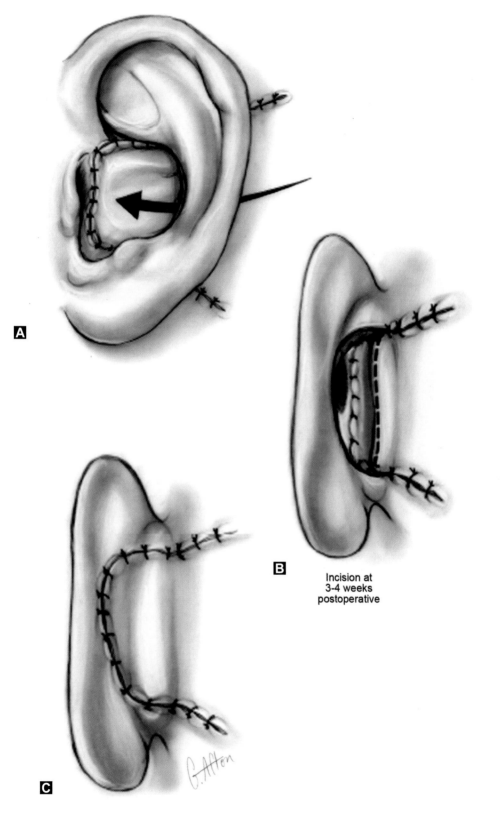

A

B

Incision at
3-4 weeks
postoperative

C

Figures 6A to C Defects of the conchal bowl. (A) Large defects repaired with a postauricular pedicled skin flap, which is elevated and laid through a slit made through the conchal cartilage; (B) The flap is sutured anteriorly, superiorly and inferiorly, leaving the posterior through-and-through slit; (C) After 3–4 weeks, the flap is released along the posterior slit and the defect is closed primarily. Loss of the ear lobe can be repaired by designing a bilobed flap based

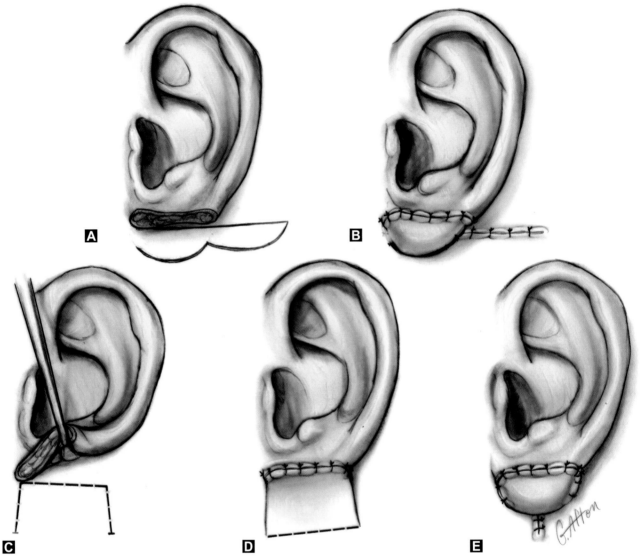

Figures 7A to E (A and B) Loss of the ear lobe can be repaired by designing a bilobed flap based anteriorly, which is lifted and folded upon itself; (C to E) An inferiorly based flap is elevated and sutured to the inferior edge of the remaining pinna. The flap is separated inferiorly and folded upon itself

repair. Too tight a dressing might compromise the blood supply. The dressing can be removed in a few days, and the bacitracin is continued for another day or two. If a takedown is necessary, it is performed after 3 or 4 weeks. After the second stage of a pedicled flap, there is usually edema of the flap side of the flap/ normal skin interface; this makes the repair more noticeable and may take several months to resolve. If after six to nine months, a depressed scar has formed (this can be especially noticeable on the helical rim), a small Z-plasty can be performed under local anesthesia.

4.3
Canalplasty: General Concepts

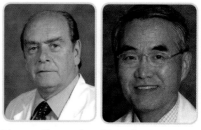

Marcos Goycoolea, Timothy Jung

INTRODUCTION

A canalplasty is a procedure that normalizes the external auditory canal by removing abnormal bony growth, such as exostosis, removing and replacing intractably infected skin of the canal, or enlarging and straightening a severely stenotic and tortuous canal. Meatoplasty (enlargement of the meatus) may be done at the same time. Canalplasty is used when there is any obstruction that blocks an adequate view of the tympanic membrane and the tympanic annulus (e.g. osseous borders, exostosis, obliterative external otitis, stenosis, tumors, etc.).

Aim

To restore the normal width and contour of the external auditory canal and, sometimes, to replace diseased with healthy skin.

Concepts

An adequate ear canal and meatus allow:
1. Adequate surgery with good visualization.
2. Good cicatrization and aeration.
3. Adequate cleansing postoperatively.
4. Good sound transmission.
   In brief, they are an essential part of middle ear and mastoid surgery.
   On the other hand, small conducts:
1. Are hard to visualize.
2. Are humid and accumulate debris.
3. Are difficult to clean.
4. Do not heal well.
5. They can ruin a well done middle ear and/or mastoid procedure.

Surgical Steps

1. Endaural or postauricular incision.
2. Elevation of canal skin flap.
3. Widening of the bony canal.
4. Placing back the canal skin flaps or skin graft.
5. Packing and closure.

Pitfalls

1. Exposing the temporomandibular joint capsule anteriorly.
2. Opening into the mastoid air cells.
3. Damaging the tympanic membrane, ossicles, or skin flaps.

Operative Procedure

The procedure usually is carried out under general anesthesia, but can also be done under local anesthesia. In either case, local injection of 1% lidocaine with 1:100,000 epinephrine is made into four quadrants of the external auditory canal. Either an endaural or postauricular approach can be used.

Exostosis

Large exostoses can cause retention of cerumen, recurrent inflammation of the canal skin, and even conductive hearing loss. An endaural approach usually is adequate. A posterior skin flap is developed from the bony cartilaginous junction to the annulus of the tympanic membrane (Figure 1A). The skin over the exostosis is elevated and preserved. When the exostoses are too large to permit a canal incision, a separate incision is made on the top of the exostoses paralleling the annulus of the tympanic membrane. Two skin flaps are developed over each exostosis, one laterally and the other medially based.

When the posterior bony canal with exostosis is exposed, the exostosis is drilled out with a cutting burr and diamond burr under continuous irrigation (Figure 1B). As the base of the exostosis is removed, the entire tympanic membrane can be visualized and the canal skin flap becomes better defined. The annulus of the tympanic membrane is left intact and the middle ear is not entered. The remaining bony canal wall is smoothened down until the canal has a normal, even contour.

Any other exostoses in the canal are removed in a similar manner. This is usually easier because the canal is less crowded and the tympanic membrane is readily visible. For an exostosis in the anterior canal, a laterally based anterior "window-shade" flap can be developed starting from an area just lateral to the anterior half of the tympanic ring. When drilling the anterior wall of the canal, care must be exercised not to enter the temporomandibular joint.

Sometimes, when drilling near the annulus is not that easy to determine where the exostosis ends, the use of curets is helpful to smooth these borders. Another method that we use all the time, but it requires experience is the use of a small chisel. If one analyzes the structure of the exostosis, one can verify that in a majority of cases they are formed in layers that can be removed gently with a chisel. The argument that one can fracture the temporal bone with a chisel is not true in our cases. We have used chisels gently for years without any problem in that regards. The drill is used primarily for smoothening borders and rough surfaces. After all the exostoses are removed and the rest of the canal wall is smoothened down, the skin flaps are laid back (Figure 1C). The external auditory canal is packed with Gelfoam saturated in antibiotic solution and "wrung out"; Owen's silk strips and pieces of cotton packing (rosebud packing) also can be used. The lateral part of the canal and the meatus are packed with ½" gauze strips saturated with antibiotic ointment.

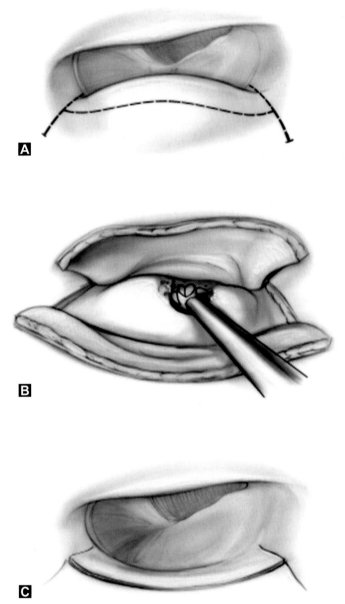

Figures 1A to C Exostosis: (A) A posterior skin flap is developed from the bony cartilaginous junction to the annulus of the tympanic membrane; (B) The exostosis is drilled out with a cutting burr and diamond burr under continuous irrigation; (C) After the removal of exostosis, the rest of the canal wall is smoothened down, and skin flaps are laid back

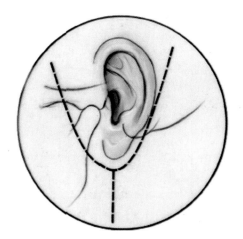

A

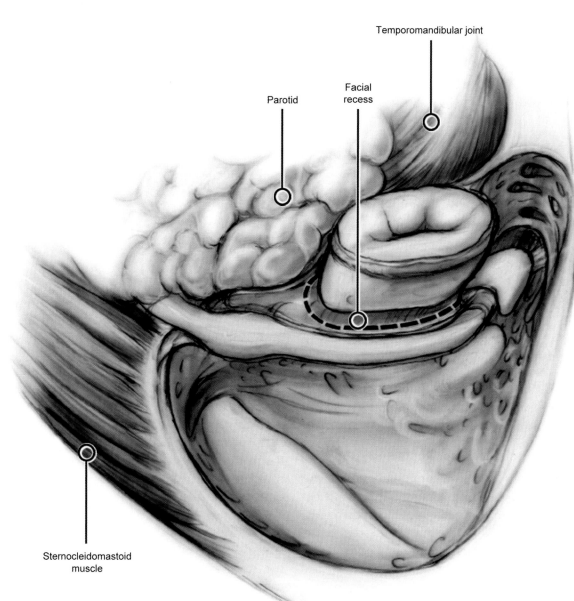

B

Figures 4A and B

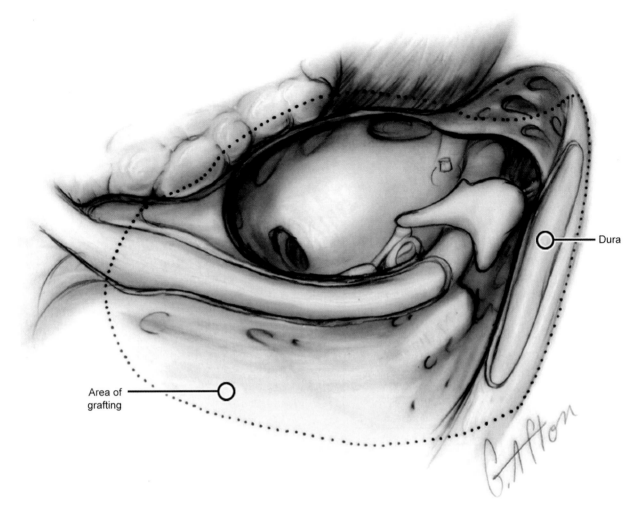

Figure 4C

Figures 4A to C Subtotal resection of temporal bone: (A) The incision is made anterior and posterior to the auricle, with the inferior extension along the anterior border of the sternocleidomastoid muscle; (B) The bony buttress of the zygomatic process of the temporal bone is drilled down, the malleus removed along with tympanic membrane, specimen separated as drilling continues just above the bony annulus; (C) After the specimen is removed, the middle ear space and exposed dura are covered by a large temporal fascial graft

is severed (Figure 5C). The internal carotid artery is exposed with a drill; during this procedure the bony eustachian tube is transected (Figure 5D). The bone over the internal carotid artery is removed with the points of the artery's entrance into the foramen lacerum defining the anterior and superior limits of the resection (Figure 6A). A mastoidectomy is performed, exposing the sigmoid sinus with a drill (Figure 6B). The specimen is removed by fracturing the temporal bone through the otic capsule with a chisel placed just posterior to the internal carotid artery. Hemorrhage is controlled with packing. The boundaries of the resection are internal carotid artery anteriorly, the middle fossa dura superiorly, the posterior fossa dura and sigmoid sinus

posteriorly, and the petrous apex medially (Figure 6C). The line of resection as seen from above, passes through the petrous portion of the temporal bone just lateral to the internal auditory canal. If the tumor extends to the dura, the involved portion may have to be resected; if there is evidence of metastasis to the neck, a radical neck dissection may be necessary. The wound is closed after the defect is filled with temporal muscle and a large meatoplasty is done (Figure 6D). A split-thickness skin graft over the temporal muscle will shorten the healing time. If the tumor extends to the auricle, the entire auricle and its surrounding skin are excised (Figure 6E). The defect is best covered with a myocutaneous flap from the greater pectoral muscle.

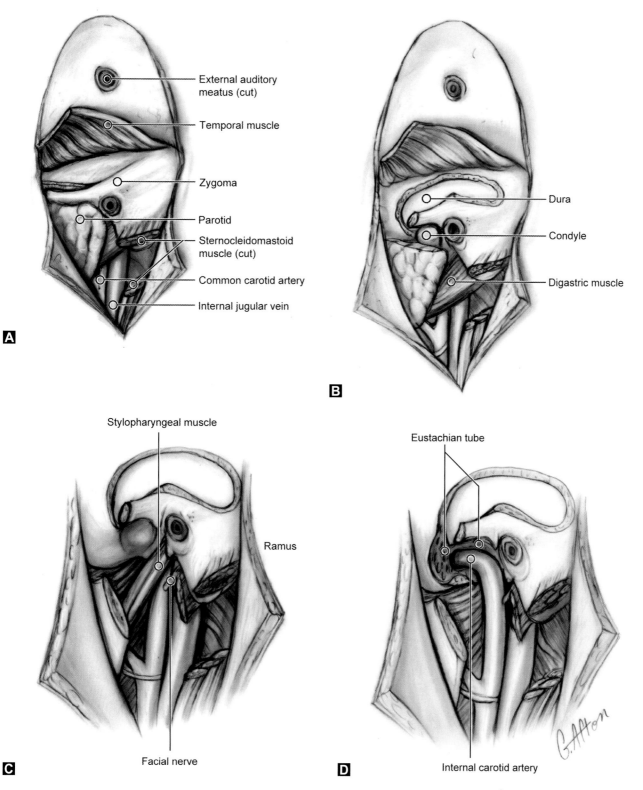

A

- External auditory meatus (cut)
- Temporal muscle
- Zygoma
- Parotid
- Sternocleidomastoid muscle (cut)
- Common carotid artery
- Internal jugular vein

B

- Dura
- Condyle
- Digastric muscle

C

- Stylopharyngeal muscle
- Ramus
- Facial nerve

D

- Eustachian tube
- Internal carotid artery

Figures 5A to D Total temporal bone resection: (A) Wide areas of the zygomatic arch, the squamous portion of the temporal bone, and the mastoid are exposed by elevating the temporal muscle; (B) Elevation of dura from the temporal bone allows the tumor to be evaluated for possible intracranial extension; (C) The head of the mandible is removed. If the tumor has invaded the anterior canal, a total parotidectomy is done; the facial nerve is resected and the posterior belly of the digastric muscle is severed; (D) The internal carotid artery is exposed with a drill; during this procedure the bony eustachian tube is transected

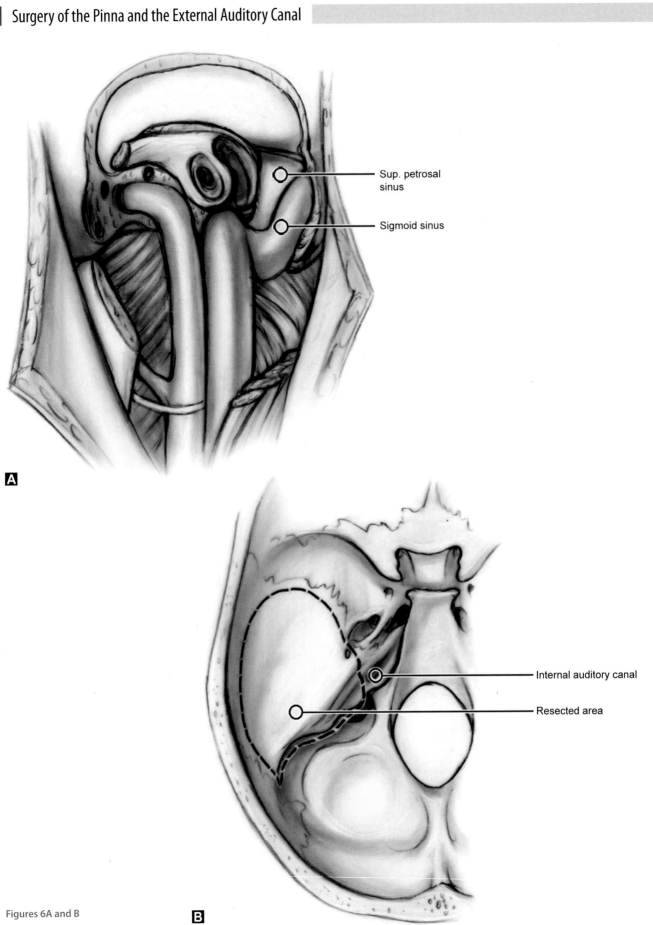

Sup. petrosal sinus

Sigmoid sinus

Internal auditory canal

Resected area

Figures 6A and B

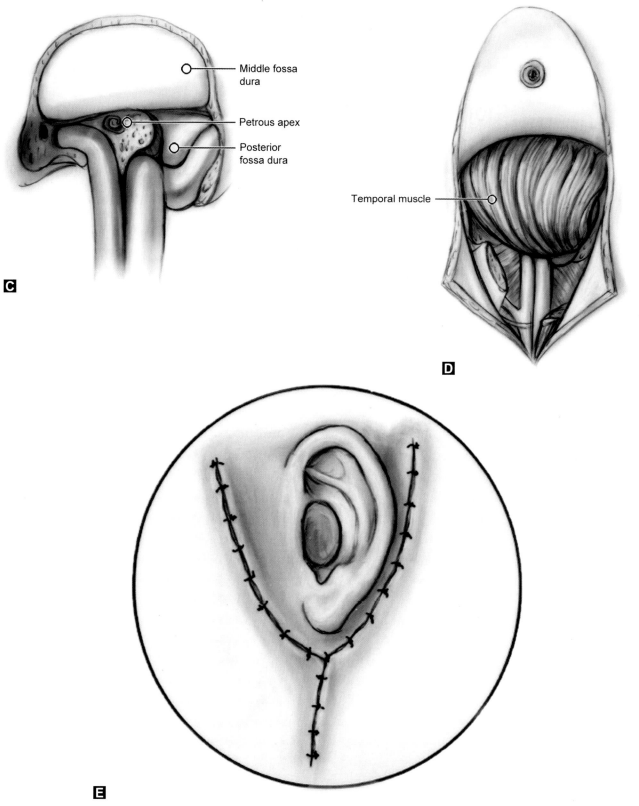

C — Middle fossa dura; Petrous apex; Posterior fossa dura

D — Temporal muscle

E

Figures 6C to E

Figures 6A to E Total temporal bone resection: (A) The bone over the internal carotid artery is removed with the points of the artery's entrance into the foramen lacerum defining the anterior and superior limits of the resection; (B) A mastoidectomy is performed, exposing the sigmoid sinus with a drill; (C) The specimen is removed by fracturing the temporal bone, boundaries of the resection are internal carotid artery anteriorly, the middle fossa dura superiorly, the posterior fossa dura and sigmoid sinus posteriorly, and the petrous apex medially; (D) The wound is closed after the defect is filled with temporal muscle and a large meatoplasty is done; (E) A split-thickness skin graft over the temporal muscle will shorten the healing time

4.4

Meatoplasty

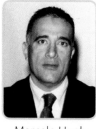

Marcelo Hueb

MEATOPLASTY

The external auditory or external ear canal (external auditory meatus, external acoustic meatus, external ear meatus) has a lateral cartilaginous one-third part and a medial osseous two-thirds part. It starts at the concha in the form of a meatus, which is a natural body opening or canal and runs towards the tympanic membrane.

Meatus acusticus externus is a Latin derived term and meatoplasty refers to procedures that restore, change or improve the form and function of the meatus. It is a technical complimentary refinement mandatorily associated with open-cavity tympanomastoidectomies, frequently performed in congenital and acquired stenosis of the external auditory meatus and eventually done in association with other surgical procedures where an inadequate postoperative view of the tympanic membrane is anticipated (e.g. closed-cavity tympanomastoidectomy with a narrow external auditory meatus and canal; in this case associated with canalplasty) (Figures 1A to D).

Aim

This surgical procedure aims to circumferentially enlarge the external auditory meatus with a fourfold achievement:

1. Provide ample 360º visualization and instrumentation of the tympanic membrane and external auditory canal.
2. Provide adequate visualization and instrumentation in cases of open cavity mastoid bowls.
3. Provide adequate aeration of this newly formed anatomy.
4. Provide adequate sound transmission.

Highlights

- Skin and perichondrium flap integrity for adequate healing.
- New meatus demarcation and cartilage removal (if necessary, in crescent strips).
- Judicious hemostasis.
- Inverted flap sutures covering conchal cartilage borders.

Surgical steps

1. Periauricular skin and external canal asepsis.
2. Endomeatal, retroauricular (or endaural) and retroconchal infiltration.
3. Skin incision, either endaural or more commonly retroauricular.
4. Exposure of the posterior aspect of the meatal skin and harvesting of a long or shorter tympanomeatal flap.
5. Retroconchal subcutaneous dissection and conchal cartilage exposure on its posterior aspect.
6. Periosteum incision near the concha and harvesting of a superiorly based periosteum flap.
7. Posterior conchal perichondrium incision and dissection of an anterior based perichondrium flap.
8. Excision and removal of conchal cartilage with preservation of the anterior conchal perichondrium.
9. Perichondrium/skin incision and creation of 3 flaps.
10. Inverted skin/perichondrium sutures.
11. Bone drilling (in cases of closed-cavity procedures) to leave an underlying large osseous aperture. This can be done at the lateral portion of the osseous meatus or a complete canalplasty can be done.
12. Packing.

Pitfalls

This procedure is not related to major perioperative complications, although careless management can predict unsuccessful

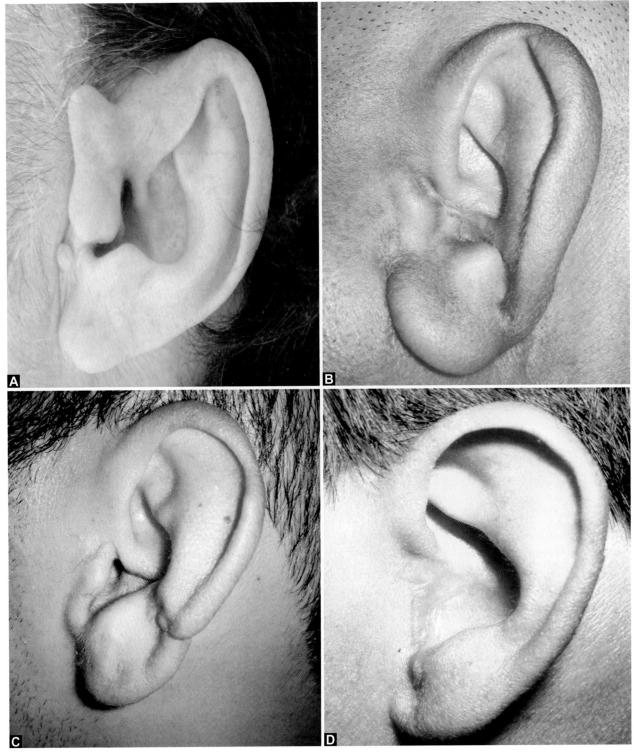

Figures 1A to D (A) Congenitally malformed meatus; (B) Infectious atretic meatus; (C) Traumatic stenotic meatus; (D) Iatrogenically atretic meatus

results. Careless dissection may result in torn skin or inadequate flap. Bleeding frequently happens and hemostasis is easily achieved with careful monopolar or preferably bipolar cauter-ization. Improper asepsis and postoperative infection of the surgical bed can be disastrous as it may lead to perichondritis, granulation tissue formation and stenosis.

Pearls of Wisdom

Although performing an open-cavity tympanomastoidectomy is commonly decided preoperatively, it is wise to anticipate this possibility and harvest an adequate tympanomeatal flap, either long or short; in this last case leaving a laterally based Koerner's flap. We prefer to leave a longer tympanomeatal flap to reconstruct the middle ear, epitympanum and antrum area, and use the lateral third of the external canal skin and exposed conchal skin/perichondrium to cover the meatoplasty area.

Before incising the cartilage, the surgical field should be washed clean with warm saline solution to wash away debris from the mastoidectomy and the meatal, conchal and retroauricular skin resterilized with a 5% or 1% chlorhexidine gluconate or a povidone-iodine solution.

To maximize results, the conchal cartilage should always be removed and its perichondrium always kept.

Conchal cartilage should be removed in an almost semicircular fashion (in crescent-shaped strips, if needed); avoid an elliptical fashion as it may facilitate postoperative retraction.

Extreme care should be taken as not to disrupt the meatal skin and conchal skin from behind.

Do not leave uncovered or exposed conchal cartilage at the margins of the newly enlarged meatus as it favors granulation tissue development and stenosis to happen.

The new meatus should be large enough as to freely allow the introduction of the surgeon's forefinger.

Procedure

As this procedure is usually associated with other major procedures, it is generally performed under general anesthesia, although it can also be performed under local anesthesia and sedation. Sterile technique should be used throughout the procedure. After adequate asepsis is done, antimicrobial surgical incise drapes with an iodophor impregnated adhesive are used (Figure 2). Retroauricular (or endaural), endomeatal and retroconchal areas are infiltrated with 2% lidocaine and 1:100,000 epinephrine solution; the endomeatal and retroconchal areas should be infiltrated using a gingival needle.

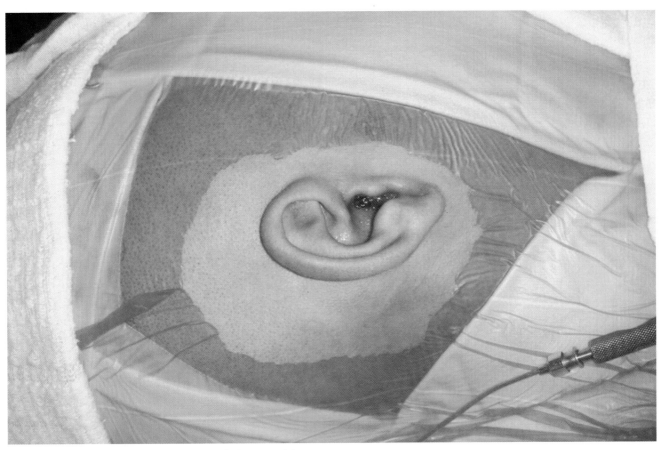

Figure 2 Immediate preoperative aspect with an iodophor surgical drape

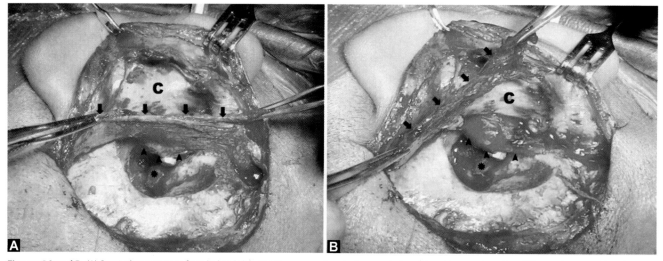

Figures 3A and B (A) Surgical aspect seen from behind showing the exposed posterior conchal perichondrium and cartilage (C), anterior mastoid periosteum (arrows), external canal skin (arrow heads) and tympanomeatal flap (*); (B) Surgical aspect seen from behind showing the exposed posterior conchal perichondrium and cartilage (C), dissected anterior periosteal flap (arrow head), external canal skin and tympanomeatal flap (*)

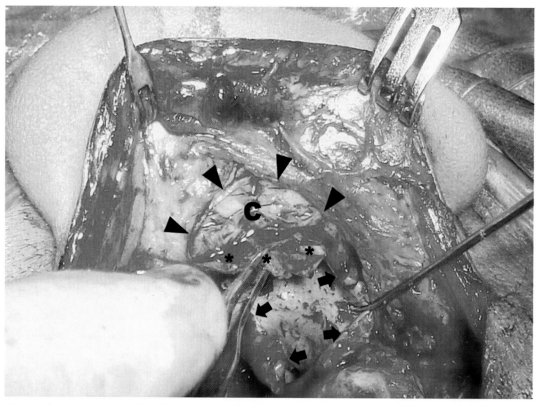

Figure 4 Surgical aspect seen from behind showing the exposed posterior conchal cartilage (C), incised posterior conchal perichondrium (arrow heads), dissected posterior perichondrial flap (*), superior and inferior external canal skin flaps (arrows)

Retroauricular incision has already been performed as part of the major procedure and at this point blunt dissection is done as to expose a large portion of the conchal cartilage and its transition to the posterior aspect of the meatal flap. The anterior periosteum flap is left intact and incised near the exposed concha to be rotated superiorly and posteriorly, and sutured to the posterior periosteum flap at the end of the pro-

cedure (Figures 3A and B). An adequate tympanomeatal flap has already been dissected and before incising the cartilage an anteriorly based flap of the posterior conchal perichondrium should also be dissected (Figure 4).

The conchal cartilage is incised posteriorly with a number 15 scalpel as to reach a size that easily allows the introduction of the surgeon´s forefinger (Figures 5 and 6); the superior and inferior limits of the new meatus are demarcated by the insertion of two needles through the concha (Figure 7). The exposed anterior conchal perichondrium is now seen in continuity with the posterior perichondrium flap with the concha skin attached anteriorly. If a Koerner's flap was not dissected this skin is somewhat shorter and should be incised in a "T" or "Y" fashion as to allow the superior flap to be inverted and sutured posteriorly, and the lateral flaps to be inverted and sutured superiorly and inferiorly (Figure 8).

The newly enlarged meatus is carefully inspected anteriorly and the retroauricular incision closed in layers with subcutaneous absorbable sutures and nylon skin sutures. Packing is performed in the mastoid bowl with rayon strips or other materials

with careful inspection as to keep the flap between the packing material and the subcutaneous tissue. The procedure through a retroauricular approach can be seen in Video 1.

In situations where Lempert's endaural incisions were made, the conchal skin is dissected posteriorly as to expose the conchal cartilage. Conchal cartilage is then removed in crescent-shaped strips in an almost semicircular fashion, and the skin repositioned and kept in place with moderate pressure packing.

Potential Complications and How to Avoid Them

- Cartilage and perichondrium infection are possible to occur, and should be prevented with a sterile technique and least

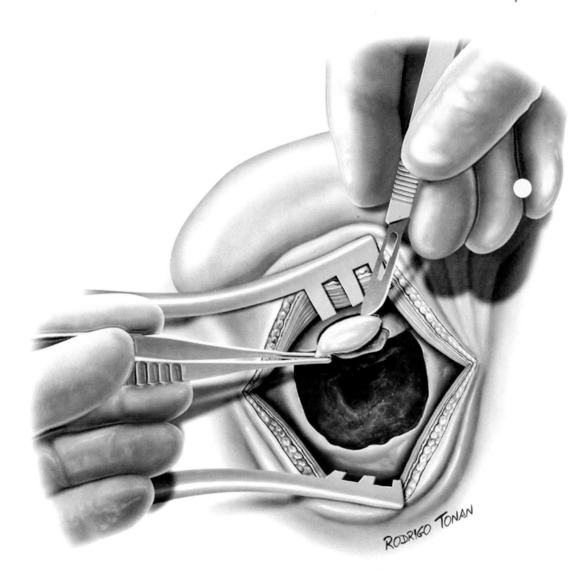

Figure 5 Conchal cartilage removal in an almost semicircular shape

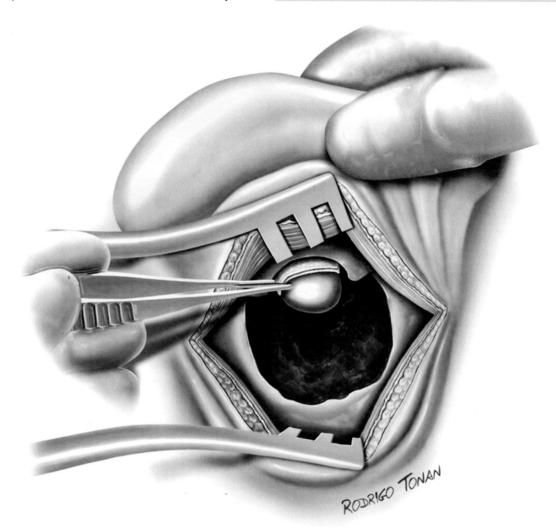

Figure 6 Surgeon's forefinger introduction method

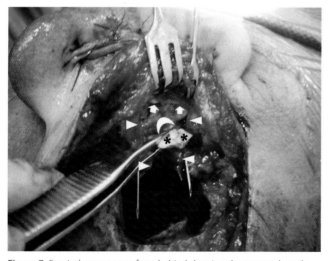

Figure 7 Surgical aspect seen from behind showing the removed cartilage (*) still attached to the perichondrial flap (crescent); arrows indicate the border or the residual conchal cartilage. Incised skin with superior and inferior flaps (arrow heads). Needles demarcate the superior and inferior margins of the new meatus

trauma possible. Sharp incision, perichondrium preservation and skin coverage helps to prevent it. Antimicrobial use is also important.

- Granulation tissue can arise in the areas of exposed cartilage at the margins of newly enlarged meatus. As above, perichondrium and skin coverage helps to prevent it.
- An inadequate sized meatus can occur when too little cartilage is removed. The surgeon´s forefinger introduction method is a "scientific" way to measure the adequate size of the meatus, and needle demarcations help achieve the upper and lower limits of the concha.
- It should be kept in mind that postoperative tissue retraction usually happens and therefore, a meatoplasty is never too large and should include most of the conchal area. Stenosis or retraction can also occur and obviously prevents the adequate functions of the meatoplasty. Care should be taken as not to leave granulation tissue and cartilage infection to

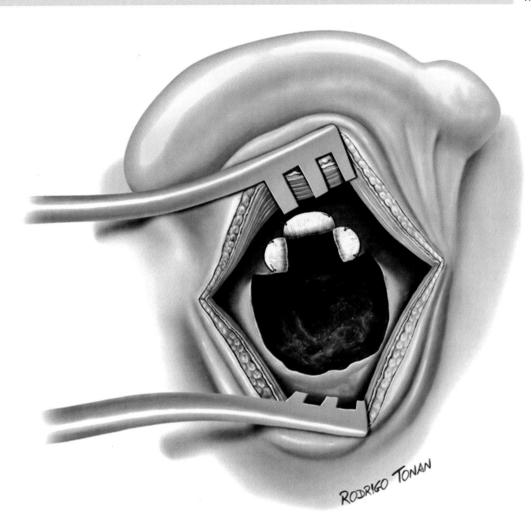

Figure 8 Skin/perichondrial flap sutured anteriorly and skin flaps sutured superiorly and inferiorly

develop. Cartilage removal should not be done in an elliptical fashion.

Postoperative Management

Packing is usually associated with packing of the newly formed mastoid bowl and it should not exert too much pressure on the walls.

Rayon strips, silastic or latex sheeting packed with antibiotic/steroids impregnated cotton or absorbable sponge pieces has a twofold function; helps structuring and achieving adequate packing positioning, and deliver drugs locally. The enlarged meatal aperture should be under light packing pressure as to avoid local ischemia.

Patients usually have a same day discharge or stay hospitalized overnight depending on the procedures that were

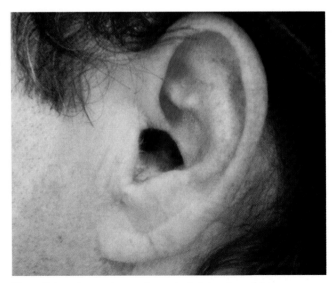

Figure 9 Long-term outcome of a meatoplasty in a 4 year follow-up

performed. Large spectrum antibiotic is initiated at the operating room and kept for a 7 day period; at this time packing is removed. Granulation tissue, if present, is gently curetted and removed, and it's bed lightly cauterized with a 5% silver nitrate solution. Patients are instructed to keep the ears dry for a one month period or until healing has completed. Regular office visits are requested as to avoid stenosis; a long-term meatoplasty is seen in Figure 9.

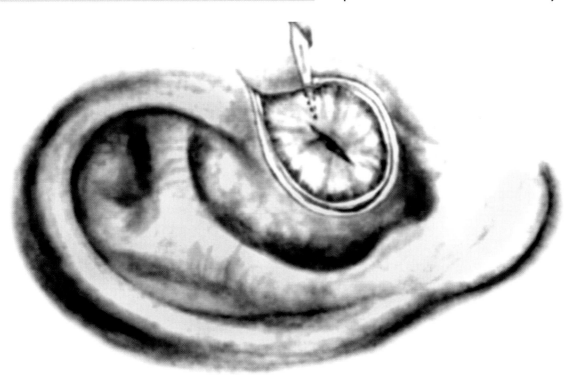

Figure 5 Meatoplasty with incision through the conchal and tragal skin with the cartilage

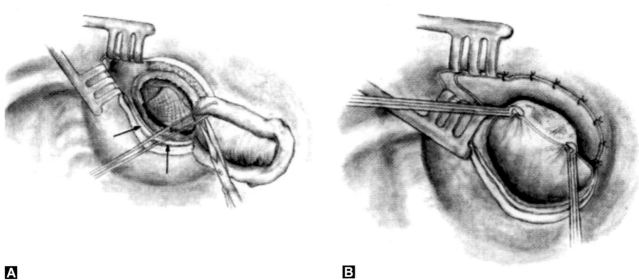

A   **B**

Figures 6A and B (A) Removal of the meatal skin and the cartilage. The gauze of the first packing becomes visible; (B) The anterior split-skin graft is sutured to the anterior tragal skin. The posterior split-skin graft is elevated to be adopted to the conchal skin

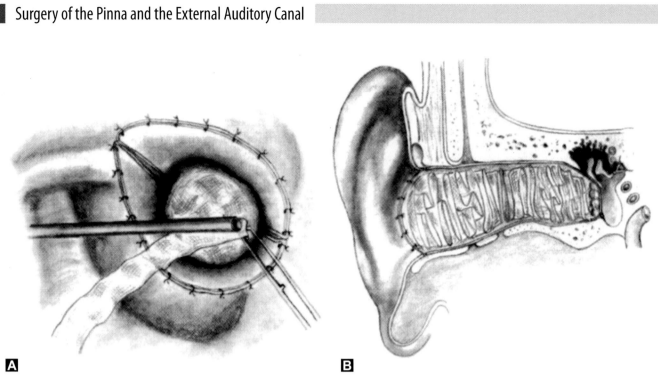

Figures 7A and B (A) The posterior split-skin graft is sutured to the conchal skin; (B) Double packing of the widened ear canal is completed

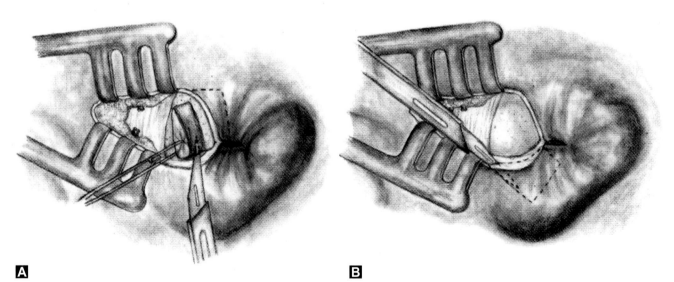

A **B**

Figures 8A and B The method of thinning and preservation of canal skin (Tos, 1997). (A) The Heermann B incision is made. The thinning of the skin is started anteriorly; (B) A wedge of the skin and subcutis is removed

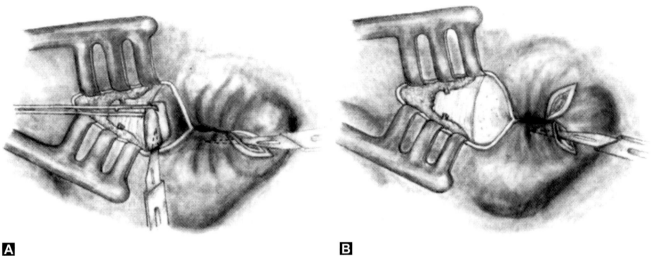

Figures 9A and B (A) The wedge of posterior part of the skin is removed and an inferior radial incision of the thick skin is performed at 7-o'clock position, and the posterior thick skin is made thinner; (B) A posterior circumferential incision and an anterior radial incision is made

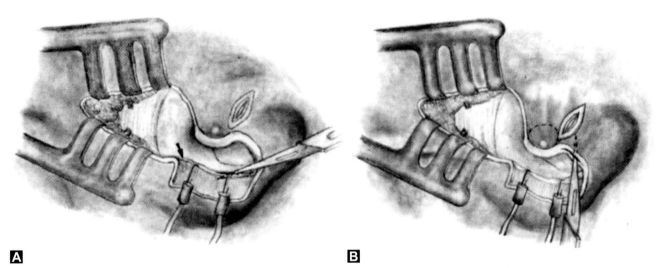

Figures 10A and B (A) The posterolateral ear canal skin is elevated outwards and thinned; (B) The inferior part of the thick ear canal skin is easily thinned

skin, which can easily be thinned (Figure 11A) and elevated (Figure 11B). Thinning of the medial part of the ear canal skin can be easy, starting with two radial incisions at the 12-o'clock and 6-o'clock positions of the posterior skin (Figure 11B). The posterior skin is thinned by introducing a scalpel tangentially along the posterior skin and dividing it into two leaves, a superficial one and a deeper one. The thin superficial epithelial

flap is turned forward to cover the eardrum (Figure 12A), the deeper layer of the canal skin is removed. Similarly, thinning of the anterior skin is completed (Figure 12B) and drilling of the bony ear canal is extensively done (Figure 13A) enlarging the entire ear canal. The thinned medial and the lateral skin flaps are replaced, and split-skin grafts are placed onto the denuded bone (Figure 13B).

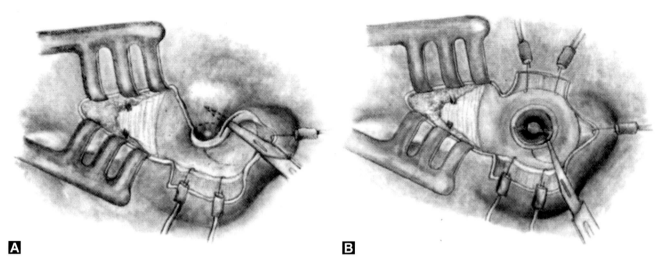

Figures 11A and B (A) Using a scalpel, the anteroinferior skin is thinned; (B) A remaining anterior circular incision is performed, and the anterior skin is elevated and thinned allowing excellent view onto the medial half of the ear canal, especially on the thinning of the median ear canal skin with a scalpel

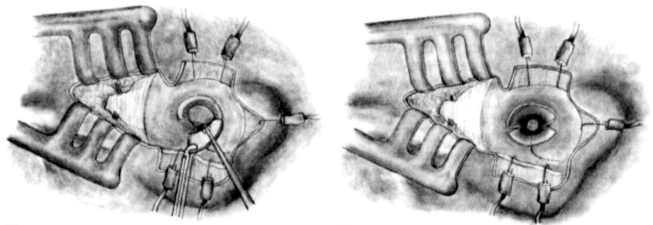

Figures12A and B (A) The thinning of the medial half of the thick ear canal skin continues with cutting and removal of the wedges, while the thinned, superficial parts of the skin are turned towards the eardrum; (B) After removing several wedges, the eardrum is not thinned

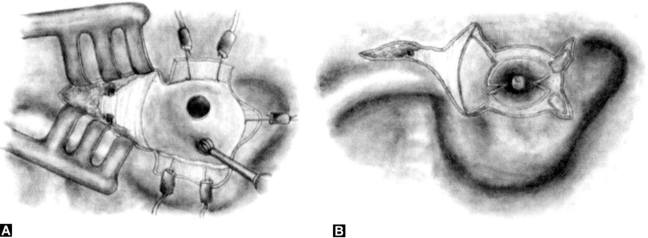

Figures13A and B (A) The thinned medial flaps are turned onto the eardrum and are protected with an aluminum cutting drill or sharp foil. The bony ear canal is extensively enlarged by drilling with diamond drills; (B) The foil is removed, the medial thin flaps and lateral flaps are replaced, and major uncovered bony areas are covered with split-skin grafts

BIBLIOGRAPHY

1. Beales PH. Atresia of the external acoustic meatus. Arch Otolaryngol. 1974;100:209-11.
2. Beales PH, Crawford BS. The treatment of post-inflammatory atresia of the external auditory meatus. J Laryngol Otol. 1966;80:86-9.
3. Heermann H, Heermann J. Endaural Surgery. Munich: Urban and Schwarzenberg; 1964.
4. Hunsacker DH. Conchomeatoplasty for chronic otitis externa. Arch Otolaryngol Head Neck Surg. 1988;114:395-8.
5. Lucente FE, Lawson W, Novick NL. The External Ear. Philadelphia: Saunders; 1995.
6. Paparella MM. Surgical treatment of intractable external otitis. Laryngoscope. 1966;76:232-45.
7. Paparella MM, Kurkjian JM. Surgical treatment for chronic stenosing exernal otitis. Laryngoscope. 1966;76:232-45.
8. Paparella MM, Goycoolea MV. Canalplasty for chronic intractable external otitis and keratosis obturans. Otolaryngol Head Neck Surg. 1981;89:440-3.
9. Proud GO. Surgery for chronic refractory otitis externa. Arch Otolaryngol. 1966;83:436-8.
10. Senturia BH. Diseases for the external ear. Springfield: Thomas; 1957.
11. Senturia BH, Lucente FE. Diseases of the middle ear: an otological-dermatological manual. New York: Grune and Stratton; 1973.
12. Shambaugh GE. Surgery of the ear. Philadelphia: Saunders; 1959.
13. Tobeck A. Operative management of bilateral stenosing chronic inflammation of the auditory canals. Monatsschr Ohrenheilkd Laryngorhinol. 1958;92:193-6.
14. Tos M. Manual of middle ear surgery. Surgery of the external auditory canal. Stuttgart: Thieme Verlag; 1997. pp. 1-167.

4.6
Congenital Atresia

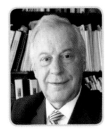

Antonio Soda Merhy, José Javier Zepeda Rodríguez

INTRODUCTION

Congenital ear atresia is a birth defect that is characterized by incomplete development of the external auditory canal (EAC). The ear canal can be absent (atresia) or partially developed (congenital stenosis). It is usually accompanied by middle ear malformations and rarely with inner ear anomalies. In 92% of the cases, there are associated malformations of the pinna (aplasia or hypoplasia), being microtia types II and III (to be described), the most commonly observed.

Microtia and atresia of the ear canal represent a unique challenge. The incidence is approximately 1 in 11,000 to 15,000 births, with a 25% bilaterality.[1] From an etiological standpoint, there are two types: (1) Congenital, secondary to teratogenic agents that act prior to the third month of pregnancy (ototoxic drugs and agents, microorganisms, etc.), and (2) Hereditary, due to the existence of genetic mutations that cause alterations in DNA codification.

In order to have a better understanding of the surgical anatomy in auricular malformations, it is important to review some embryological concepts.[2,3] The external, middle, and inner ears have an independent development. Although their development is interrelated, the malformation of one of them does not mean that it will be accompanied by malformation of one of the others.

The period between the fourth and eighth week of development is the fastest growing period of the facial and auricular structures; therefore, it is in this period that congenital or hereditary factors cause the malformations.

DEVELOPMENT OF THE EXTERNAL EAR

The auricle develops from six protuberances from the mandibular and hyoid arches that fuse at the third month of fetal life.

Microtia, anotia and malpositioned auricle are caused by failure in the differentiation of the first and second branchial arches. By the end of the third month of intrauterine life, the auricle is formed and majority of the middle and inner ear structures are well differentiated.

The EAC develops from the first branchial groove. During the second month, a solid epithelium migrates from the rudimentary auricle and is the precursor of the formation of the EAC, which forms at the sixth month and becomes canalized at the seventh month; originating the development of the mastoid and its separation from the mandible, which causes the ear and the facial nerve to acquire their normal position. Mastoid pneumatization continues until the postnatal period. If the process of canalization is interrupted prematurely, it is likely that the osseous portion of the canal and the tympanic membrane (TM) become associated with marked stenosis of the EAC; a situation that predisposes the formation of a cholesteatoma of the canal due to entrapment of squamous epithelium that keeps on desquamating.

The tympanic bone can be present with modifications that range from mild hypoplasias to absence. When the tympanic bone is absent there is a bony wall termed atretic plate that constitutes the lateral wall of the middle ear. When superior portion of the Reichert's cartilage is hypoplastic, an osseous process from the squamous portion of the temporal bone and the hypotympanum fuse, and close the lateral wall of the middle ear. It is here where the chorda tympani can be found traversing through the atretic plate and in rare occasions, with the third portion of the facial nerve.[4,5]

DEVELOPMENT OF THE MIDDLE EAR

When the first branchial arch (ectoderm) invaginates, it comes close to the tubotympanic cavity, which is endodermic above and below (in between) appears the mesoderm. From this fusion will develop the TM and middle ear structures.

The first pharyngeal pouch (covered by endoderm) expands to originate the Eustachian tube and the middle ear cavity. In patients with atresia, the middle ear cavity is smaller than normal.

With the exception of the vestibular portion of the footplate, which is derived from the otic capsule, the ossicular chain is derived from the first and second branchial arches.

The second arch will originate the handle and external process of the malleus; the long process of the incus and stapes (except the already mentioned vestibular portion of the footplate).

Ossicular deformities usually accompany deformities of the external canal; however, they can also be present as isolated ossicular deformities with the rest of the ear structures being normal.

Abnormalities of the facial nerve are common in cases of aural atresia, especially the dehiscence of the Fallopian canal and with less frequency there are alterations in the second genu, which provides a more anterior position in the mastoid portion and also more lateral in its exit at the level of the stylomastoid foramen. This represents a risk when a new canal is surgically created in the posteroinferior portion. There is also a correlation between facial nerve anomalies and the degree of microtia.[6]

CLINICAL PICTURE

The essential symptom is hearing loss, which can be unilateral or bilateral, depending on whether one or both the ears are involved. Hearing loss is conductive and ranges from 45 to 60 dB in complete atresia and from 30 to 40 dB in partial atresia. In approximately 10% of cases, there is associated sensorineural hearing losses of variable degrees.

The majority of major malformations are evident at birth because of the microtia; however, in patients with a discrete auricular unilateral malformation and stenosis of the ear canal, the diagnosis can be made later.

When cases are bilateral the two main priorities are: (1) To perform audiological studies and fit hearing aids in order for the child to have adequate language development, and (2) To develop treatment strategies and timings with other specialists (e.g. plastic surgeons) for the necessary recommendations for rehabilitation and possible surgical treatments.

Physical examination is essential in order to evaluate craniofacial development and to determine if there are abnormalities or syndromes of the first and second branchial arch that can be associated with microtia-atresia, such as Treacher Collins, Crouzon's, Klippel Feil, Pierre Robin and Goldenhar.[1]

Patients with congenital atresia of the ear can be classified according to the degree of development of the auricle, EAC and middle ear.

The deformity of the auricle can be divided into three degrees.

Grade I: Microtia with small malformations, the auricle is of a smaller size than normal, but has all the structures and these are well defined.

Grade II: The auricle is formed by a fragment of soft tissue and cartilage, with a slight curvature similar to a primitive helix and generally there is a "rotated" lobule.

Grade III: There are only rudiments of soft tissue[7] (Figures 1A to C).

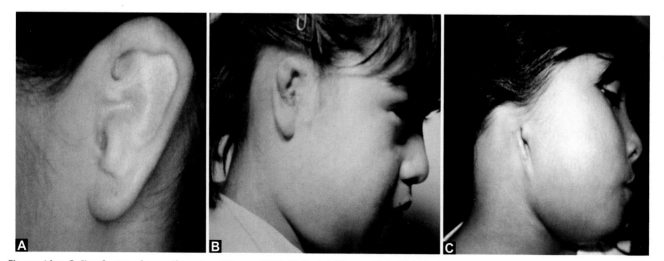

Figures 1A to C Classification of ear malformations (Altmann 1965). (A) Grade I, Discrete; (B) Grade II, Moderate; (C) Grade III, Severe

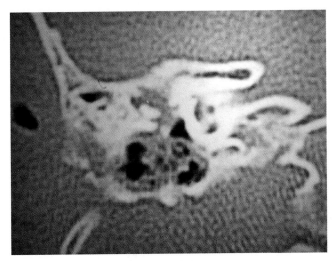

Figure 2 CAT scan showing atresia and cholesteatoma

The classification of the EAC and the middle ear has been more difficult and different parameters have been used, such as findings in clinical examination, radiologic findings, surgical observations or histopathological studies, resulting in numerous classifications.[7-9] One which we use because we consider it the simplest and most useful is the classification of Ombredane that classifies them in two groups: major and minor malformations.[10]

Major Malformations

In this group the EAC and TM are usually nonexistent; however, in this group severe stenosis of the EAC is also included. Occasionally, a rudimentary TM that is adherent to the atretic plate can be observed. The size of the middle ear is diminished and the malleus-incus complex is deformed, fused and adherent to the atretic plate. In severe cases, the middle ear space is very small and the ossicular chain is absent. There can be dehiscence or displacement of the facial nerve. The inner ear is usually normal. The auricular malformation is usually microtia type II or III.

Minor Malformations

The main defect in this group is in the middle ear. There is conductive hearing loss because of absence, fixation or deformities in the ossicular chain. The most common abnormalities are those of the stapes. The tympanic membrane and the middle ear space are normal or slightly reduced in size. The EAC is present, but it can be slightly stenosed. The displacement or

dehiscence of the facial nerve is present in some patients. The auricle has a normal development or is slightly deformed.

LABORATORY STUDIES

Audiological Evaluation

In the initial evaluation of patients with microtia-atresia, it is necessary to investigate the functional and anatomic integrity. Functional integrity is evaluated with audiological studies. Auditory evoked potentials (ABR) are used in the first weeks and months after birth. In bilateral cases hearing aid fitting is essential, not so in unilateral cases. In older children, conventional audiological studies are indicated.

Imaging Studies

Tomography (CAT Scan) is used in order to evaluate anatomic integrity; however, we do it at 5 or 6 years of age once the mastoid pneumatization is completed, the child cooperates and it is not necessary to subject him to general anesthesia. In addition, surgery is done after this period of time. However, if cholesteatoma is suspected because of infection or facial paralysis, the tomographic study is done (Figure 2).

In addition to providing anatomical integrity, CAT studies must be oriented towards defining the structural elements of the EAC and middle ear in order to determine the degree of malformation and surgical risks. This is essential for the evaluation of benefits versus risks of an eventual procedure, and the selection of the treatment approach. Jahrsdoerfer developed a system to evaluate surgical candidates and to determine a functional prognosis according to radiological criteria by assigning points according to fixed parameters.[11] Martín and Soda,[12] based on this system, described a classification that is based exclusively on radiological findings in order to determine prognosis and risk. They assign 1 point for each of the following elements:

- Complete pneumatization
- Incomplete atretic plate
- Presence of middle ear space
- Presence of malleus-incus complex
- Presence of stapes
- Presence of oval window
- Mastoid portion of the facial nerve in normal position (Figures 3A to C).

The sum of all these factors totals 8 points. We consider that 8 points has an excellent prognosis, 7 very good, 6 good, 5 regular, 4 or less poor.

DIFFERENTIAL DIAGNOSIS

In cases of isolated malformations of some of the ossicles (Figure 4), a differential diagnosis must be made with otosclerosis, otitis media sequelae, middle ear tympanosclerosis and otitis media with effusion. All of these entities are capable of causing conductive hearing loss; however, with the current diagnostic tools the diagnosis can be made precisely.

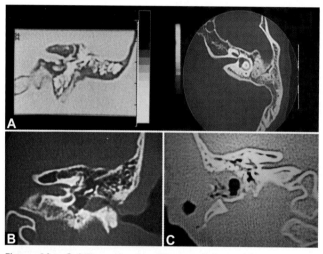

Figures 3A to C CAT scan showing different pathologies. (A) Atresia of the external auditory canal; (B) Congenital stenosis; (C) Atresia and cholesteatoma

TREATMENT

The management of these patients must be multidisciplinary and includes the participation of the audiologist, radiologist, otologist and plastic surgeon.

There is some controversy as to who operates first—the otologist or the plastic surgeon. The otologist wants to drill an ear canal in a site that is dictated by the position of the middle ear and not where the plastic surgeon created the auricle (Figure 5). The plastic surgeon does not want incisions and scarring that can interfere with the blood supply of flaps. In order to solve these problems, since 1978, both operate together and the results have been better than when a specialist operates alone.[13-15]

According to the radiological criteria, the patients with a low grade will be offered hearing devices and auricular reconstruction. The hearing device that offers the most benefits is the bone anchored hearing aid (BAHA), and is indicated in patients with nonsurgical malformations, in failures of conventional surgery and in recurrent stenosis of the meatoplasties (Figures 6 to 8).[16-18]

If there is a major perceptive component, the BAHA is more efficient than the bone conduction aids (Figure 9).

In cases with adequate grades (points), a cosmetic and functional reconstruction is conducted (Figures 10A to D).

In recent years, implantable hearing aids have been placed in the middle ear in cases of external and middle ear abnormali-

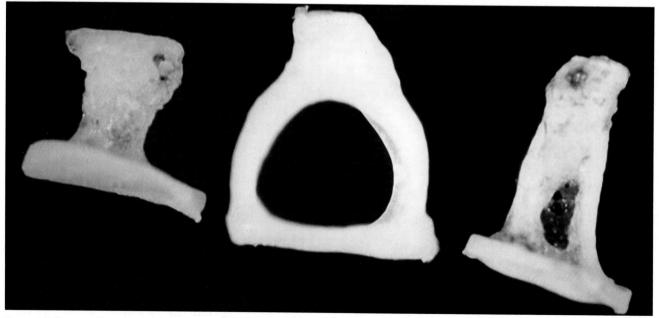

Figure 4 Different malformations of the stapes

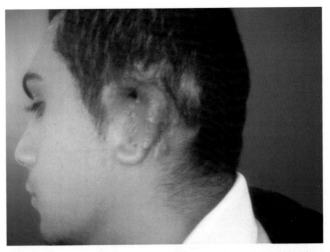

Figure 5 External auditory canal and auricular framework do not coincide in position

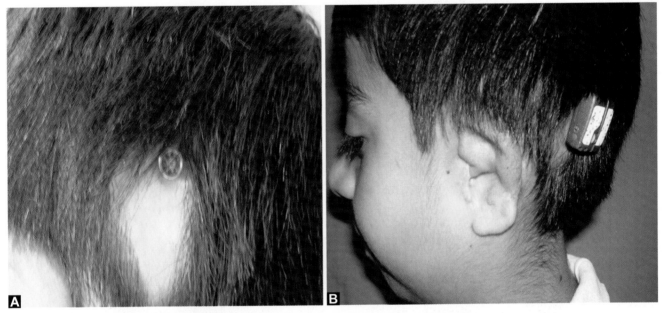

Figures 6A and B Pedestal of the BAHA and Processor

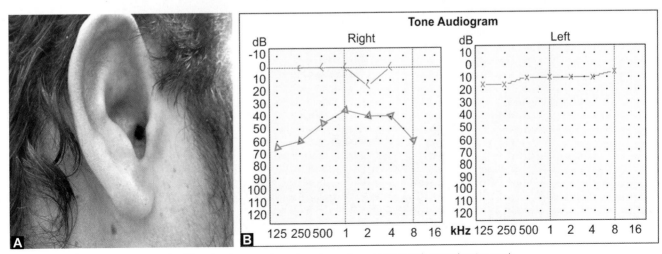

Figures 7A and B Postoperative results of functional surgery. A good meatus and ear canal but with a poor hearing result

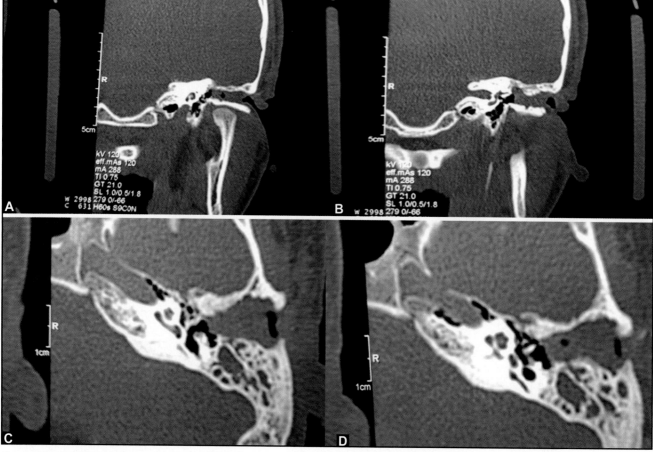

Figures 8A to D CAT scans showing failure of conventional surgery

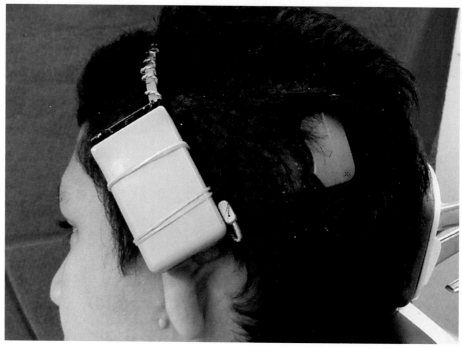

Figure 9 Comparison of the size of the bone vibrator that the patient used and the BAHA

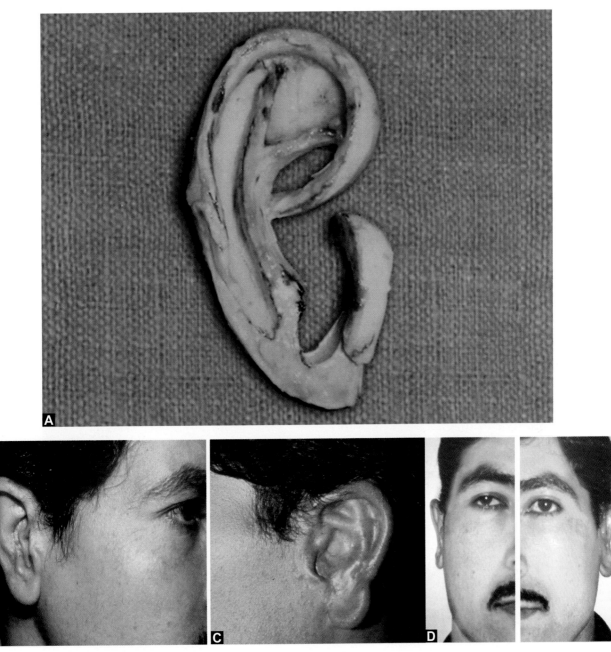

Figures 10A to D Cosmetic and functional reconstruction

ties. At present, we do not have enough follow-up to provide results in mid- and long-term results.

In unilateral cases, there are authors that delay surgery until the patient can make his/her own decisions. We offer surgery at early age when we consider that there is a low risk like in the case of minor malformations, where we can perform a safe surgical procedure with the consent of the parents.

In cases of unilateral major abnormalities, we consider that the patient should make the decision as an adult, once the pros and cons have been described and evaluated.

The reconstruction of EAC atresia with microtia requires many surgical steps:

1. Development of an auricular framework and rotation of the lobule (Figures 11 and 12).

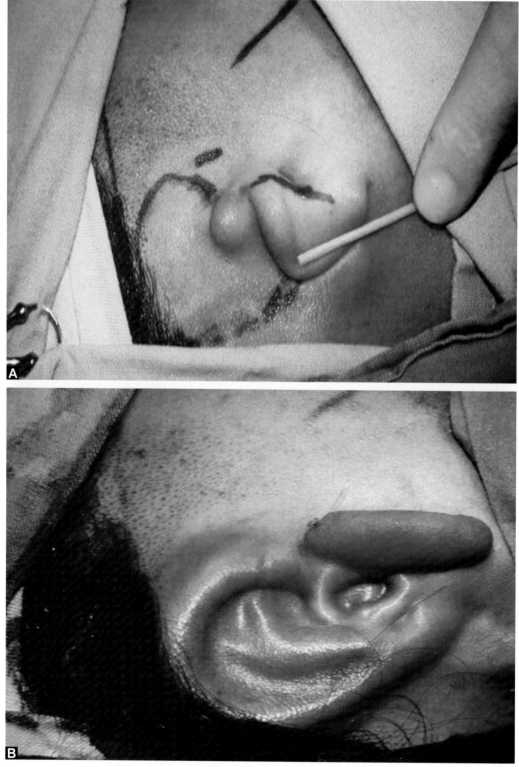

Figures 11A and B Placement of the auricular framework

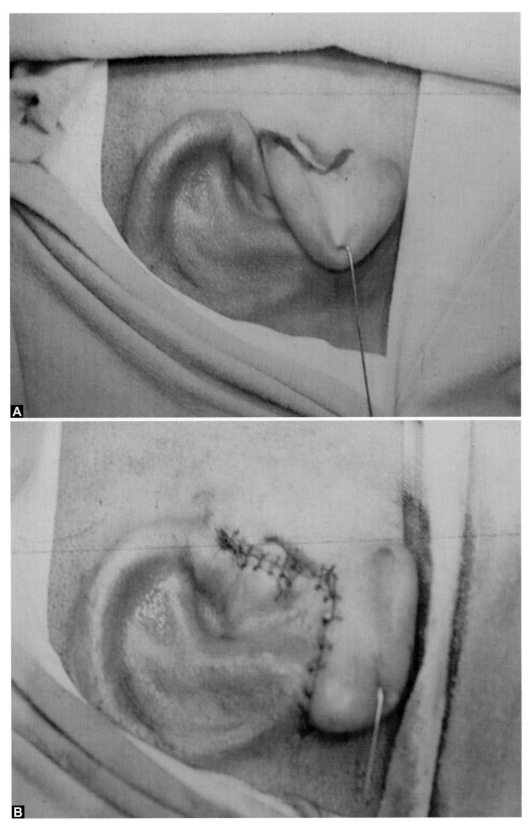

Figures 12A and B Rotation of the lobule

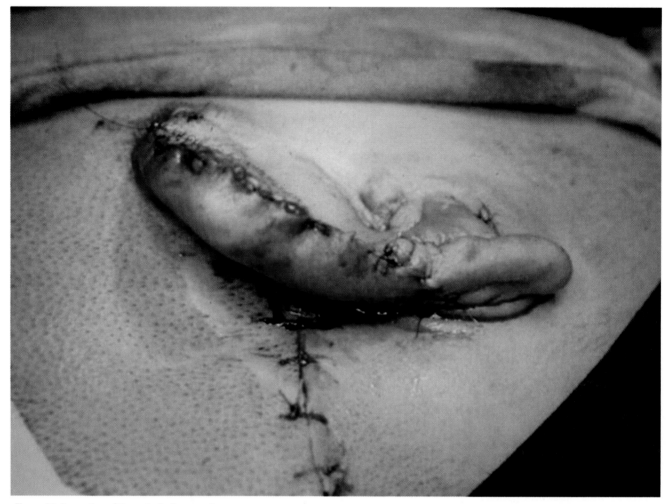

Figure 13 Separation of the auricular framework

2. Functional step with the creation of a new EAC, tympanoplasty and meatoplasty.
3. Release of the auricular framework (Figure 13).
4. Formation of the tragus, deepening of the concha.

These steps or stages are done with a difference of four months. We will first describe the cosmetic steps and then the functional steps.

RECONSTRUCTION OF THE AURICLE

In relation to formation of the auricular framework, we have had important stages of development and learning. Among these we have the four reconstructive stages developed in the 80s by Burt Brent.[19,20] In the 90s, Satoru Nagata developed two reconstructive stages and precise techniques in the development of the cartilaginous framework.[21] At the beginning of this century, Francoise Firmin surprised us by giving more impor-

tance to the quality of the skin coverage, anatomical details of the cartilaginous framework and a simple classification of the skin approaches.[22]

One of the most difficult anatomical structures to create is the auricle because it has a complex framework with grooves and creases that are hard to emulate, such as the helix, antihelix, triangular and scaphoid fossa, tragus, etc. Many materials have been proposed, e.g. silicon, proplast, homologous cartilage, etc. However, only homologous cartilage has provided good long-term results. We prefer costal cartilage at the level of synchondrosis of the sixth to ninth ribs (Figures 14A to D).

The costal cartilage can be ipsilateral or contralateral. The aim is to have enough cartilage to reproduce a three-dimensional anatomic framework. The incision in the thorax is done horizontally, following the lines of Langer. Intense pain postoperatively is due to incision on the rectus anterior muscle of the abdomen. We separate the muscle from the fascia and on occasions we

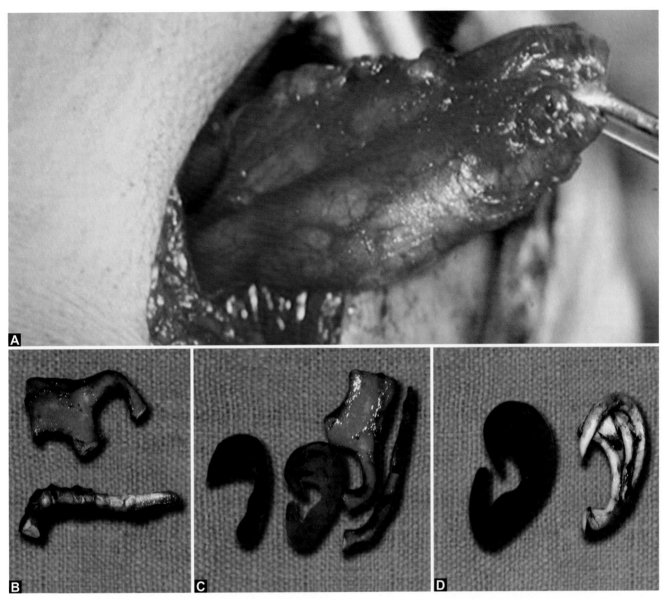

Figures 14A to D Obtaining costal cartilage and making the auricular framework

disinsert it in the upper (cephalic) portion and move it to the midline, thus removing cartilage without damaging the muscle. We are very careful not to cut at the level of osteocartilaginous junction in order not to interfere with thoracic growth.

The age of the reconstruction is determined by the thoracic perimeter of around 60 cm. We obtain a mold or framework of the contralateral ear or from a close relative (anthropometrically similar) in bilateral cases. The framework is divided into four parts: the base, helix, antihelix, and the tragus-antitragus. We bring them together with 3-0 or 4-0 prolene with sufficient sutures in order to have a firm framework. We then evaluate the skin (alopecic) that we have and use Dr Firmin's classification

in order to determine the surgical approach: Type 1—z-plasty, rotating the lobule; Type 2—an incision through the auricular remnant, using it to cover the inferior third of the framework; Type 3—incision in a strategic place when the ear is of an almost normal size, but with an abnormal contour, or when there are no auricular remnants.

Once the framework is done, it is placed subcutaneously in an appropriate position. The contralateral ear is used as reference and we measure the distance from root of the helix to canthus of the eye and the inclination of the nasal dorsum. Suction is generated with syringes and #8 suctions (we use feeding tubes) thus, avoiding formation of seromas, hematomas, or dead spaces for 4–6 days allowing the skin to adhere to the framework, while reproducing the anatomical details of the framework (Figures 15 and 16). Six months after the first surgery the framework is lifted in order to form the new auriculocephalic crease.

FUNCTIONAL STAGE

The functional stage consists of creating a new EAC with removal of the atretic plate and re-establishment of the conduction mechanisms by means of tympanoplasty procedures. Skin grafts are used to cover the new ear canal and meatoplasty.

There are two types of approaches to the middle ear:

1. The transmastoid approach through which the antrum is approached, and then the aditus and antrum until reaching the middle ear (Figure 17).
2. The anterior approach that approaches the ossicular chain through the epitympanum (Figure 18).

In the transmastoid approach we use an approach that is posterior to the middle ear and the atretic plate. Dissection starts by using the anterior wall of the mastoid as a reference, the linea temporalis from above, and the angle in between both structures, which is the center of the fossa cribrosa where the drilling is done. The tegmen and sinodural angle are used as references. By following them medially, the antrum is reached and the horizontal semicircular canal is identified. The canal is at times abnormal, being flattened and at the same level of the second portion of the facial nerve. Thus, the nerve must be monitorized and identified at this stage. The atretic plate must be carefully removed with a diamond burr in order to avoid acoustic trauma to the inner ear by vibration. The disadvantage of this approach is the creation of an open mastoid cavity. We use this technique occasionally, when we are not able to reach the middle ear directly.

In the majority of cases we use the anterior approach. This approach consists of removing the atretic plate in order to reach the middle ear. The dissection is initiated in the linea temporalis, immediately posterior to the temporomandibular joint. In this approach, the mastoid air cells are not opened and the posterior wall of the new EAC is left intact. In this technique, the references are the tegmen (superiorly) and the glenoid fossa (anteriorly). These are followed medially through the atretic

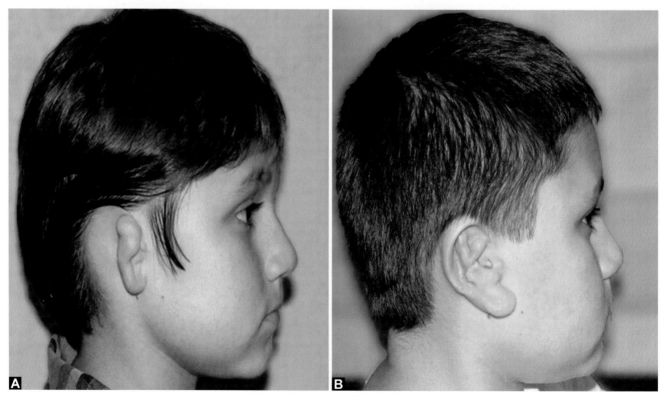

Figures 15A and B Pre (A) and post op (B) of auricular reconstruction

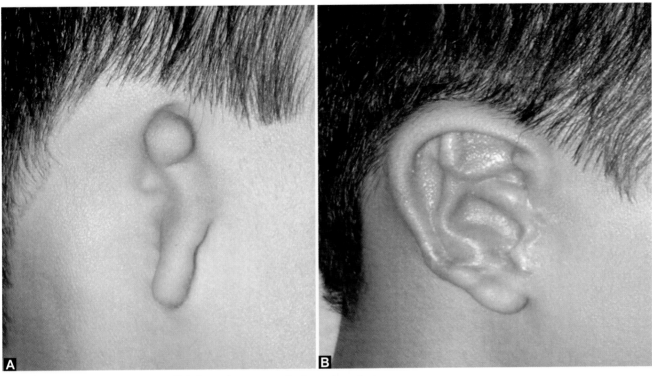

Figures 16A and B Pre (A) and post op of (B) of auricular reconstruction in another patient

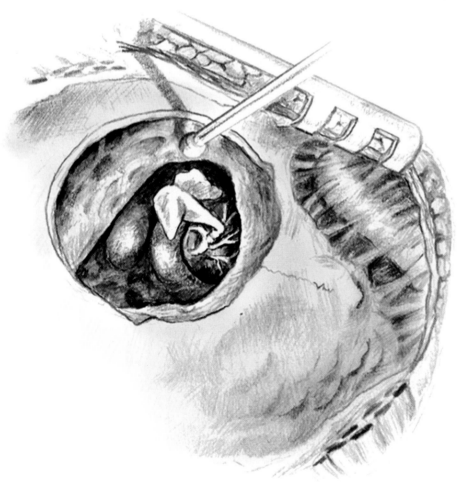

Figure 17 Transmastoid approach

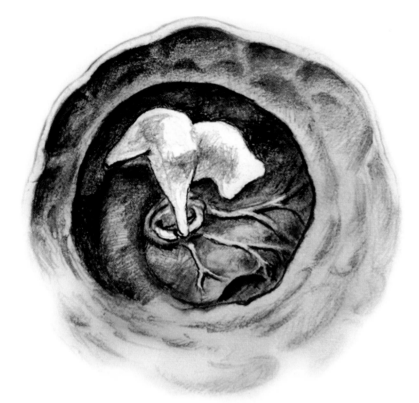

Figure 18 Anterior approach

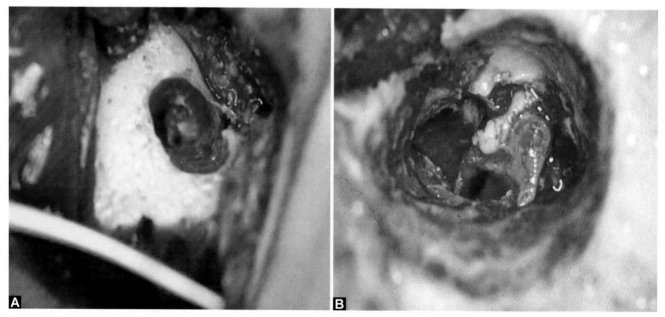

Figures 19A and B Removal of atretic plate

plate up to the epitympanum, allowing identification of the ossicular complex (Figures 19A and B). This approach avoids harming the facial nerve in its vertical portion, which is medial to the ossicular complex.

After removing the atretic plate, the mobility of the ossicular chain is evaluated. Particular attention should be given to

stapes. In general, hearing results are better when the ossicles are respected, as long as there is continuity between them, even if they are malformed. However, in cases of discontinuity, reconstruction has to be done (e.g. with interpositions). On rare occasions, we use PORPS or TORPS made of alloplastic materials. We use temporalis fascia to create a new tympanic membrane and then place it directly over the ossicles. In order to avoid lateralization, we drill a small bony groove anteriorly and when there is no malleus handle, the fascia is incised with two parallel incisions from the center to the periphery, developing a belt that is placed under the long process of the incus and rotated over it, while the middle ear is sealed with the rest of the tissue.

The final step consists in covering the exposed mastoid or the new ear canal with skin grafts obtained from the internal part of the arm or thigh. The canal is packed with a silastic button medially, followed by Gelfoam® and umbilical tape saturated with antibiotics in order to maintain the skin in place (Figures 20A and B) and finally the meatoplasty (Figure 21).

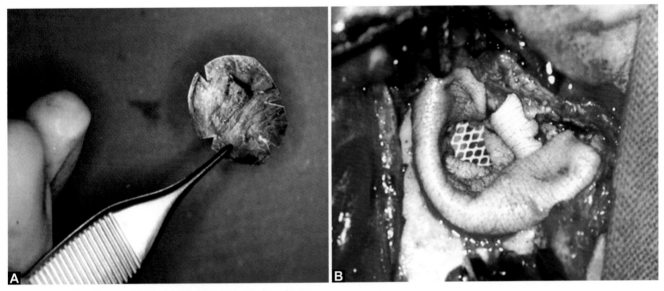

Figures 20A and B Placement of temporalis fascia skin and silastic button

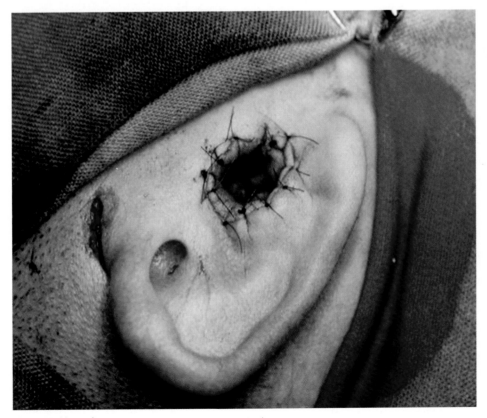

Figure 21 Meatoplasty

Surgical Techniques in Cases in which we Use BAHA

Placement of the BAHA in one surgical stage: After shaving 10 cm of the area of hair implantation, the patient is placed in a supine position, the usual skin preparation is done and the area where the screw will be placed is marked. This area is 5.5–6 cm pos-terosuperior to the posterior wall of the temporomandibular joint (Figures 22A and B). A rectangular area of 24 x 30 mm is marked with methylene blue and the area is then elevated as a pedicled flap of partial thickness (Figures 23A to C) either with a dermatome or a scalpel. The soft subcutaneous tissues are removed until reaching the pericranium and the periosteum is elevated. Drilling is done for screw placement (Figures 24A

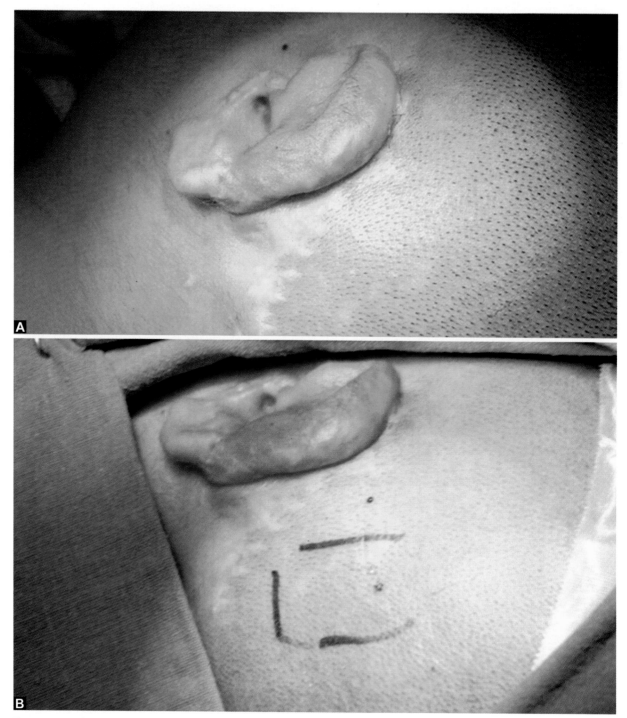

Figures 22A and B Anatomical site for the location of the flap

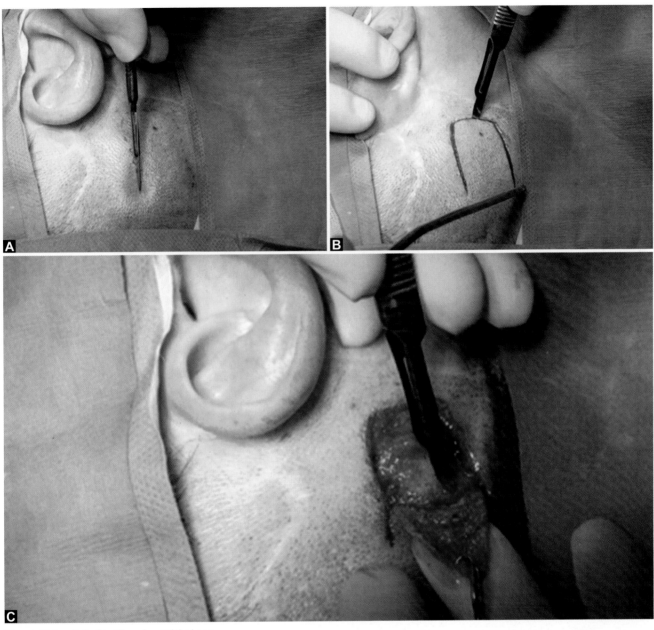

Figures 23A to C Pedicled flap of partial thickness

to C), with a 3 mm and 4 mm burr, respecting the inner table. The titanium screw is placed (Figures 25A and B) and the flap is fixed with sutures fixing skin and periosteum (Figures 26A and B). A skin punch is used in order to expose the screw (Figures 27A and B). A gauze saturated with antibiotics is placed around the pedestal of the screw and a silastic protector is placed (Figure 28).

Placement of the BAHA in two surgical steps: The following variations are done:

- Burrs and screws of 3 mm are used
- Drilling can traverse the inner table and the screw can be in contact with the dura
- The first surgical stage concludes with the reposition of the flap
- After 4 months of osteointegration, the second stage is performed.

At this stage the skin is perforated (skin punch) around the screw and the pedestal is placed (Figures 29A to F).

COMPLICATIONS

The two main potentially serious complications in surgery for atresia are sensorineural hearing loss and facial nerve paralysis. However, the most common ones are meatal and EAC stenosis, chronic infection, graft failure and conductive hearing loss. The majority of these complications can be avoided with meticulous technique.

POSTOPERATIVE CARE

The first check-up in functional surgery is done between the eighth and tenth postoperative day. It consists of removal of the external dressing. If part of the ear packing is adherent, it must be "softened" with hydrogen peroxide (10 volumes) until it loosens up. Analgesics and antimicrobials, such as second generation cephalosporins are used as long as there is packing in place.

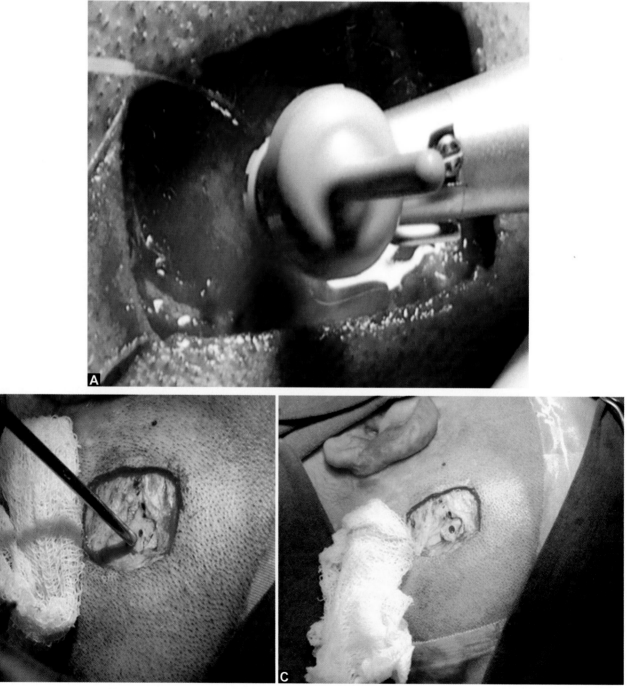

Figures 24A to C Preparation of the site for titanium screw placement

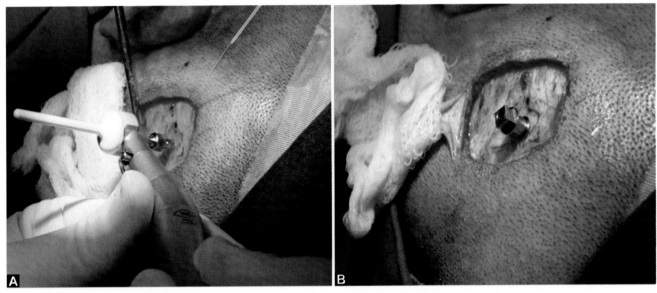

Figures 25A and B Placement of the titanium post

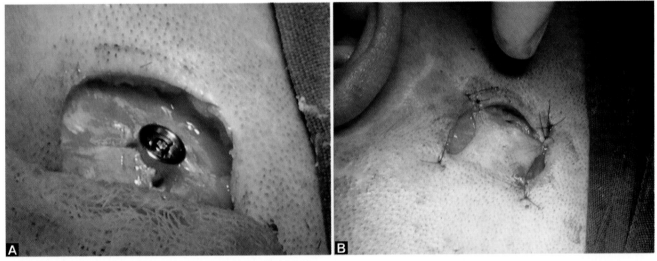

Figures 26A and B Pedestal has been placed and the flap is repositioned

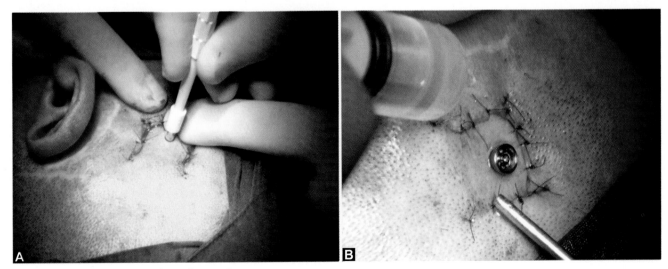

Figures 27A and B Opening in order to allow coupling

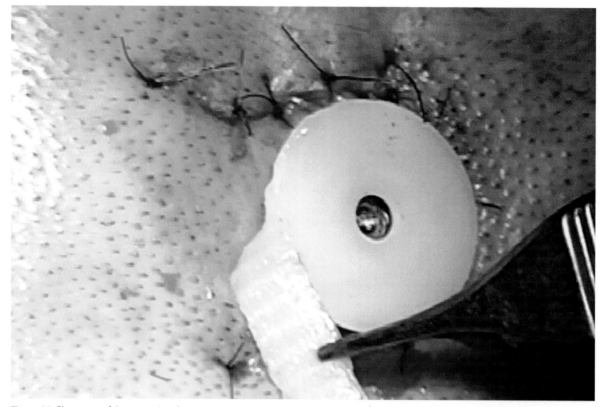

Figure 28 Placement of the protection device

During the first month, there is no suctioning over the grafts. Small moist (saline) cotton balls can be used for cleansing.

Sutures from the meatus and from the incisions are removed after 10–12 days.

In BAHA cases, the first cleansing is done after 5 days and the condition of the flap is checked.

OUR INSTITUTIONAL EXPERIENCE

Our experience consists of 190 cases operated upon between 1978 and 2009, and are divided into a first stage from 1978 to 1991 with 47 patients who were operated with different techniques, and a second stage from 1992 to present who were operated upon with standardized technique. These were 131 patients and in 22 we did the auricular framework and the functional surgery in one surgical stage. From 2007 to 2009 we placed BAHA in 12 patients.

In the patients subjected to functional surgery, the youngest was 5 years old and the oldest 48 years old. Fifty-one percent were 5–10 years old, 27% were 11–15 years old, 13% were between 16–20, and 9% over 20 years. Fifty-one percent had bilateral involvement, while 49% were unilateral. Fifty-five percent had atresia and 45% had stenosis. In relation to the radiologic point scale of Martin and Soda: 14% (8 points) were

excellent, 35% (7 points) very good, 35% (6 points) good, 43% (5 points) regular, and 4% (4 points) were poor. The poor cases were operated upon because they had cholesteatoma.

Congenital stenosis of the EAC predisposes to cholesteatoma. The destructive changes secondary to cholesteatoma start showing up during adolescence. These lesions can be significant, if they go undiagnosed. Cole recommends surgery for all cases of stenosis that measure 2 mm or less in order to avoid irreversible damage and complications.[23]

In this group, 12 patients had cholesteatoma and had congenital stenosis. The audiological results based in pure tone audiometry. In frequencies of 500 Hz, 1000 Hz, and 2000 Hz, they had an average gain of 29.8 dB in the first group (first stage) and 32.4 dB in the second group. These results are similar to those reported by other authors. Schuknecht reported a 30 dB improvement in 50% of patients followed for 5.5 years. Teufert and de la Cruz[24] in a six month follow-up noted that 53% had a conductive deficit of 20 dB or less. Jahrsdoerfer[25] reported that 65% had an average of 30 dB or less with follow-up of 8 years. Lambert[26] reported that 67% had a level of 30 dB at one year.

The most common complication is restenosis of the EAC. This alters the audiological results and has been reported in 7%, 15% and 31% in different series.[9,27]

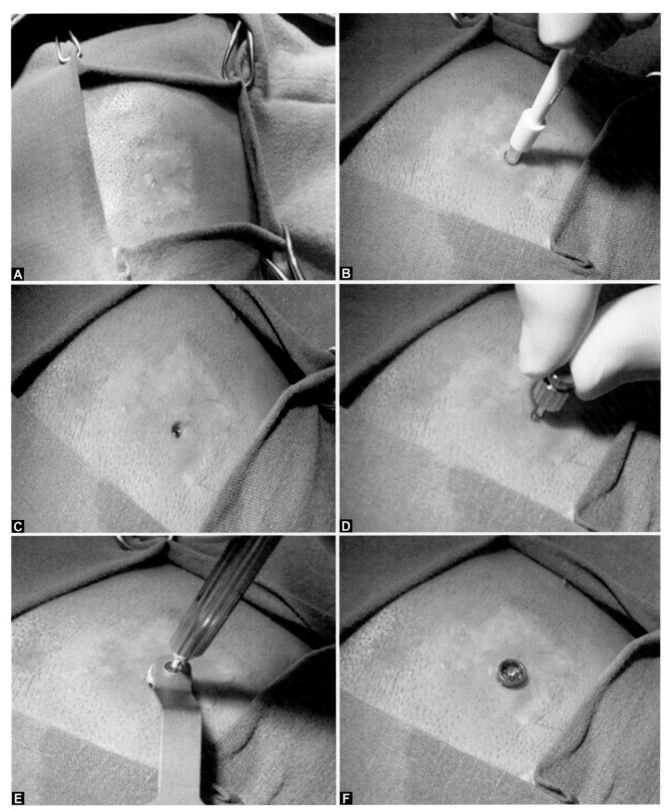

Figures 29A to F BAHA second step. Four months after the first

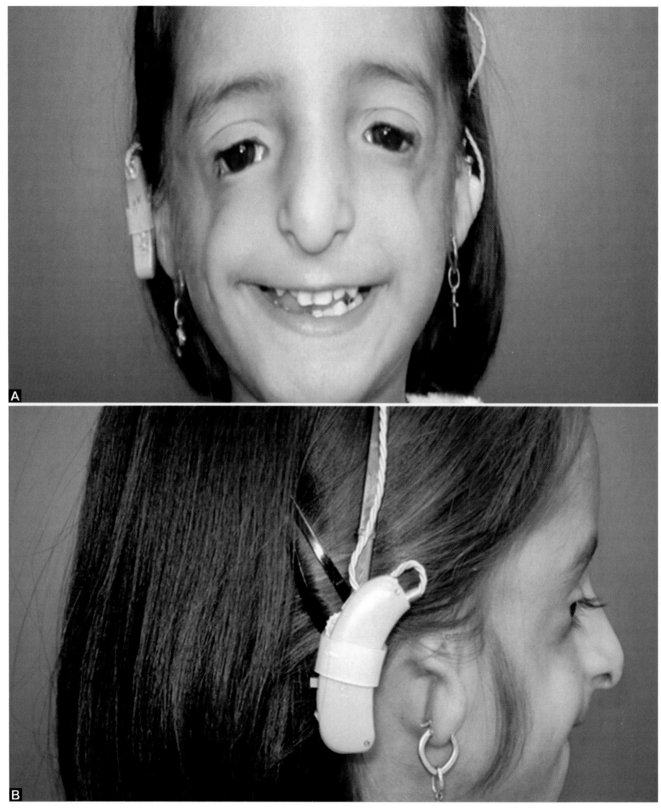

Figures 30A and B Treacher Collins syndrome

Section V

Middle Ear and Mastoid Surgery

Adriana Severina, Alejandro Rivas, Alejo Suárez, Andréa Felice dos Santos, Angel Lede Barreiro, Angel Ramos, Axel Christensen, Bernard Ars, Carlos Curet, Carlos Ruah, Carlos Sttot C, Carlos Young, Claudia Romani, Edgar Chiossone Lares, Elisa Gil-Carcedo, Enrique Valenzuela, Ernesto Ried G Jr, Ernesto Ried Undurraga Sr, Fábio André Selaimen, Fernando Mendonca, Gloria Ribalta, Gonzalo Bonilla, Hamlet Suárez, Héctor Rondón Cardoso, Joel Lavinsky, Jorge Caro Letelier, Jorge E Spratley, José Antonio Rivas, José Miguel Contreras, Juan A Chiossone Kerdal, Leticia Petersen, Luis María Gil-Carcedo, Luis Ángel Vallejo, Luis Dentone, Luis Henrique Motta, Luiz Lavinsky, Manuel Bernal, Marcelo Hueb, Marcos V Goycoolea, Marcus D Atlas, Mauricio A Cohen, Mauricio Noschang da Silva, Michael Gluth, Michael M Paparella, Michelle Lavinsky, Miguel Aristegui, Miguel Caballero Borrego, Mirko Tos, Nicolás Albertz, Primitivo Ortega, Rafael Urquiza, Raquel Levy, Ricardo F Bento, Ricardo Larrea, Ricardo M Vaz, Richard Gacek, Rick Fox, Rodrigo Posada Trujillo, Sady Selaimen da Costa, Santiago Arauz, Sten Hellstrom, Timothy K Jung, Ugo Fisch, Victor Slavutsky, Viviana Orellana

5.1.1

Exploratory Tympanotomy

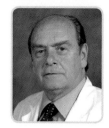

Marcos Goycoolea

GENERAL CONCEPTS

The exploratory tympanotomy (exploration of the middle ear cavity) is highlighted in this chapter as an extremely helpful and innocuous diagnostic and often, therapeutic procedure. As an integral part of a tympanoplasty, it is therapeutic. Used in the presence of an intact tympanic membrane when a diagnosis of ear disease is in doubt, it is diagnostic. This exploration can be performed as a transcanal procedure (when suspected disease is limited to the middle ear) or as an endaural procedure (when suspected disease involves the attic or mastoid, or both). The tympanotomy can be done under local or general anesthesia (depending on the case) and can be used under many different clinical circumstances, such as in cases of unexplained conductive hearing loss and occasional sensorineural hearing losses (for example, if there is suspicion of perilymphatic fistulae) or when the presence of adhesions or a loculated middle ear effusion is suspected. This chapter discusses the use of the exploratory tympanotomy for possible perilymphatic fistulae and for tympanic neurectomy. The essential concept is that exploratory tympanotomy, which can be used routinely as a safe and simple diagnostic procedure for a variety of middle ear conditions is also potentially therapeutic.

EXPLORATORY TYMPANOTOMY FOR PERILYMPHATIC FISTULA

Perilymphatic fistulae have no consistent pathognomonic signs. Although some patients may have clearly suggestive symptoms, such as hearing fluctuations associated with vestibular disturbances, tinnitus, and a positive fistula test, more often than not the symptoms are isolated and require a high degree of suspicion on the part of the surgeon.

Fistulae can involve the round window or oval window, or both, and at times even the lateral semicircular canal. They can be caused by implosive or explosive forces; thus they are not entities by themselves but manifestations of an underlying or causative problem. Fistulae caused by granulation tissue, cholesteatoma and other factors constitute different clinical entities from those discussed here; they are described in different chapters and can involve structures other than the oval and round windows.

Round window fistulae do not necessarily imply a flow of perilymph as an essential element for the diagnosis. Since the approximate average volumes of perilymph and endolymph are 78.3 µl and 2.76 µl respectively, "a free flow of perilymph from the round window" or "a free flow of endolymph after

opening the endolymphatic sac" can only be accounted for by other explanations. Free "fluid" gushing from the round window is not perilymph but cerebrospinal fluid and requires a patent cochlear aqueduct and modiolus. At the same time, when this anatomic pathway is not present there is no "free flow," although a fistula still exists.

Procedure

Local or general anesthesia can be used. Exploratory tympanotomy flaps and entrance into the middle ear beneath the annulus have been described in previous sections. The posterior canal is lowered with curettes or burrs in order to clearly visualize the round and oval windows. (If involvement of the lateral semicircular canal is suspected, an endaural approach is preferred).

The middle ear cavity, including both windows, is completely inspected. It should be noted whether the round window membrane is visible or in a covered position in the niche. It is also important to distinguish the membrane itself from mucosal folds in the niche (the so-called "false membrane").

A fistula may be obvious at this point (Figure 1A). If not, the ossicular chain is mobilized and gently palpated and the windows are observed for leaks. The presence or absence of a round window reflex (when mobilizing the ossicular chain) is to be noted; if the window is not visible, a few drops of saline solution can be placed in the niche in order to observe such a reflex. In the presence of obvious leaks or if the reflex is absent, a patch of connective tissue (collagen or fat) is placed over the window and reinforced with Gelfoam® (Figure 1B). We have evaluated the use of connective tissue as a seal for the round window and it works nicely resulting in a great seal that remains

in place. (The round window membrane is three-layered, with a central layer of connective tissue.) In unclear cases, small pieces of Gelfoam® are used to cover such areas since small fistulae may not be visually evident. (If the procedure is being done under local anesthesia, the patient can be asked to perform Valsalva's maneuver).

The flaps are repositioned, the ear canal is packed and a dressing is applied.

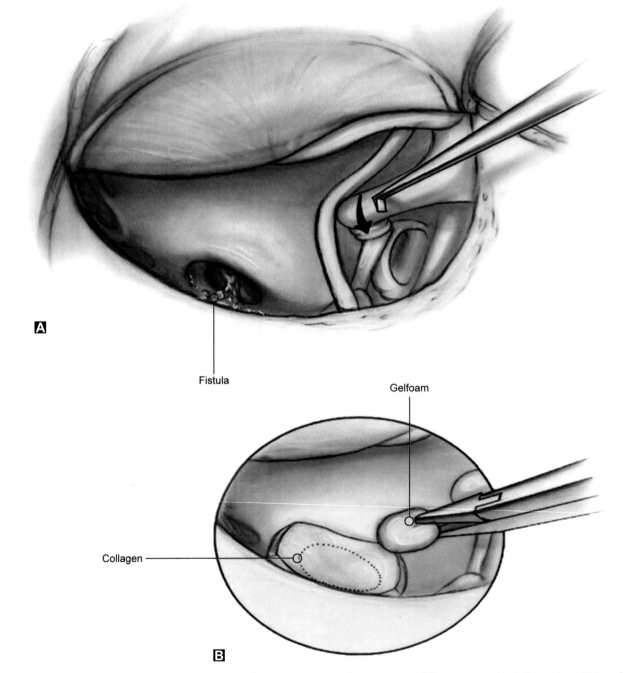

Figures 1A and B Exploratory tympanotomy for perilymphatic fistula. (A) Fistula seen after inspecting middle ear cavity and both the windows; (B) A patch of connective tissue (collagen or fat) is placed over the window and reinforced with Gelfoam®

5.1.2

Anterior Bony Overhang

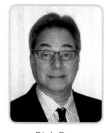

Rick Fox

Aim

An essential part of performing a tympanoplasty is complete visualization of the entire tympanic membrane and annulus. A frequently encountered problem at the time of surgery is blockage of the anterior tympanic membrane by an anterior canal wall bony overhang. Failure to achieve complete exposure will compromise surgical results.

Highlights

- Proper vasoconstriction
- Adequate patient positioning
- Availability of correct drills
- Protect canal skin flap
- Complete removal of debris and bone dust

Pitfalls

- Breaching the temporomandibular joint
- Tearing or drilling skin flap
- Failure to remove bone dust and debris
- Drilling on tympanic membrane

Procedure

The patient is prepped in a sterile fashion, usually under general anesthesia. The ear canal is injected with 1% lidocaine with 1:100,000 or 1:200,000 epinephrine.

A choice of two anterior skin flaps may be used either medially based or laterally based (anterior window shade), which may be elevated. In the medially based anterior canal skin flap begins with an incision at the bony cartilaginous junction and is then joined to the vertical incisions (Figures 1A and B). The anterior flap is thus elevated medially towards the annulus until all relevant bone is exposed (Figure 1B). Canal skin is gently elevated laterally with a curved round canal knife or duckbill elevator.

Anterior bone removal is carried out working in a lateral to medial direction always under direct vision using diamond drills (Figures 1C and D). When the bone has been maximally thinned, the area adjacent to the temporomandibular joint will appear bluish.[1] If the temporomandibular joint is inadvertently breached and is extracapsular, the anterior canal skin flap will suffice for coverage.

Special care must be taken to prevent injury to the delicate canal flap. This will be facilitated by coverage with silk gauze after positioning the flap as far as possible from the drill site.

The laterally based anterior skin flap, canal incisions are made at 6 o'clock and 12 o'clock positions, and connected by an incision 1–2 mm from the anterior annulus (Figure 2A). The canalplasty is carried out in a similar manner (Figure 2B).

Regardless of which technique is employed, it is essential to meticulously remove all bony fragments and bone dust to prevent future tissue reaction.

The thickest part of the anterior bony wall is superiorly towards the zygoma root and inferiorly toward the thick part of the tympanic ring. The degree of bone removal may be up to 5 mm in the anterior part of the canal bone and up to 13

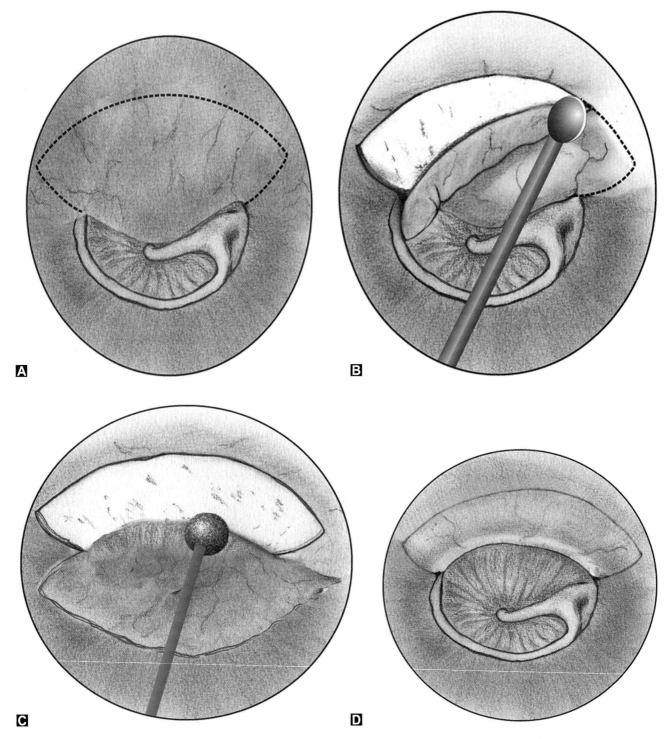

Figures 1A to D Medially based anterior canal skin flap elevation. (A) Incision made at the bony cartilaginous junction and then joined to the vertical incisions; (B and C) The anterior flap is elevated medially toward the annulus till all relevant bone is exposed; (D) The flaps must be carefully repositioned after the procedure

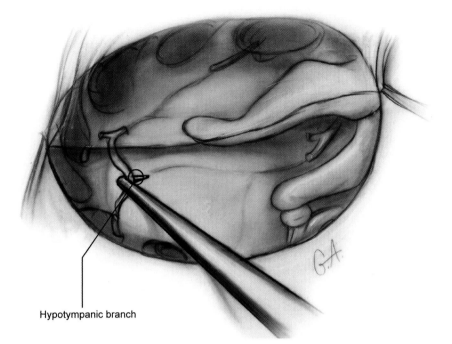

Figure 1C

Figures 1A to C The tympanic nerve: Its origin and distribution

Hypotympanic branch

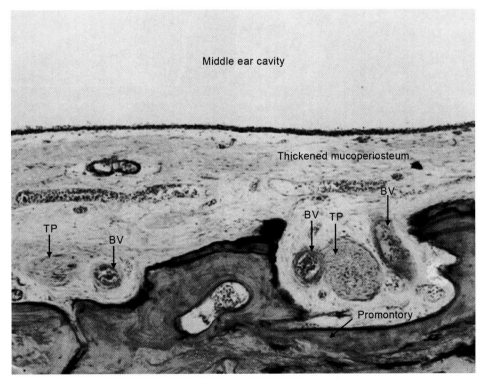

Middle ear cavity

Thickened mucoperiosteum

BV

BV TP

TP

BV

Promontory

Figure 2A

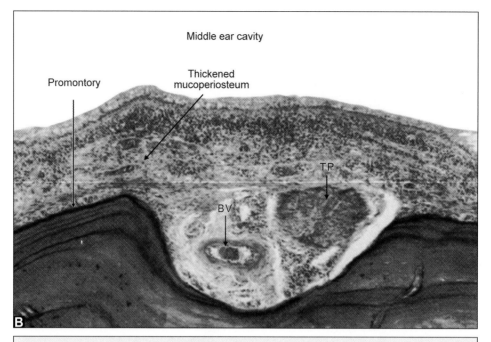

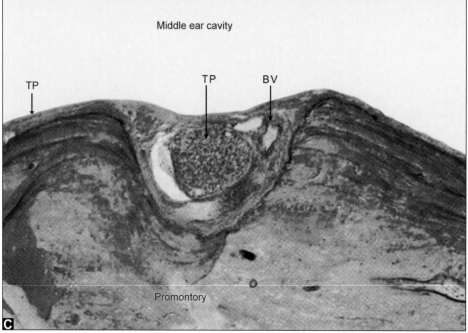

Figures 2B and C

Figures 2A to C Photomicrographs of horizontal sections of temporal bones show the nerves of the tympanic plexus (TP), accompanied by their corresponding blood vessels (BV) in bony canals within the promontory. Additionally, figures are showing a thickened mucoperiosteum overlying the promontory, making identification of these grooves very difficult. The surgeon must "peel" this mucoperiosteum

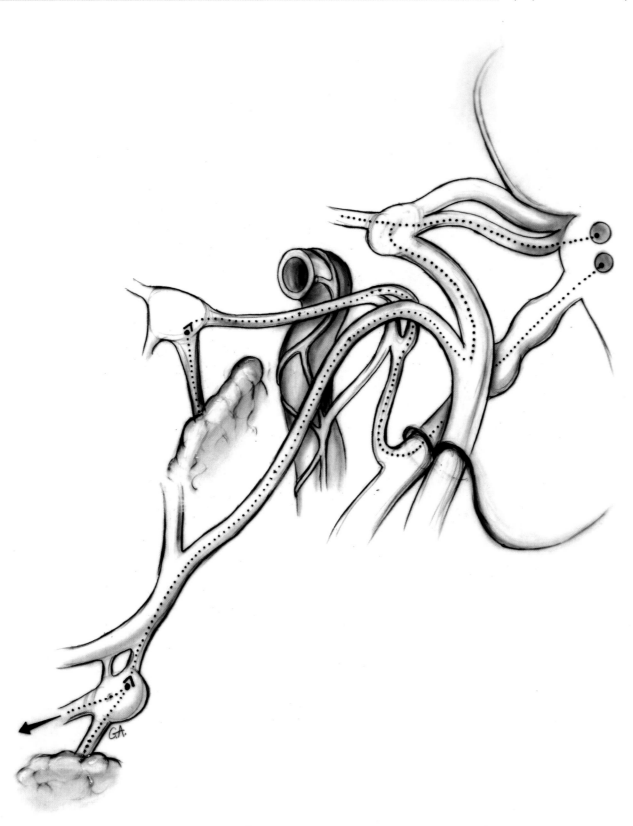

Figure 3 Caroticotympanic canaliculi (located anteriorly), incorporating sympathetic branches from the internal carotid plexus

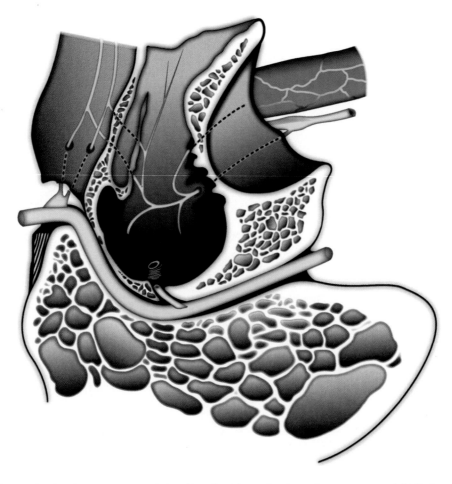

Figure 4 Jacobson´s neurectomy: surgical position of a right ear that shows the emergence and distribution of the tympanic plexus

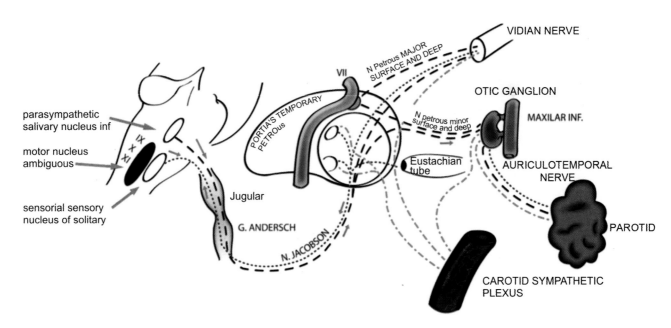

Figure 5 Tympanic neurectomy: schematic drawing of the anatomy of Jacobson´s nerve

5.1.4

The Use of Otic Drops and Antiseptics in Otologic Surgery

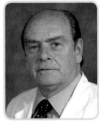

Marcos Goycoolea

Since otic drops and antiseptics that are commonly used in otology have a potential for ototoxicity, it is essential to review the evidences available in order to develop rational means of avoiding these complications. Ototoxicity due to these agents involves the concept that in specific circumstances, when placed in the middle ear, some of the components of these preparations can reach the inner ear and cause sensory damage.

AIMS

1. To review the evidences available for ototoxicity due to ear drops and antiseptics.
2. To develop an understanding of the pathophysiology.
3. To develop rational means of prevention and treatment in order to try to avoid this potential complication.

MAIN QUESTIONS AND CONCERNS

1. Can substances placed in the middle ear reach the inner ear?

It is well established that substances placed in the middle ear can be recovered in perilymph (directly or indirectly) and/or observed to cause morphologic inner ear changes, and/or noted to cause detectable neurophysiologic changes, and/or can be localized in the perilymph, cochlea, vestibular labyrinth and endolymphatic sac.[1,2] In fact, pharmacologic labyrinthectomy (placement of vestibulotoxic drugs through a ventilation tube); one of the established treatment modalities for severe Meniére´s disease is based on the passage of these substances from middle to inner ear.

2. Which are the potential pathways and the passage (permeability) factors?

Possible routes from middle to inner ear include round and oval windows, bony fistulas, microfissures, blood and/or lymph vessels. Bony fistulas, microfissures and oval window do not seem to play a role, and lymphatics, which are abundant in the round window membrane, seem to participate in a peripheral rather than in a central direction. This is because the inner ear is of neurectodermal origin, therefore, it should not have prominent lymphatic conduits.[1] Blood vessels are an important route to consider (which requires further investigation) because of the abundant vascular connections between the middle and inner ear in the round window.[1,3,4]

The predominant pathway and the most evaluated (I have dedicated 25 years of research to this subject) seems to be the round window membrane. This membrane is the only soft tissue barrier between the middle and inner ear. It is located inferiorly in the medial wall of the middle ear and lies in a niche, being therefore susceptible to exposure by fluids in the middle ear cavity.

Ultrastructural studies of the round window membrane of humans, monkeys, felines and rodents have disclosed three basic layers: (1) an outer epithelium; (2) a middle core of connective tissue; and (3) an inner epithelium. Despite being formed by three layers, experimental evidence has suggested that it behaves like a semipermeable membrane. Such evidence suggests that the layers of the round window participate in resorption and secretion of substances to and from the inner ear. Different substances, including antibiotics and tracers, when placed in the middle ear traverse the membrane. Permeability is selective. Factors affecting permeability include size, concentration, electrical charge, thickness of the membrane and facilitating agents.[5,6] (histological evidences are described in "Permeability of the round window membrane" under Section VI).

3. Which components of commonly used ear drops which when placed in the middle ear have been demonstrated to pass to the inner ear?

Components of commonly used ear drops, which when placed experimentally in the round window niche have been detected directly or indirectly in the inner ear and are listed in Table 1.[6,7]

Table 1 Components of commonly used ear drops which can be detected directly or indirectly in the inner ear after placing them experimentally in the round window niche[8,20]

Antibiotics	Solvents	Corticosteroids	Local anesthetics	Antiseptics
Chloramphenicol	Propylene glycol	Hydrocortisone	Lidocaine	Acetic acid
Ciprofloxacin		Betamethasone		Ethanol
Gentamicin				
Neomycin				
Polimyxin B				

Components of commonly used ear drops, which when placed in the middle ear of humans have been reported to cause an effect in the inner ear and are listed in Table 2.[9,10]

4. Are there evidences to suggest which of these ear drop components, when instilled transtympanically, can be toxic or nontoxic to the inner ear?

I. Evidences available from experimental animal studies

Chloramphenicol, neomycin and polymyxin B have been shown to cause hair cell damage.[1,7,11] Installation of gentamicin[11,12] has also resulted in labyrinthine changes. On the other hand, ciprofloxacin traverses the membrane from middle to inner ear and seems to be nontoxic.[13] Local anesthetics diffuse across the round window membrane and can act as facilitating agents for an increase in permeability.[1,14] In addition, it is a well established clinical fact that local anesthetics instilled in the middle ear of patients can cause significant vertigo.

Propylene glycol has not only been shown to be ototoxic, but also causes significant inflammatory reactions in the middle ear mucosa.[15]

Antiseptics that are used in ear surgery, such as chlorhexidine, povidone iodine scrub and ethanol can also cause labyrinthine changes and they are listed in Table 3.[6,7]

Dexamethasone, hydrocortisone and methylprednisolone have been also documented to traverse the round window membrane.[10] When used intratympanically in humans (for the treatment of inner ear disorders), methylprednisolone and dexamethasone[10,16] appear to be safe.

II. Evidences available from human clinical studies

Non otitis media cases (normal membranes): Gentamicin has well known toxic effects in the inner ear. When this drug is placed transtympanically (in normal middle ears), its effects are manifested in the inner ear. This has been extensively documented and is so well established that it is currently used as a standard form of therapy for severe Meniére´s disease. Similar findings have been reported with streptomycin.[1]

Otitis media cases: There are at least 9 reports totaling 165 documented patients who have developed sensorineural hearing loss due to the use of otic drops for otitis media.[9] Moreover, in a survey that comprised 2,235 otolaryngologists, 3.4% reported having seen irreversible cochlear damage due to otic drops.[17] If each of these otolaryngologists would have seen at least 1 case, this would represent 76 additional cases.

5. The experimental permeability evidence presented so far represents studies in normal membranes and middle ears. Is it valid for otitis media cases?

The round window membrane in otitis media undergoes the same histopathological changes than the mucoperiosteum of the middle ear mucosa (it is part of it). These changes are suggestive that in early stages, there may be an increase in permeability but that, as the inflammatory process develops, the membrane becomes thicker and develops protective mechanisms in terms of decreased permeability. As the active inflammatory process decreases, so does the thickness and the protective mechanisms developed by the membrane. Experimental evidence in cats, chinchillas and guinea pigs, using tracers and neomycin has confirmed this suggestion.[5,7]

6. The experimental evidence available through animal studies is fine, however, what occurs in animals does not occur in humans and is not valid in the clinical setting?

I was of the same opinion when I started working on this subject (25 years ago). After all, clinical and experimental conditions differed, and the round window membrane was thicker in humans, decreasing gradually in monkeys, felines and rodents. In fact, the degree of passage of tracers was directly related to the thickness of the membrane, being higher in rodents and decreasing in felines and primates. In addition, the round window membrane is more exposed in animals and the degree of inner ear changes was always more significant in animals with thinner membranes. However, despite these differences, as time went by, two constant facts remained: (1) the thickness of the membranes was different, but the anatomical structure was the same; (2) the degree of passage and of inner ear changes differed, but passage and inner ear changes equally occurred in humans. When our systematic and progressive studies started including humans, and our observations started to be corroborated by clinical experience and clinical reports on

Table 2 Components of commonly used ear drops which when placed in the middle ear of humans have been reported to cause an effect in the inner ear[8,20]

Antibiotics	Local anesthetics
Chloramphenicol	Lidocaine
Framycetin	Corticosteroids
Gentamicin	Dexamethasone
Gramicidin	
Neomycin	
Polymyxin B	

Table 3 Antiseptics commonly used in surgery that have been reported to cause labyrinthine changes

Ethanol
Chlorhexidine
Povidone iodine scrub

the subject, I reached my current impression that is, "In round window membrane permeability studies, despite the differences in thickness and the differences between clinical and experimental conditions, what occurs in animals, for the most part occurs in humans, but with a lesser degree of severity." (What I have also learned is that research and clinical work are not opposed but complimentary).

7. Otologists have used otic drops in patients with draining ears with and without ventilating tubes for years, and cases of sensorineural hearing loss as a result of treatment are not seemingly common. How can we explain this discrepancy based on the multiple animal studies available which consistently show inner ear damage?

The apparent discrepancy between experimental studies and clinical reports is, in my opinion, only apparent. My impression is as follows:

Otitis media is an inflammatory process of the middle ear cavity, mastoid and Eustachian tube. It involves all anatomical structures and the mucoperiosteal layer that covers them.[18] The round window membrane as part of the lining of the middle ear is involved in this process. As this gradual reaction develops, the histopathological changes also involve the round window membrane. As they occur, the permeability of the membrane changes. Therefore, when we talk about passage of a substance through the membrane, it is essential to define at what stage of reactivity is the middle ear mucosa (the round window membrane included). In normal round window membranes, passage of tracers and ototoxic drugs to the inner ear is well established in animals and humans. As mentioned earlier, the clearest example in humans is transtympanic pharmacologic labyrinthectomy, where a vestibulotoxic drug (e.g. gentamicin) is instilled in the middle ear with the purpose of causing a toxic effect in the inner ear. Animal studies have shown that during an established active inflammatory process ("draining ears"), round window membrane permeability drastically decreases. This is possibly due to an increase in thickness of the membrane,

defensive mechanisms in the membrane[19] and dilution effects by the middle ear effusion. In my opinion, this is what happens in the cases of "draining ears" (which are seen by the physician once the active inflammatory process is already established). Therefore, in light of the available experimental evidence it comes to as a no surprise to me that in these cases, ototoxic drugs do not traverse the membrane and do not cause inner ear damage. Once the active inflammatory process decreases or subsides, the defensive mechanisms decrease and the membrane becomes more permeable. Moreover, if one reviews the clinical reports available (see question number 4), these tend to coincide with this explanation. Most of the reported cases are related to prolonged use of drops and/or in patients who continued their use once the drainage had subsided. That is to say, ototoxicity occurred once the active inflammatory process had subsided, the defensive mechanisms had decreased and the membrane had become more permeable.

The apparent discrepancy that there are multiple experimental studies showing ototoxicity due to ear drops, whereas in clinical studies these reports are virtually nonexistent, is also only apparent. If one reviews the number of experimental studies reported in ototoxicity due to ear drops in otitis media (<10 drops), these are less than those reported in clinical cases in humans.[9] The vast majority of experimental studies are reports in animals with normal middle ears. Moreover, if one compares the number of these reports with the published clinical studies in humans using vestibulotoxic drugs (normal human middle ears) the numbers are similar.

8. What do you do with your own patients?

1. Prophylactic use of otic drops when placing ventilation tubes in order to prevent or reduce postoperative infection: I seldom use them. For the most part (exceptions are beyond this chapter) we insert tubes after a prolonged course (21 days) of antibiotics at full dose (plus yoghurt with *Lactobacillus acidophilus* and/or *Saccharomyces boulardii*), since with this modality we reduce the need of insertion of tubes by 60%. The 40% that fail (and require insertion of tubes), uncommonly have an active infection. They usually have abundant seromucoid effusion. Prior to the procedure, we rinse the canal with an alcoholic iodine solution. Once the myringotomy is done, we "wash" the middle ear

with saline and diluted hydrogen peroxide and then insert a tube. If the effusion is cloudy, purulent or has a hemorrhagic component, we obtain a culture and additionally wash with ciprofloxacin drops. No other types of otic drops are used. We then prescribe 4–6 ciprofloxacin drops three times a day for 3 days and check the patient at the third day with the results of the cultures in hand. Depending on the culture and findings, an antibiotic (if needed) is prescribed. Our overall postoperative infection rate is 2%. It is to be mentioned that: (1) we are only discussing use of otic drops; our overall management of the patient and our conduct with adenoidectomy (essential in adequate treatment) are beyond the purpose of this chapter; (2) the 60% response to antibiotic treatment refers to "regular fluid ears" and does not include other stages of otitis media, such as atelectasis or membranes with retraction pockets.

2. Use of otic drops in patients with a perforation of the tympanic membrane or a ventilation tube and a draining ear: It is very important to establish that a draining ear in a patient with a ventilation tube is a totally different clinical entity than a chronic draining ear in a patient with a perforated tympanic membrane (chronic otitis media). Management is therefore, different. A patient with a ventilation tube and chronic drainage is considered as having chronic otitis media. A draining ear in a patient with ventilation tubes usually represents an acute exacerbation of an otitis media process or contamination by water (swimming, showering, etc.).

Exacerbations are treated primarily with systemic antibiotics, like for an acute otitis media; the drainage is suctioned periodically (every 3 days on the average) and topical drops of ciprofloxacin are used (4–6 drops three times a day). I doubt the effectiveness of the drops for these middle ear processes (in prophylaxis too) and the reason we use them (and suction the canal periodically) is mainly to cleanse the canal and avoid skin irritation by the middle ear secretions (on occasions we insuflate ciprofloxacin powder). By seeing the patient every 3 days we follow the process and the response very closely. On the other hand, in chronic draining ears, topical treatment is our main modality. If there is no response, a culture is obtained and antibiotics and drops are used according to the culture. If the culture is negative (not infrequently) the antibiotic is changed and we switch to gentamicin drops, since the chances of ototoxicity in an active infection are minimal. In our group, the patient is seen by one physician during the whole treatment. If the physician is out of town, the patient is followed by only one associate staff member. Unusual or unresponsive cases are seen by the group, however, the patient remains in the care

of one doctor. Neomycin-polymyxin drops are reserved only for external otitis. This classic combination has not been that useful in these or in our chronic otitis cases. In cases of drainage after water contamination, we treat them in the same manner. For prevention of this occurrence, we insist the use of ear plugs and a head band. The parents are instructed that if despite the use of plugs, definite water contamination occurs, they should use ciprofloxacin drops three times a day for 3 days regardless of the symptoms. In these cases, the ciprofloxacin (since there is no fluid pouring out, ciprofloxacin can reach the middle ear) and the water absorption capabilities of the vehicles seem to be useful.

3. Intraoperative use alone or with a Gelfoam® saturated with an otic preparation follows the same principles and conducts described in 1 and 2. We commonly do middle ear and mastoid washings with saline solutions and diluted hydrogen peroxide. They help us to cleanse debris and epithelial remanents as well as to remove biofilms. Following washings we use ciprofloxacin solution and in draining ears we might use gentamicin. However, if we leave Gelfoam® saturated with an antibiotic solution, the solution is always with ciprofloxacin. Ciprofloxacin is amazingly non-ototoxic. We have tested it in rodents again and again in Lars Lundman´s laboratory as well as in ours.

4. Antiseptics that are used to prepare the skin of the periauricular area and pinna in the operating room should be used with caution when there are tympanic membrane perforations. These solutions can be extremely ototoxic in a middle ear with a permeable round window membrane.[6,7]

5. A word of caution with local anesthetics, such as lidocaine. When these agents reach the middle ear and traverse to the inner ear, the patients might develop severe vertigo. If this occurs in the outpatient clinic, not uncommonly the symptoms are so severe that it might be necessary to admit the patient (a patient who went to the office for a "minor" procedure "under local anesthesia"). Intraoperatively one might be tempted to use it with epinephrine as a vasoconstricting agent only to have (on occasions and not always) an extremely vertiginous patient in the recovery room that does not respond that well to the usual medication (e.g. ondansetron, granisetron) and might require droperidol drip.

In addition to having a patient that feels miserable, a number of doubts ensue in terms of a possible vestibular damage secondary to the surgical procedure (e.g. in case of a stapedectomy). It is very useful to have a solution with diluted epinephrine and without anesthetics for use as a "vasoconstricting" agent in the operating room.

the capacity or potential to develop a complication. For example, granulation tissue is a sequela, but erosion of bone by granulation tissue is a complication.

4. The line between complications and sequelae is at times very tenuous, therefore, the reader is allowed to switch cabinets ad libitum.

5. Acute otitis media (acute suppurative otitis media, acute purulent otitis media), refers to a clinically identifiable infection of the middle ear with sudden onset and short duration (with or without tympanic membrane perforation).

6. Recurrent otitis media, refers to repeated episodes of acute otitis media in between periods of apparent remission (3 episodes in 6 months or 4 episodes in 1 year).

7. Otitis media with effusion (chronic otitis media with effusion, secretory otitis media, nonsuppurative otitis media, catarrh, tympanic mucositis, serous otitis media, serotympanum, mucoid otitis media, mucotympanum), refers to the presence of middle ear effusion behind an intact tympanic membrane without acute signs or symptoms. This broad term includes clinically noninfectious forms of otitis media. However, evidence suggests that effusions are, for the most part infectious. Cultures of serous effusions yield between 22 to 52% positively, percentages that increase to 77.3% if PCR is used. The type of effusion reflects a dynamic process in which some forms evolve into others depending on the interaction of defensive versus aggression forces (e.g. the aggression forces prevailing in the more infectious phases; the defensive forces prevailing in the noninfectious phases).

10. Chronic otitis media (chronic suppurative otitis media, silent otitis media), refers to a chronic inflammatory process, with or without tympanic membrane perforation; with or without drainage. Chronic suppurative otitis media refers to a chronic process with tympanic membrane perforation and drainage. A chronic otitis media with perforation can also occur without drainage. Silent otitis media refers to a chronic process behind an intact tympanic membrane.

11. Histopathologically, the term acute refers to infiltration by polymorphonuclears and classic signs of acute inflammation. Chronic otitis media implies infiltration of the mucoperiosteum by round cells or the cells of chronic inflammation.

12. The presence of the arrows in the Figure 1 reflect the concept that otitis media is a dynamic inflammatory process in which some forms lead to others.

HISTOPATHOLOGICAL RESPONSE OF THE MIDDLE EAR

What is involved and how does the ear react to the aggression? How does the ear react to aggression?

The ear responds with histopathologic defensive changes that are gradual, systematic and universal, and have variations which are adaptations to the different forms of aggression. Their forms of presentation and their severity will depend on the balance of aggression versus defense, with a direct influence of the environment, the genetic conditions of the host and his general defensive status at the time of aggression.

The inflammatory process involves all the walls, cavities and anatomical structures that these contain as well as the mucoperiosteum that lines these cavities and structures. Multiple factors play a role in the defensive mechanisms of the middle ear. The most important nonspecific factor (nonimmunologic) is an adequate Eustachian tube function and the mucociliary system.

Once the aggression is established, the result is the nonspecific universal reaction of inflammation that is the starting point of the sequential steps that will be described later in this chapter. Among the initial nonspecific cellular factors are the epithelial cells, the fibroblasts and with certain reserve the endothelial cells.

With the understanding that the reaction is simultaneous at all levels, for practical reasons, the epithelial changes will be initially described.

CHANGES IN THE EPITHELIUM

The epithelial cells participate in the inflammatory reaction by themselves and also as part of the mucociliary system.

The epithelial cells (Figure 2) become taller and have an increased secretion. In early stages, the secretory cells stain positively for Periodic acid Schiff [(PAS) (Figure 3)]. There is also some new gland formation. Cells become hyperplastic and there is also an increase in goblet cells.

Cells secrete different defensive substances, such as lysozymes (Figures 4A to D). The epithelial cells of middle ear also have the capacity of synthesizing the secretory piece of IgA [(secretory IgA) (Figure 5)].

All these secretions plus the cellular elements that fall into the middle ear cavity contribute to develop the middle ear effusion (fluid ear) (Figures 6 and 7). In some areas and depending on the degree of aggression, epithelial rupture occurs.

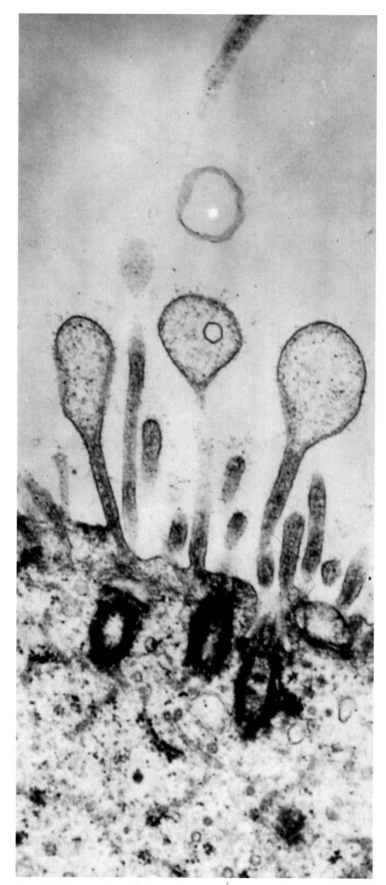

Figure 2 Changes in the epithelium with increased secretion

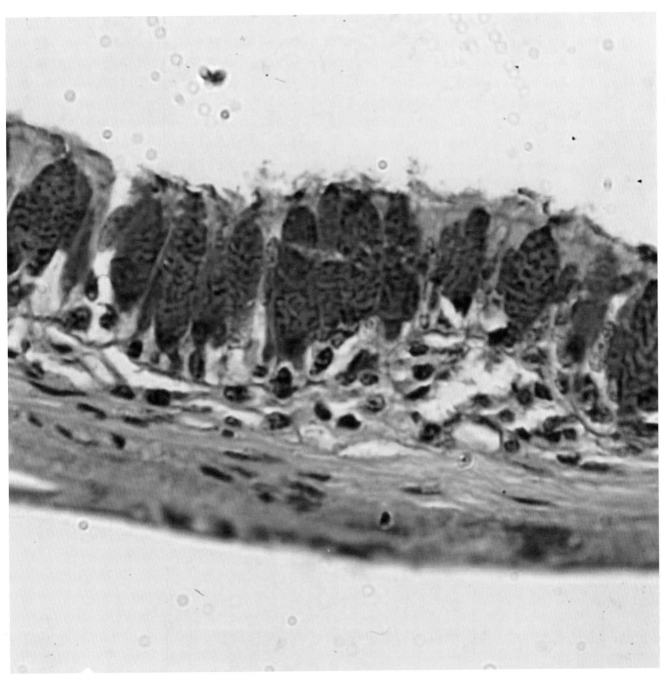

Figure 3 Epithelial secretory cells stained with Periodic acid Schiff (PAS)

In some chronic cases, there are metaplastic changes of the epithelium toward squamous epithelium, however, these are only isolated occurrences without an apparent pathological significance. Cholesteatomas seem more likely to be migration of the epithelium of the tympanic membrane (and/or ear canal) rather than the result of metaplastic changes of the middle ear mucosa.

This statement is supported by histopathological findings described in temporal bones in which cholesteatomas do not seem to have any relationship with these isolated metaplastic island.

CHANGES IN THE CONNECTIVE TISSUE AND PERIOSTEUM

Changes in the connective tissue are characterized by the following:

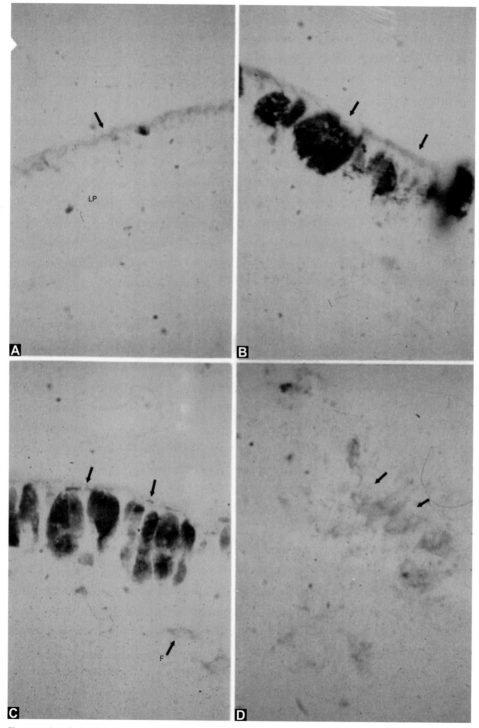

Figures 4A to D Epithelial secretory cells stained positively for lysozymes

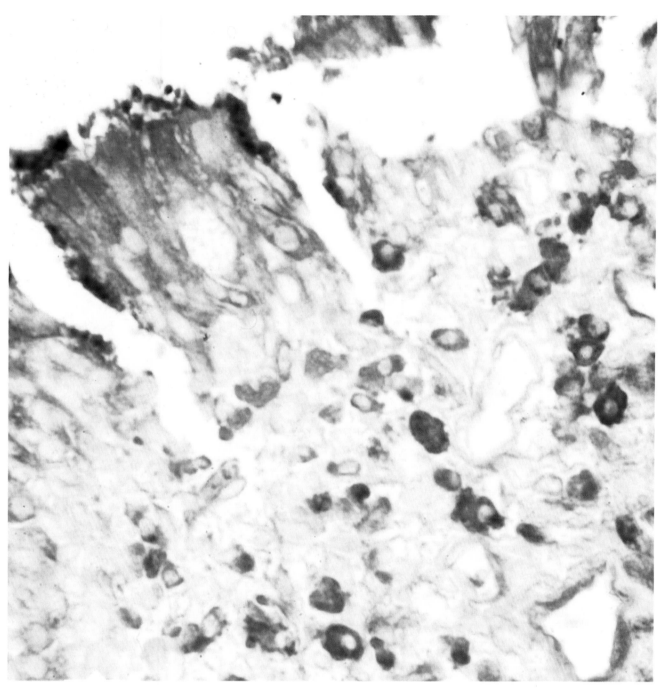

Figure 5 Epithelial secretory cells positively stained for IgA secretory piece

- Thickening
- Edema; and
- Increased vascularity

Cellular changes are characterized by the following:
- Gradual cellular infiltration (Figures 8 to 10)
- Changes in the type and numbers of cells
- Changes in the shape and numbers of fibers

- Inflammatory reaction of the periosteum
- Inflammatory reaction of the underlying bone. (Figures 11 A to D)

In early stages of the inflammatory process, the initial infiltration is based on polymorphonuclears (Figure 12) that respond rapidly and traverse the capillaries toward the connective tissue. From there some migrate through the

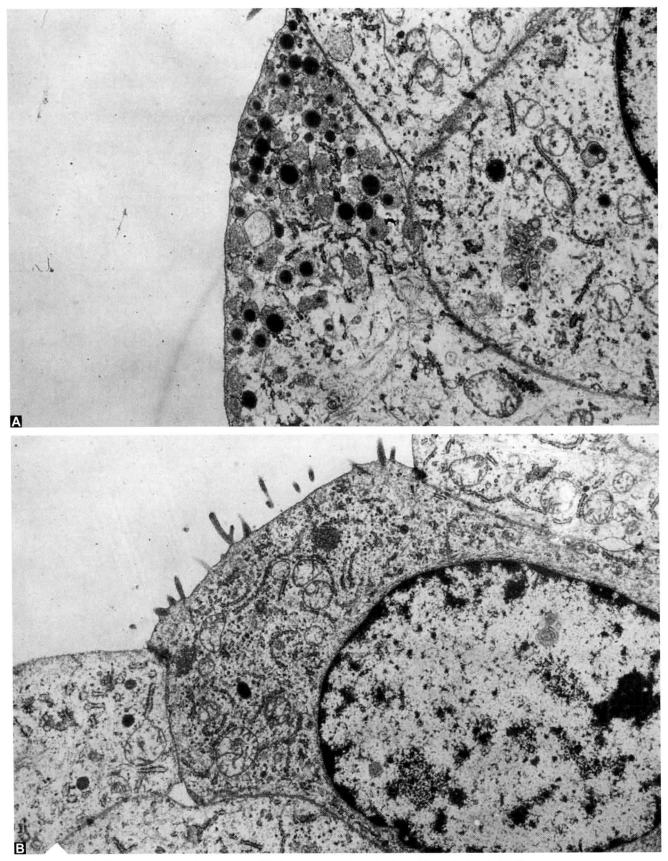

Figures 6A and B Epithelial secretory cell with a cytoplasm full of secretory granules and with an active endoplasmic reticulum

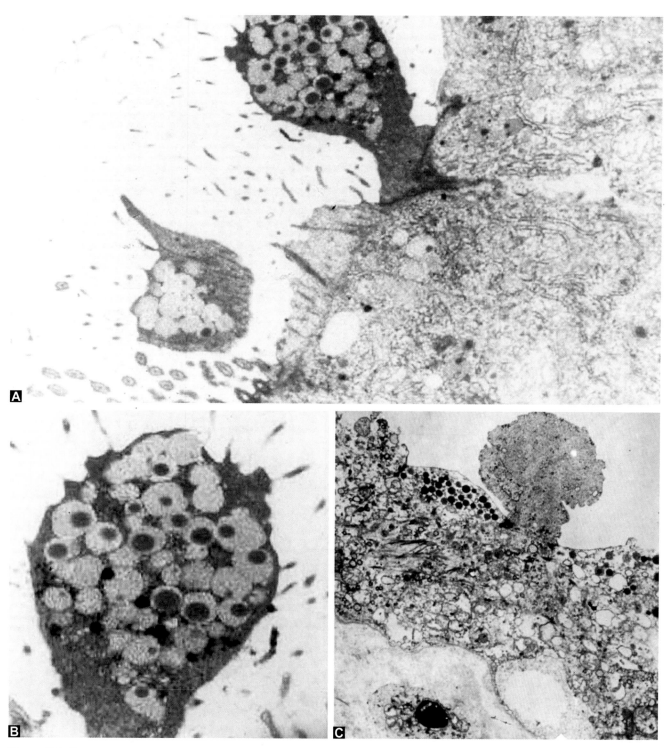

Figures 7A to C

epithelium toward the middle ear cavity (Figures 13A to E). The majority are neutrophils, but there are occasional eosinophils. Their primary function is engulfment of particles and microorganisms.

The second cells to appear active are macrophages (Figure 14) and fibroblasts. Macrophages, despite being nonspecific,

mark the starting point toward a specific immunological reaction mediated by T and B lymphocytes (Figures 15A and B).

Macrophages play a role in processing antigens and interacting with B lymphocytes (humoral immunity) and T (cellular immunity), which are the cells with capacity for specific recognition. B cells develop toward antibody-secreting cells.

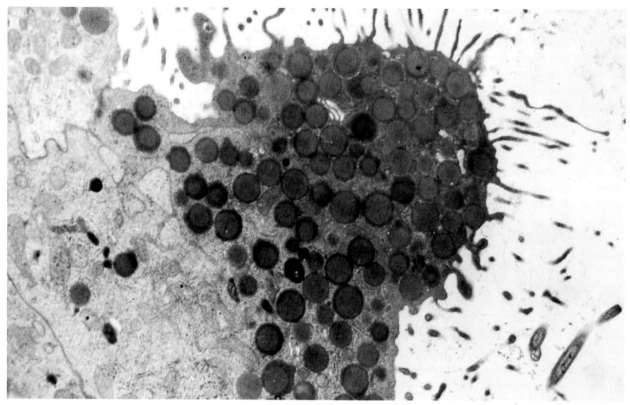

Figure 7D

Figures 7A to D Extrusion of different types of secretory granules

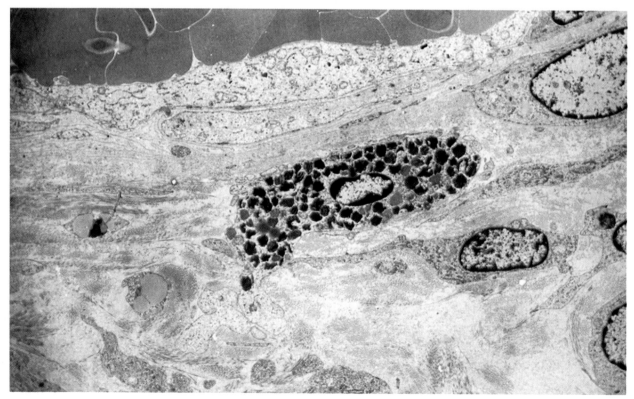

Figure 8 Mast cell in connective tissue layer

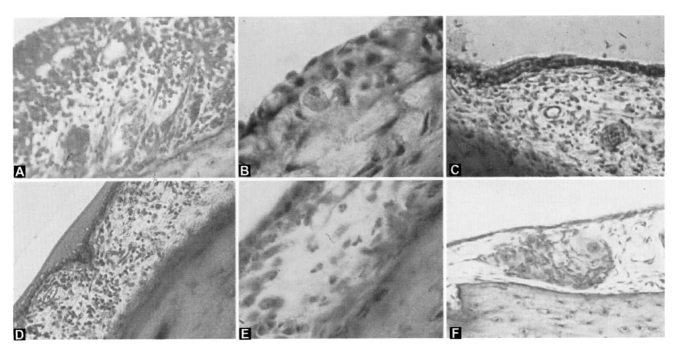

Figures 9A to F Composite slide at the promontory level that shows a normal section followed by the different stages of cellular infiltration that occur over time

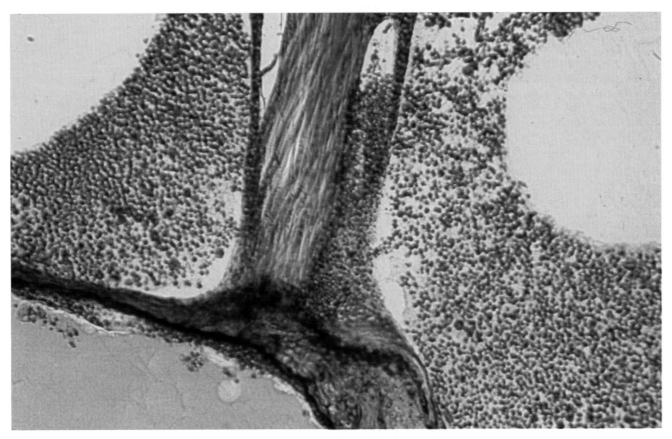

Figure 10 The cellular infiltration also involves the stapedius muscle

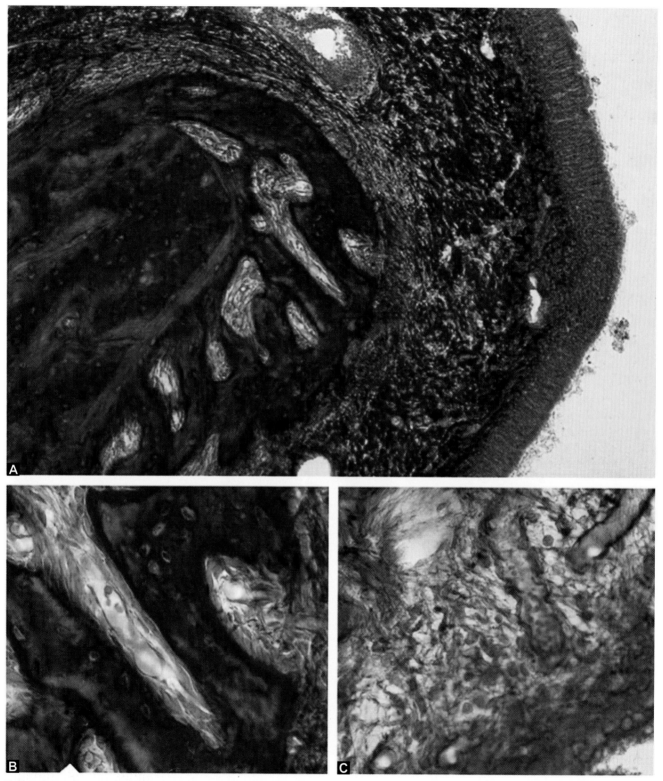

Figures 11A to C

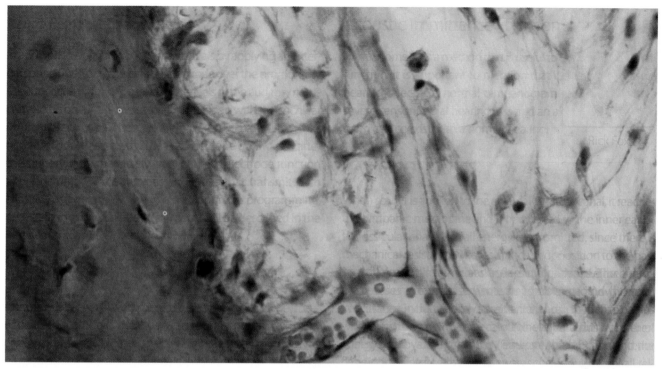

Figure 11D

Figures 11A to D Promontory with inflammatory reaction of the underlying bone (osteitis) with new vessel formation. Azan stain.

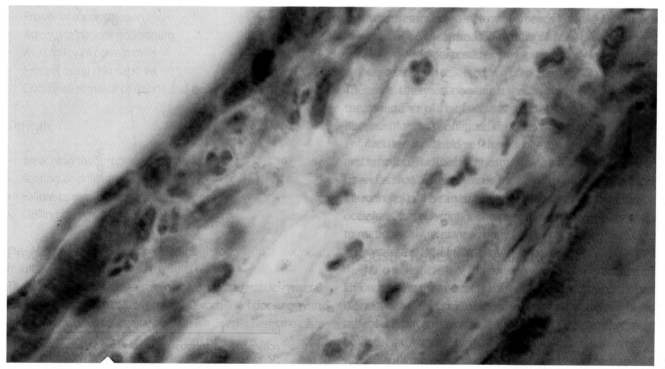

Figure 12 Promontory with early infiltration by polymorphonuclears

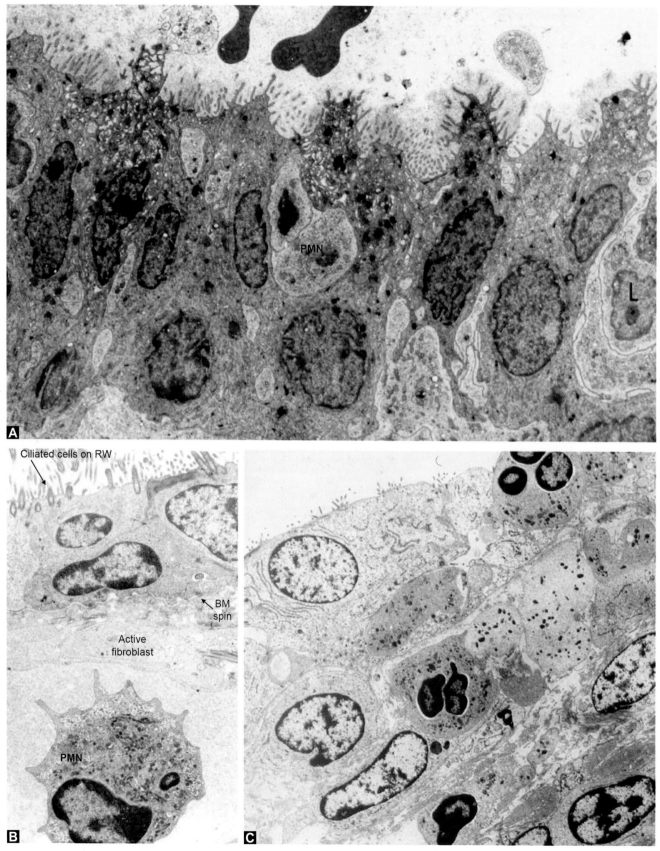

Figures 13A to C

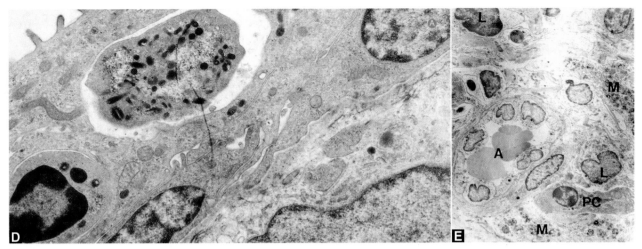

Figures 13D and E

Figures 13A to E Electrón micrographs showing infiltration by different cells and polymorphonuclear (PMN) migration through the epithelium toward the middle ear cavity

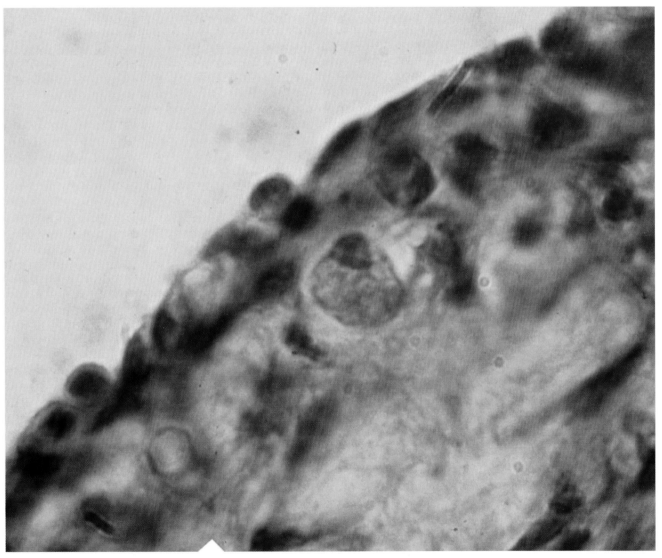

Figure 14 Promontory with infiltration by macrophages (processing antigens)

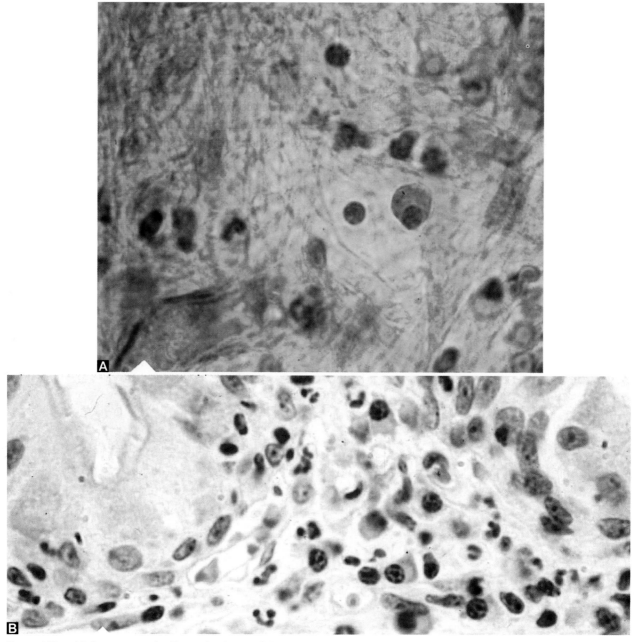

Figures 15A and B Promontory with infiltration by plasma cells (immunoglobulin synthesis)

The middle ear mucosa also has a local immunological system via secretory IgA in which IgA is secreted by the plasma cells (B cells) and the epithelial cells add the secretory piece. IgG and IgM could also be considered secretory since they are also synthesized by plasma cells and secreted toward the mucosal surface (Figures 16A to C).

Fibroblasts become active at early stages of the inflammatory process. They become larger and start secreting fibers. This is also evident in chronic cases. The reaction of these cells at early stages (Figures 17A to L) is so prominent that these early stages could be described as a fibroblastic-macrophagic reaction with fiber and amorphous substance secretion. Over

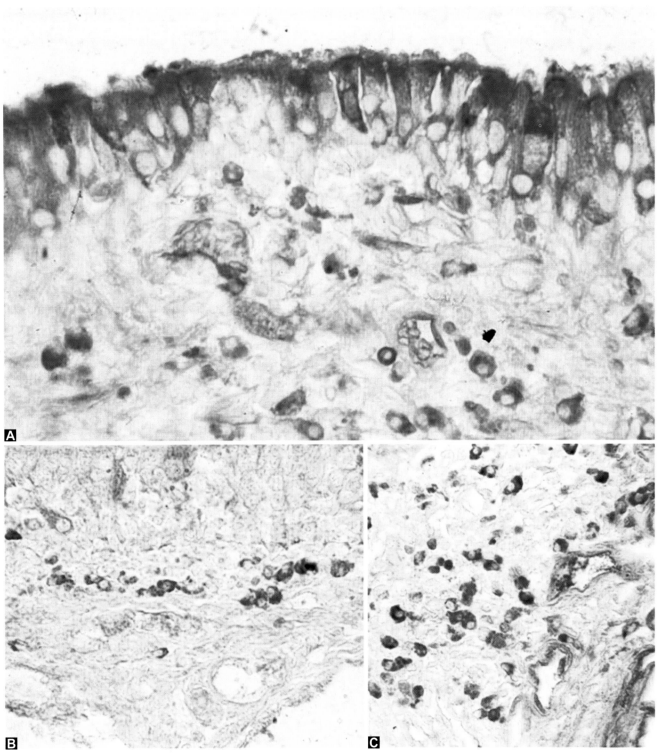

Figures 16A to C Plasma cells positively stained. (A) for IgA; (B) for IgM; and (C) for IgG. It also shows positive staining for IgA secretory piece

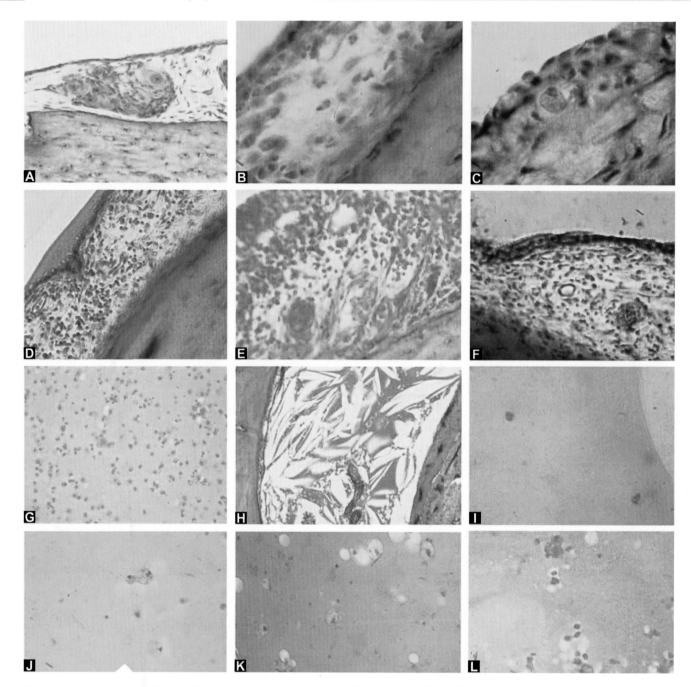

Figures 17A to L Composite slides that show a normal mucoperiosteum and different types of cellular infiltration according to inflammatory stages and the equivalent section of the middle ear effusion showing a similar cellular composition in all these stages

time the collagen fibers become thicker and better organized (Figures 18A to C).

MIDDLE EAR DEFENSE SYSTEM

- An epithelium that is continuous, regenerative and constitutes a mechanical barrier

- Mucociliary transport system (mucus, lysozymes, ciliated and secretory cells)
- A patent and functional Eustachian tube
- Inflammatory reaction of the connective tissue
- Edema
- Fibroblasts (collagen, amorphous substance)
- Polymorphonuclears (macrophages, lysozyme)

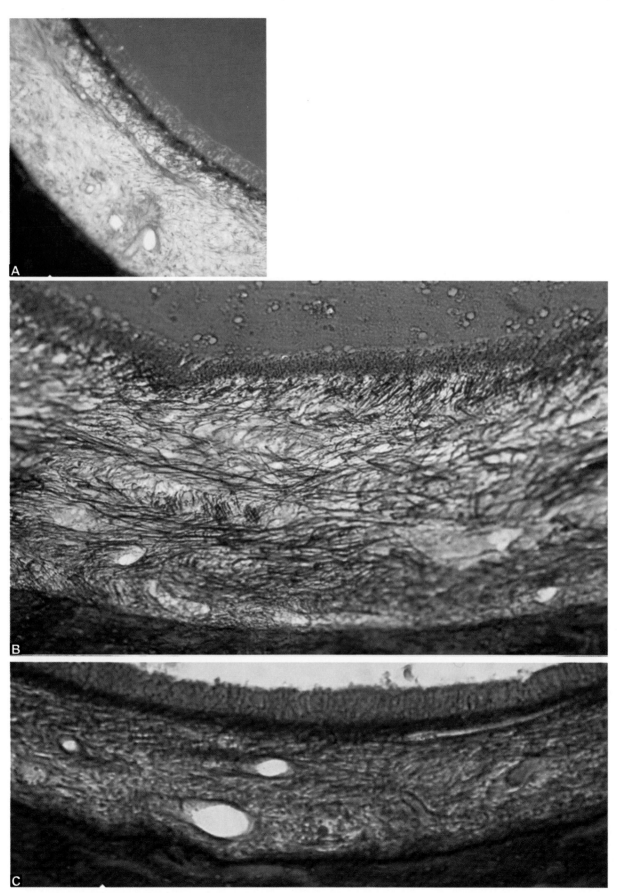

Figures 18A to C Thickened promontory with abundant collagen fibers stained with Azan stain (at three different stages)

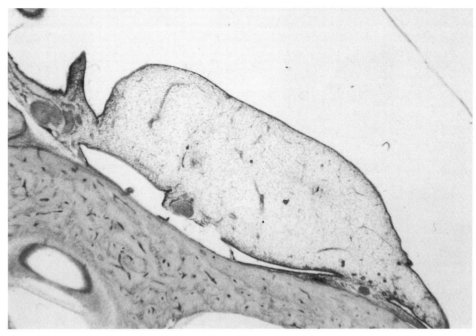

Figure 19 Polypoidal formation

- Lymphocytes (small and large T and B cells, respectively)
- Plasma cells
  - Immunoglobulins (IgA, IgG, IgM, IgE)
  - Complement system.

EFFUSION FORMATION

Absorption?	Transudate
Lymphatics	Exudate
Blood vessels	Cells
Secretion	Macrophages
Epithelial cells	Plasma cells
Glands	Mononuclears
Connective tissue cells?	Epithelial cells

CHANGES IN THE MUCOSA AS A WHOLE

The middle ear mucosa develops polypoidal (Figure 19) changes with areas that are prominent and areas that are depressed. Gland formation (Figures 20A to C) as well as new blood vessel formation can be more commonly observed in the depressed areas. It is quite likely that the basal cells play an important role in these processes.

Participation of All Structures

The inflammatory process involves all the cavities and structures of the middle ear, mastoid and Eustachian tube. The inflammatory process is dynamic. The middle ear effusion (fluid) is also dynamic and tends to follow the histopathologic changes that are occurring in the middle ear mucosa (Figure 21). The different

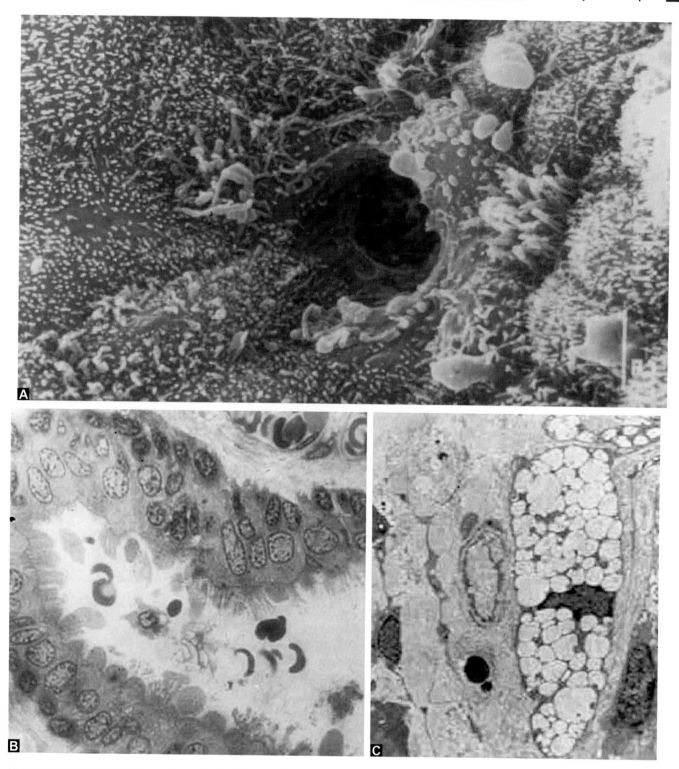

Figures 20A to C (A and B) Electron micrographs showing mucosal invagination leading to gland formation; (C) New gland formation

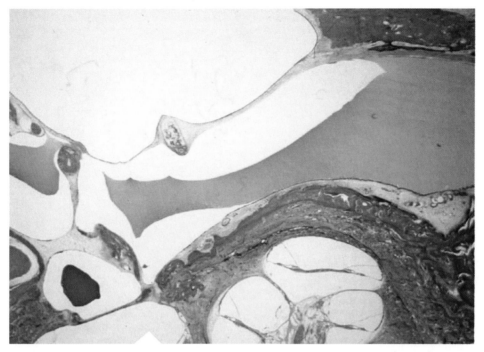

Figure 21 The middle ear effusion suggests a simple serous otitis, however, there is a significant inflammatory reaction of the mucosa with osteitis of the underlying bone

forms of presentation of the otitis media process are therefore moments or instants of this dynamic process.

If the process is seen in this manner, otitis media is much more than middle ear fluid and the histopathological changes described are a reflection of the stage of confrontation between the aggression and the defensive factors.

COMPLICATIONS AND SEQUELAE

Epithelial ruptures (Figures 22A and B) occur in some areas of the mucosa (the degree will depend on the magnitude and type of aggression).

These ruptures allow:

- Pockets with serous content
- Adherence formation (Figures 23A and B): These originate when granulation tissue that persists become epithelized. Adherences serve at times as bridges for cellular migration as is the case for cholesteatomas.
- Inflamed connective tissue without epithelial covering (granulation tissue) can migrate through these openings (Figures 24A to C). This tissue can disappear or persist. Persistance can be alone (by itself) or associated with a cholesteatoma leading to complications. Local tissue destruction by these entities is caused by erosion

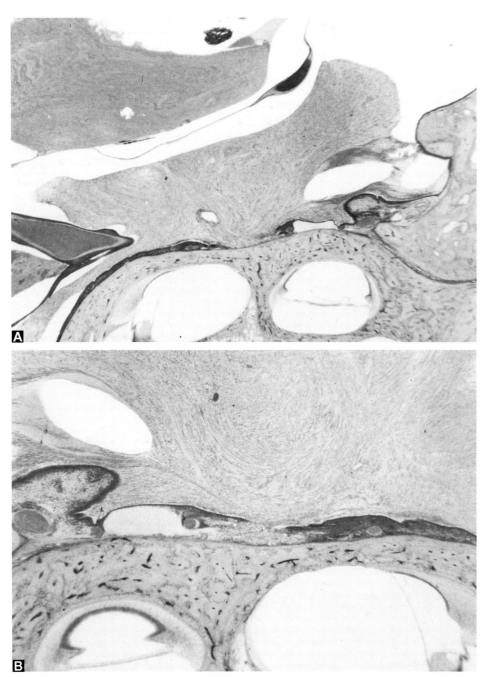

Figures 22A and B Epithelial rupture at the promontory level

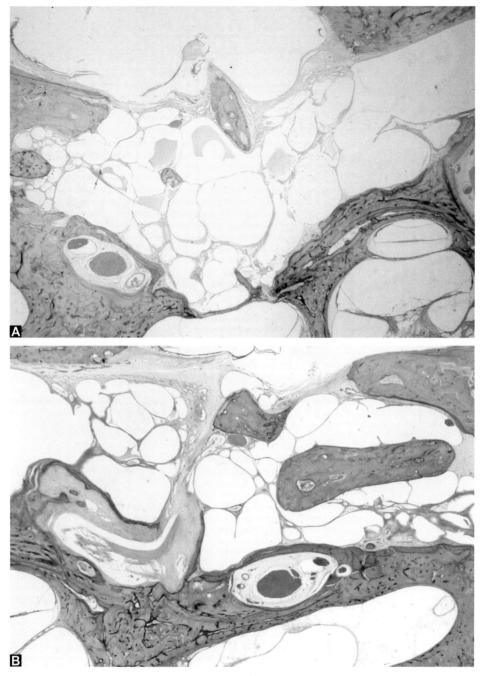

Figures 23A and B Adherence formation

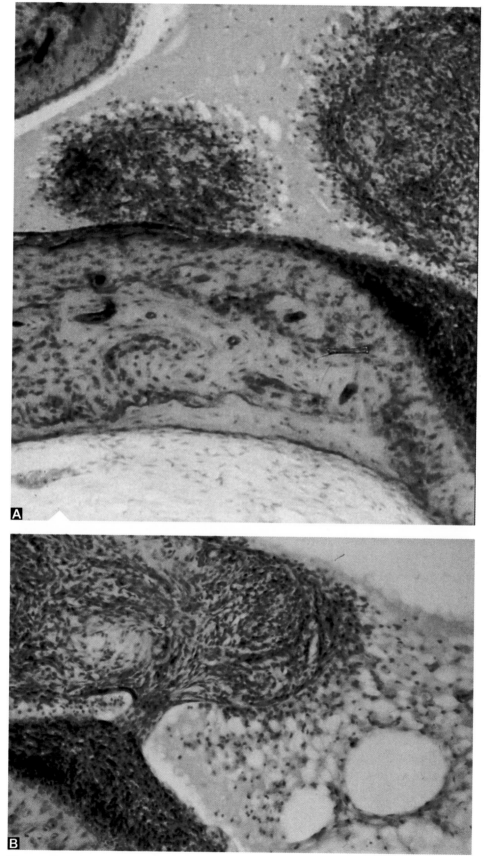

Figures 24A and B

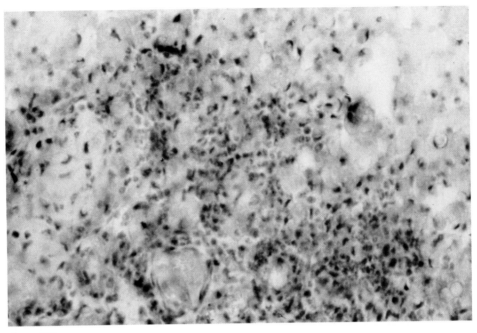

Figure 24C

Figures 24Ato C Granulation tissue formation at an epithelial rupture site (without epithelial coverage)

BIBLIOGRAPHY

1. Aschan G. The eustachian tube. Acta Otolaryngol (Stockh). 1954; 44:295-311.

2. Bendick GA. Histopathology of transudatory secretory otitis media. Arch Otolaryngol. 1963;73:33-8.

3. Chung MH, Griffith SR, Park KH, Lim DJ, De Maria TF. Cytological and histological changes in the middle ear after innoculation of influenza A virus. Acta Otolaryngol (Stockh). 1993;113: 81-7.

4. Daly KA. Epidemiology of otitis media. Otolaryngol Clin NAm. 1991;24:775-86.

5. Farrior EJ. Histopathologic considerations in treatment of the eustachian tube. Arch Otolaryngol. 1943;37:609-21.

6. Friedmann 1. The pathology of acute and chronic infections in the middle ear cleft. Ann Oto Rhinol Laryngol. 1971:80:390-6.

7. Goycoolea HG, Goycoolea MV, Farfan CR. Racial and familial factors in otitis media. Arch Otolaryngol Head Neck Surg. 1988; 114:147-9.

8. Goycoolea MV, Hueb MM, Ruah CB. Definitions and terminology. Otolaryngol Clin NAm. 1991;24:757-61.

9. Goycoolea MV, Paparella MM, Carpenter AM, Juhn 5K. A longitudinal study of cellular changes in experimental otitis media. Otolaryngol Head Neck Surg. 1979;87:685-700.

10. Goycoolea MV, Paparella MM, Juhn 5K, Carpenter AM. Cells involved in the middle ear defense system. Ann Otol Rhinol Laryngo 1. 1980;89:121-8.

11. Goycoolea MV, Ruah CB, Bequer N. General surgical approach based on pathogenesis. Otolaryngol Clin NAm. 1991;24:957-66.

12. Goycoolea MV. Otitis media: definitions and pathogenesis. In: Paparella MM, Goycoolea MV (Eds). Clinical problems in otitis media and innovations in surgical otology (Ear Clinics International, vol 2.) Baltimore: Williams and Wilkins; 1982. p. 154.

13. Goycoolea MV. Pathogenesis of otitis media; an experimental study in the cat (PhD Thesis): University of Minnesota, June, 1978.

14. Gundersen T, Gluck E. The middle ear mucosa in serous otitis media. Arch Otolaryngol. 1972;96:40-4.

15. Hentzer E, Jorgensen MB. The submucous layer of the middle ear in chronic otitis media 1. Secretory otitis media. Arch Exp Ohr NasUKehlkHeilk. 1972;201:108-18.

16. Hentzer E, Jorgensen MB. The submucous layer of the middle ear in chronic otitis media. II. Chronic suppurative otitis media. Arch Klin Exp Ohr Nas Heilk. 1972;201:119-26.

17. Hentzer E. Ultrastructure of the middle ear mucosa. Ann Otol Rhinol Laryngol. 1976; 85 (Supp 25): 30-5.

18. Hussl B, Welzi-Mueller K. Secretory otitis media and mastoid pneumatization. Ann Otol Rhinol Laryngol. 1980;89(Suppl 68):79-82.

19. Klein JO, Tos M, Hussl B, et al. Definition and classification. Ann Otol Rhinol Laryngol. 1989;98(Suppl 139):10.

20. Lim DJ, Klamer A. Cellular reactions in acute otitis media. Scanning and transmission electron microscopy. Laryngoscope. 1971;81:1772-86.

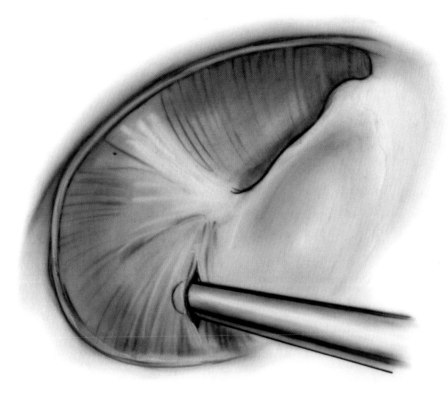

Figure 5 A no. 5 suction tip can be used; placed barely through the incision while trying to avoid enlarging the incision or causing localized bleeding

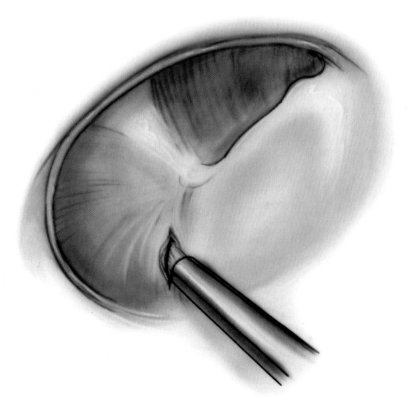

Figure 6 A no. 7 suction tip placed immediately above (not through) the incision can be used for literally pulling the thick mucoid effusions

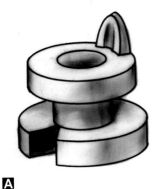 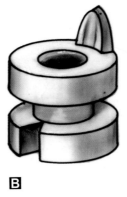 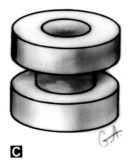

Figures 7A to C Types of tubes

less epithelial debris than long-term tubes protruding from the tympanic membrane. In general, however, most well-designed tubes work well if they are properly used.

Cost of the tubes is also a factor. Variations in price sometimes seem illogical. The authors have designed and used 18 karat gold tubes handmade in Chile that are 200% cheaper than the least expensive custom sold plastic tube.

Placement of the Tube

Using baby-alligator forceps, the tube is grasped gently from its outer border or from its special lip. The incision should be clean and free of blood. The inner flange is laid sideways on the incision (proximal end) (Figure 8A). Sometimes it can be "popped" or "screwed" in with a gentle motion (Figure 8B). Usually, it can be laid over the proximal lip of the incision and then pushed in with a blunt pick, either by pressing it from its superior surface or by gently twisting it around (Figures 8C and D). Once the tube has been inserted, it is a good idea to rotate it to ensure that it is in position.

Once it has been verified that the tube is in place, it is a good idea to place a no. 20 (or smaller if needed) suction tip through the opening of the tube (Figure 8E). Any middle ear fluid or blood should be suctioned and a few drops of hydrogen peroxide should be left in place. Postoperatively, the authors tend to recommend neutral pH drops for 2 or 3 days to ensure that patency is maintained. The bottle with the drops is warmed in closed hands for a few minutes before instilling them; gentle body temperature of the drops when instilled to reach the inserted tube can make a whole difference, especially in babies and small children. If there is any pain or discomfort with the drops, they are discontinued. If the fluid is cloudy or shows any signs of infection, do not hesitate to culture the effusion and keep the patient on antibiotics. These apparently small details

in technique can make a big difference in ventilation tube insertion and its follow-up.

Potential Complications

As in most surgical procedures, the best treatment for complications is to prevent them. Excessive desire for speed is a potential surgical enemy, particularly harmful in tube insertion. Many unnecessary problems arise in training programs because this "simple procedure" is left to the most junior and inexperienced surgeons. It takes time to learn how to use an operating microscope properly and to see all that must be seen. Mutual coordination and understanding with the anesthesiologist are essential. The resident should ask for help if his or her orientation and timing are inadequate. The anesthesiologist should understand that the purpose of the procedure is to protect the patient's ears, not the anesthesiologist's hand.

Intraoperative Complications

1. A small and narrow ear canal can make visualization of the entire tympanic membrane difficult. Extreme care should be taken to avoid damaging the friable skin of the ear canal; bleeding will further obscure vision. A small ear speculum can be gently "screwed" in and the speculum size can be gradually increased.
2. For lacerations, bleeding or hematoma of the ear canal, carefully irrigate with hydrogen peroxide or apply small cotton balls saturated with epinephrine, or both. Just take time until the bleeding stops.
3. Facial paralysis due to injection of local anesthetics is a temporary phenomenon of no consequence, but the surgeon must be aware of this annoying possibility. A detailed and careful explanation to the patient and/or his relatives is mandatory.

5.2.3B

The Marquet Technique to Remove Non-Fixed Retraction Pockets at the Time of Tube Placement

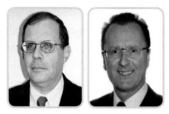

Carlos Ruah,   Bernard Ars

INTRODUCTION

According to Tran Ba Huy and Herman, a retraction pocket is a partial invagination of the tympanic membrane (TM) towards an aerated middle ear space.[1] This allows the distinction between a retraction pocket and a middle ear atelectasis or an adhesive otitis media. Furthermore, one may distinguish between a simple retraction of the TM in which the diameter of the external aperture is larger than the inner portion and a retraction pocket in which the diameter of the external aperture is much smaller than the inner diameter.[2]

For a retraction pocket to occur, it requires two main factors:
1. A structural weakness of the TM, which may be constitutional or acquired. In relation to the pars flaccida, it is not inserted in a bony sulcus, lacks an organized fibrous layer, is very rich in elastic fibers and vessels, and in 3.5% of cases presents congenital defects in its fibrous layer.[3] In relation to the pars tensa, the posterior superior quadrant is larger than all the other quadrants, has a wider vibration swing[3] and is the most vascularized of the quadrants.[3] The insertion of this quadrant in the bone is shallow because of the lack of a well defined bony sulcus at this level and because the direction of the radial fibers of the TM is perpendicular to the direction of the Havers canals of the tympanic bone.[4] In the inferior quadrants, the bony sulcus is well-defined and the direction of the radial fibers is the same as the Havers canals, allowing a deeper penetration and anchorage in the tympanic bone. Acquired weakness results from recurrent or persistent inflammation of the middle ear leading to the progressive destruction of the collagenic and elastic components of the TM. This inflammatory reaction is greatest in the most vascularized areas, which includes the pars flaccida and the posterior superior quadrant of the pars tensa.[5] Repetitive placement of ventilating tubes may also lead to a localized weakness of the TM.[7]
2. Presence of a persistent negative middle ear pressure leading to a persistent stretching of the fibrous layer with progressive rupture of the connecting bridges among the collagen fibers.[3]

PATHOLOGY

Biopsies of the tympanic membrane with otitis media with effusion during the placement of a ventilating tube has allowed for the staging of the progressive TM changes.[8] In stage 1, there is a submucosal edema with preservation of both fibrous layers. In stage 2, the inner circular fibrous layer has disappeared. In Stage 3, a greater part of the outer radial fibrous layer has disappeared. In stage 4, the TM is thin with no fibrous layer, which was replaced by connective tissue (Figures 1A to E).

A simple retraction or a retraction pocket was never observed in normal temporal bones (TB) or with mucoid otitis media.[2] Simple retraction was seen in 2.1% of TB with serous otitis media and both simple retractions and retraction pockets were seen in 19.5% of TB with chronic otitis media.[2]

The most frequent location of the retraction pockets vary in different studies. Wells and Michaels see them more often in the pars flaccida.[6] Ars and de Craemer,[3] and Edelstein et al.[9] see them more frequently in the pars tensa. Yoon et al.[2] found an equal frequency in the pars flaccida and pars tensa in TB. It appears, however, that simple retractions are more frequent in the pars tensa[2] and in this location, retraction pockets occur more often in the posterior superior quadrant.[3]

No retraction pockets are seen before the age of 3 years.[2,3,5,9,10] The majority of the mesenchyme in the middle ear and TM disappears or differentiates during the first year of life. Nevertheless, it may persist in large quantities beyond 2 years of age in the presence of recurrent or persistent otitis media and beyond 3 years of age in the presence of congenital malformations[5] Both conditions lead to a marked delay in the formation of the Prussak's space and in the maturation of the collagen and elastic fibers, preventing pars flaccida retraction. It also allows for the posterior superior quadrant of the pars tensa to remain too thick to retract.[5,10]

CLASSIFICATION

Many classifications of retraction pockets have been proposed over the last 30 years.[11-15] Because of the clarity, simplicity and respect for the pathological evolution of the disease, retraction pockets of the pars flaccida and pars tensa can be classified as follows:[14,15]

1. Mobile retraction pockets, which may protrude with the Valsalva or Politzer maneuver.
2. Fixed but controllable retraction pockets in which the bottom of the pocket can be easily observed, is usually self-cleaning, nonkeratinizing nor infected, or can be easily cleaned under the microscope.
3. Fixed noncontrollable retraction pocket, too deep to accurately be observed or cleaned under the microscope, may still be self-cleaning with or without recurrent infection.

Once the retraction pocket is fixed, it may be considered a precholesteatoma stage. Once this pocket shows keratin debris with or without infection or an inflammatory polyp, it may be considered a cholesteatoma.

Using the same evolutionary criteria, Ars[16] defines three levels of retraction pockets:

1. Level 1 in which the pocket is safe and stable, the histological characteristics of the TM remain unchanged with time and are potentially reversible. Hearing remains normal. There is no risk of cholesteatoma formation.
2. Level 2 in which the behavior of the pocket is uncertain. Progressive morphological changes in the TM may be seen over time with further deepening of the pocket, but hearing remains normal. The development of cholesteatoma is uncertain.
3. Level 3 in which the pocket is unstable, adhering to neighboring structures, erodes the ossicular chain or tympanic bony frame, looses its capacity for self-cleanliness and may be the source of recurrent bouts of infection with otorrhea, bleeding, discomfort and the appearance of a polyp. Con-

ductive hearing loss is usually present. The risk of developing cholesteatoma is very high.

TREATMENT

In Level 1 pockets, the treatment is conservative with periodic observation and cleaning, if necessary.

In Level 2, a tympanostomy tube may be inserted and the pocket is excised by the Marquet technique described later in this chapter.

In Level 3, a reinforcement tympanoplasty may be performed using composite cartilage-perichondrium grafts with ossicular reconstruction, if necessary. The status of the mastoid is important to evaluate and treat, since it may lead to failure of any middle ear reconstruction. It includes the removal of mastoid and middle ear inflammatory tissue, the restoration of the role of the mastoid as a buffering chamber in middle ear cleft pressure variations balance.[17]

If cholesteatoma has developed, treatment should follow the standard surgical techniques specific for this pathology and described elsewhere.

SURGICAL PROCEDURE

The aim of the procedure is to restore the structure of the TM, maximizing vibration and sound transmission and prevent recurrent retraction pocket after extrusion of the tympanic ventilating tube.

The surgical steps include:

1. Myringotomy and placement of ventilating tube. The tube should be placed in an area of healthier TM avoiding the retraction pocket (Figure 2).
2. The retraction pocket is suctioned, becoming an outpocket (Figure 3).
3. The outpocket is twisted or pressure is applied to the opening of the pocket (Figure 4).
4. The pocket is excised (Figure 4).
5. If the TM opening due to the removal of the pocket is small and the edges are in close contact, the TM will heal well (Figure 5).
6. If the edges are far apart and a large hole is left with its edges falling into the middle ear cavity, it is necessary to raise these edges and keep them in close contact, for which two options may be used:
   i. With a small hook entering through the perforation, the TM annulus is raised with part of the skin of the external auditory canal, allowing for the junction of the edges of the perforation (Figure 6).

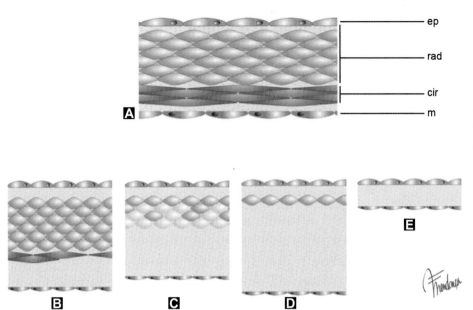

Figures 1A to E Normal histology and progressive changes in TM to become thin and retracted. (A) Normal histology of TM with an outer epithelial layer (ep), outer radial fibrous layer (rad), inner circular fibrous layer (cir) and mucosa (m). (B) Stage 1—submucosal edema with both fibrous layers present; (C) Stage 2—disappearance of circular fibrous layer; (D) Stage 3—disappearance of most of radial fibrous layer; (E) Stage 4—Thin TM without fibrous layers

Source: Illustrated by Fernando Vilhena de Mendonca MD, Otolaryngologist and Medical Illustrator, Director of Circulo Medico

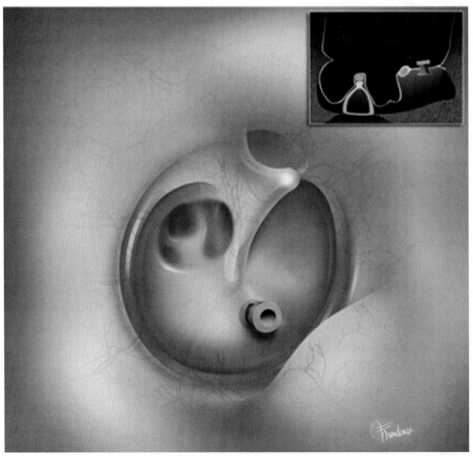

Figure 2 Myringotomy and placement of ventilating tube. The tube should be placed in an area of healthier TM avoiding the retraction pocket

Source: Illustrated by Fernando Vilhena de Mendonca MD, Otolaryngologist and Medical Illustrator, Director of Circulo Medico

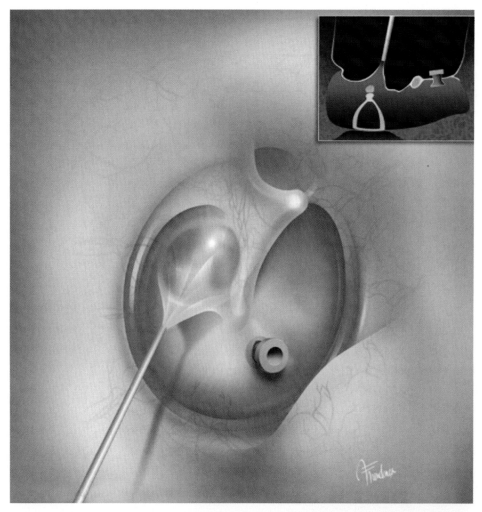

Figure 3 The retraction pocket is suctioned, becoming an outpocket

Source: Illustrated by Fernando Vilhena de Mendonca MD, Otolaryngologist and Medical Illustrator, Director of Circulo Medico

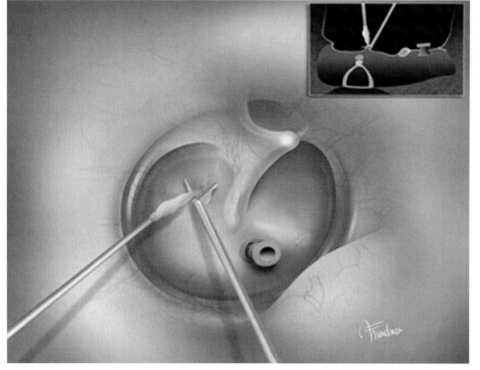

Figure 4 The outpocket is twisted or pressure is applied to the opening of the pocket and the pocket is excised

Source: Illustrated by Fernando Vilhena de Mendonca MD, Otolaryngologist and Medical Illustrator, Director of Circulo Medico

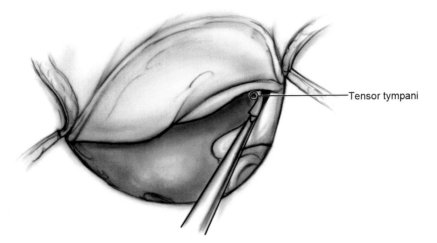

Tensor tympani

Figure 3 Sectioning of the tensor tympani tendon

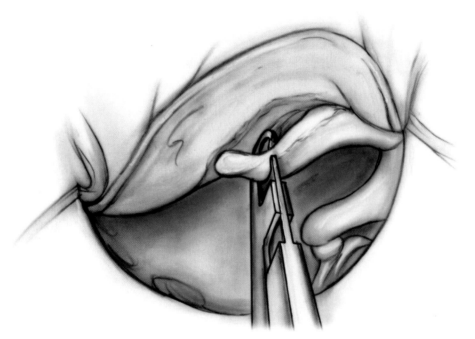

Figure 4 The distal tip of the long process of the malleus is severed after being carefully separated from the overlying TM

thread a small piece of synthetic nonabsorbable suture through the tube and into the canal in order to avoid plugging of the tube with packing and debris. The authors have not observed plugging to be a problem in these cases. The ventilation tube helps to ensure postoperative aeration and healing of the middle ear. The ear canal is packed, the Lempert II incision is closed in two layers and a mastoid dressing is applied.

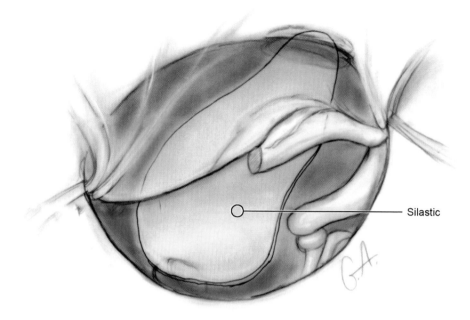

Figure 5 Placing of a piece of thin Silastic sheeting extending from the Eustachian tube to the tympanic sinus and round window niche

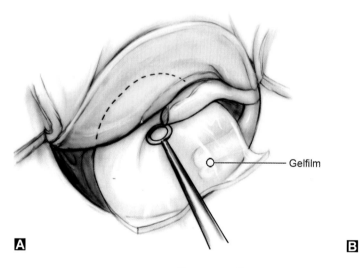

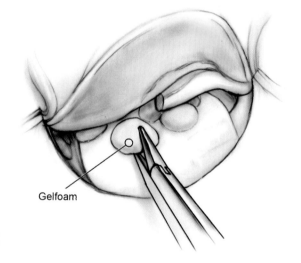

Figures 6A and B Placement of Gelfilm® and Gelfoam®

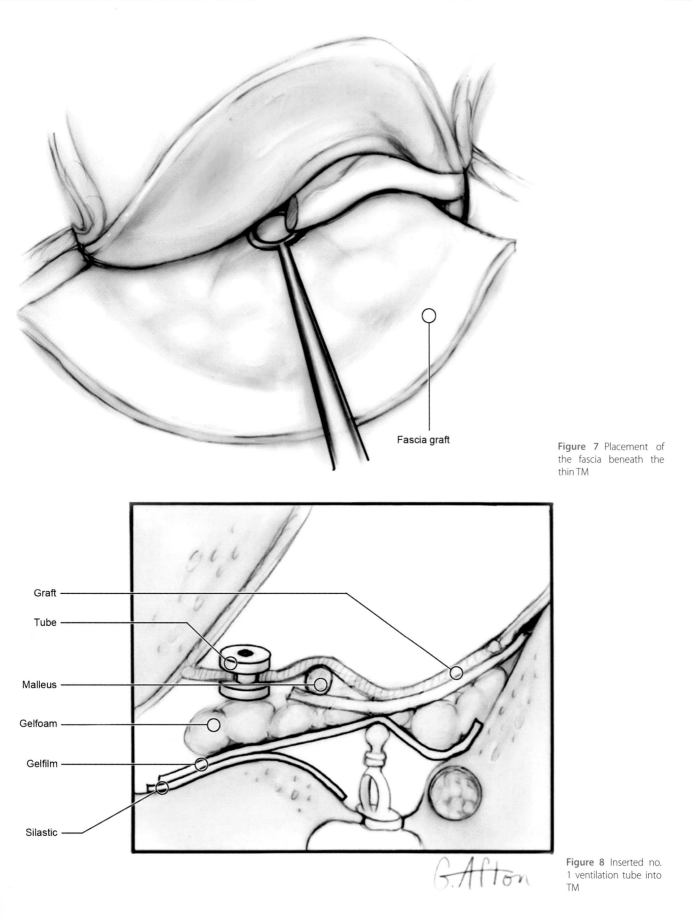

Fascia graft

Figure 7 Placement of the fascia beneath the thin TM

Graft

Tube

Malleus

Gelfoam

Gelfilm

Silastic

Figure 8 Inserted no. 1 ventilation tube into TM

G.Afton

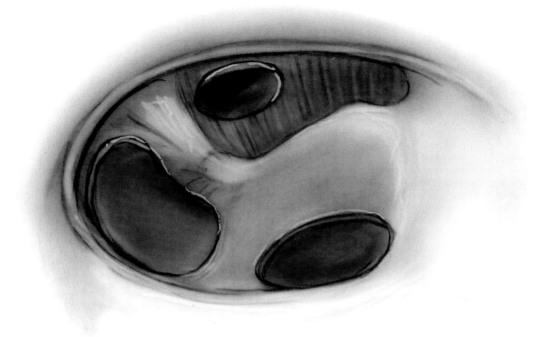

Figure 2E

Figures 2A to E Tympanic membrane perforation. (A and B) Involving more than one quadrant; (C) Perforation may be total central or marginal; (D and E) Several perforations, for example in tuberculosis

Once the approach has been selected and performed, and the tympanic membrane is visualized, the next decision is the canal incisions to use. Before elevating the flaps, any tympanic membrane work (such as trimming the edges) should be performed, since it is simpler at this time and the membrane is in its natural position. The basic principle is to enter the middle ear cavity (type I tympanoplasty) in a way that allows adequate inspection of the cavity and efficient placement of a graft. The alternatives are many and vary according to need and prefer-ence, as well as imagination of the surgeon. A classic posterior canal flap (1 and 6 o'clock vertical incisions) offers adequate exposure in most (if not all) cases and is a good alternative. An anterior or an inferior flap might suffice (Figures 3A to C), or a "swinging door" technique can be used (Figures 3D and E). If skin reinforcement is needed, a pedicled flap can be utilized. Some of the most commonly used flaps will be described in the discussion of specific procedures. They are simply alternatives and are not necessarily the only choices.

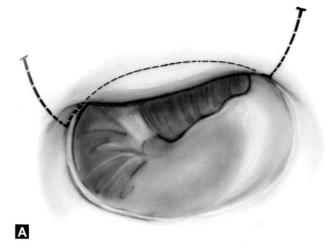

A

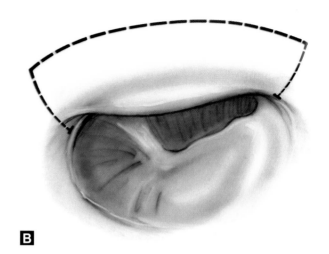

B

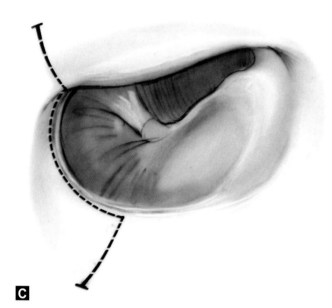

C

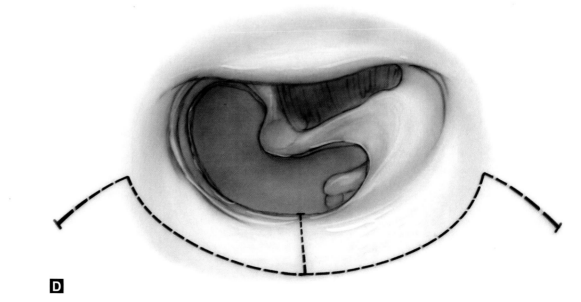

Figures 3A to D

D

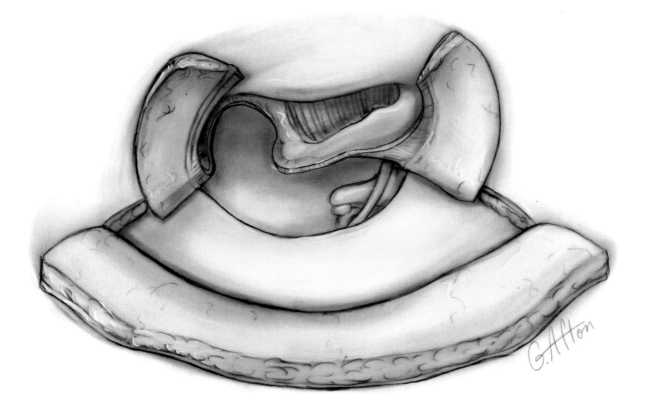

Figure 3E

Figures 3A to E   Approach to type I tympanoplasty. (A to C) Anterior or inferior flap; (D and E) "Swinging door" technique

5.2.4A(I)

Influence of the Mechanoacoustic Factors in Tympanoplasty Results

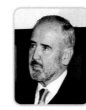
Elisa Gil-Carcedo

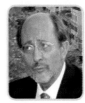
Luis María Gil-Carcedo

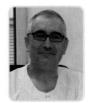
Luis Angel Vallejo

Primitivo Ortega

INTRODUCTION AND PURPOSE

The structural changes that occur in the ear, secondary to surgical manipulation have a direct influence in the hearing results. The hearing results must be considered not only on quantitative, but also on qualitative characteristics. In this chapter we will review the influence of the surgical procedure on the mechano-acoustical behavior of the ear components and how these manifest in the functional result of tympanoplasty.

The end result in hearing will depend on the mechano-acoustical efficiency of the new ear configuration secondary to the surgical procedure.

The functional usefulness of ear after tympanoplasty depend on the surgical act performed in the following three stages:

1. The participation of external ear canal in the hearing process is commonly forgotten. Surgical manipulation in the ear canal can have a significant influence in the impact of the sound wave on the tympanic membrane.

2. The functional capacity of a reconstructed tympanic membrane is essential. The reception of sound energy in first functional step in the middle ear and its transference to the malleus handle is a very important step.

3. For a final functional result, it is essential that the mechanical energy transfer through the ossicular chain is most efficient. Therefore, the technique of ossicular chain reconstruction is essential for transmission.

Surgical techniques end up always being less efficient than the natural structures. There are also other factors such as the underlying pathological process. Firstly, an adequate reconstruction has to be performed in order to replace the ossicular chain. Secondly, a well ventilated middle ear and an adequate volume is required, as well as a functioning Eustachian tube. Otherwise adhesions and atelectasis might compromise the tympanoplasty results.[1]

The great variety of prostheses available is related to different degrees of biological acceptance of these materials, and to their design and physical characteristics.

Their incidence of disarticulation and extrusion is the best indication of their overall quality.

The persistence of inflammatory process and the middle ear mucosal changes will also be responsible for surgical failures and these failures keep recurring if the underlying process is not resolved (medically or surgically).

Decrease in mobility of the ossicular chain is clearly reflected in the functional results. Surgical scarring can lead to significant fixation as well as tympanosclerosis; however, the latter does so in the long range. A fixed stapes or malleus head is easily detected; however, there are failures in mobility that are partial but they diminish the transference of sound energy to the endocochlear fluids. Different degrees of sclerosis of the annular ligament of Rudinger, hardly detectable, can cause a poor functional tympanoplasty result in an otherwise fine procedure.

Surgical ability and experience are also of paramount importance. In addition, there are measures that are to be considered, such as coffee and stimulants that might have a negative influence on the pulse. Previous physical activity as well as of hypoglycemia have a detrimental effect. The importance of a comfortable chair and sitting position cannot be emphasized enough. The chair should allow reclining both arms and spatial distribution of the instrumentation should be adequate. Instruments should be of optimal quality and so should the magnification (surgical microscope).

The authors have developed a 3D model of finite elements (3D FE) that is quite useful for tympanoplasty training.

EFFECTS ON THE SOUND TRANSMISSION CAUSED BY THE MORPHOLOGICAL CHANGES IN THE EXTERNAL EAR CANAL BY THE TYMPANOPLASTY PROCEDURE

Modifications of the Pinna

The pinna operates as a linear filter whose transference function depends on the direction and distance from the sound source. Due to its physical characteristics, the pinna causes distortion of the linear sound signals, but not in the same manner for all directions and distances. In this manner, the pinna translates spatial characteristics of the signal. This "codification process" is due to physical phenomena of the sound waves (reflection, diffraction, refraction, interference and resonance formation). However, sound amplification by the pinna is minimal, and is very slightly observed in different frequency ranges.[2] In other words, there is no evidence that modifications of the pinna have a significant influence in auditory function in humans. On

the other hand, meatoplasty can have a significant cosmetic influence.[3]

Although in tympanoplasty the peripheral area of pinna is usually not involved; the area of the auditory meatus, "entrance area or inlet area," can be significantly affected. In radical cavities, if width of the area is increased the resonant frequency is changed. A 20% increase in width decreases the resonant frequency in 1 kHz. This implies that the compression of consonants, in which the 3–4 kHz frequencies have great importance, can decrease around 10 dB.[4]

Modifications in the inlet areas caused by meatoplasty, especially in more radical procedures, have significant changes in amplification of the sound wave (energy) over the tympanic membrane.[5]

Modifications in the External Auditory Canal

In practical terms, it is difficult to determine the exact degree of loss because in these procedures there are alterations of different areas of the external and middle ear, and the surgical modifications usually involve these different areas.[6]

The ear canal has a role coupling an external sound that propagates in waves toward the tympanic membrane (Figure 1). The behavior of acoustic signal in the ear canal is different depending on the segment that is considered. The first segment (its extent

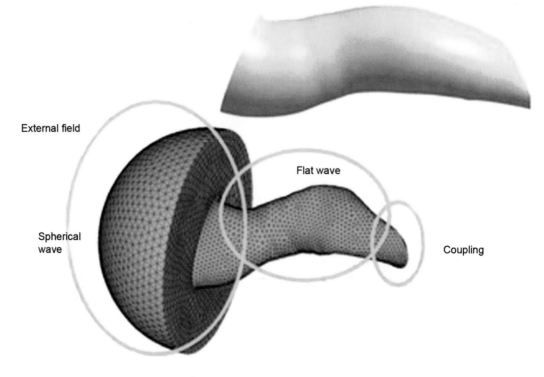

External field

Flat wave

Spherical wave

Coupling

Figure 1 External auditory canal (EAC). Modeling of the EAC using the method of finite elements (3D FE)

is not precise) of 2–3 mm constitutes the point of connection between the pinna and the ear canal, and is considered as part of the "inlet" to which we have already referred.

In the second segment, the sound wave acquires a form that approaches a flat wave that propagates in a similar way as that of acoustic energy in a cylindrical tube (Figure 2). In frequencies between 1 kHz and 4 kHz, the canal can be modeled as a tube with a uniform section that ends in a perpendicular surface, represented by the tympanic membrane. This can be valid even up to 8 kHz, but after this frequency it is necessary to design a new model (Figure 3) that considers the curvature and caliber variations of the canal as well as the tympanic membrane in an inclined position that is not exactly perpendicular to the axis of the tube.[2]

These data are even harder to interpret if the individual variability in length, caliber and form are considered.[7]

In the third zone which connects the ear canal and the tympanic membrane (drum coupling region or DCR), the acoustical events secondary to sound wave interaction with the tympanic membrane are hard to evaluate (Figure 4).[8] The gain in this area is minimal in low frequencies and of a maximum of 10 dB around the 4 kHz (Figures 5A to C).

Surgical changes in the DCR and particularly in the anterior tympanomeatal angle (Figure 6) can alter the levels of sound pressure in the tympanic membrane in high frequencies.[9]

Considering the ear canal as a whole, the resonance causes an amplification of 20 dB in the 2.8–3 kHz, depending on the length and diameter of the canal.[10]

In general, changes in volume and shape of the canal are not innocuous since they have, even if discrete, a functional incidence (Figure 7).

In radical cavities, the significant change in resonances has an effect that is significant for the low frequencies. The irregularity of the cavity causes only small changes of amplitude of the resonance (6 dB), but does not alter the resonant frequency.[11]

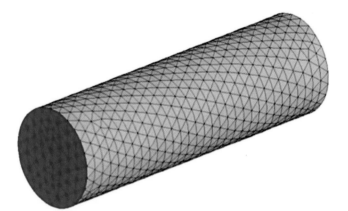

Figure 2 Modeling of a cylindrical tube of the dimensions of the EAC, in order to simulate its acoustical characteristics

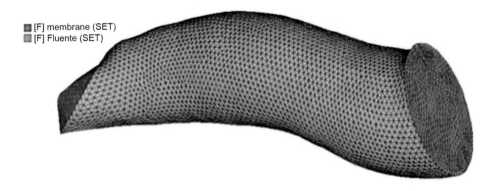

■ [F] membrane (SET)
■ [F] Fluente (SET)

Figure 3 3D FE model of EAC with its curvatures and caliber variations

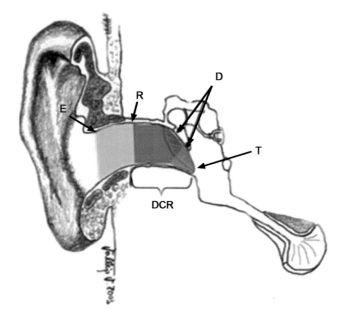

Figure 4 Areas in which Hudde and Engel[42] divide the external auditory canal according to its acoustical behavior
Key: E: entrance; R: reference section; DCR: region of sound wave coupling; D: tympanic membrane; T: tympanomeatal angle

Practical Suggestions

Based on what has been exposed it is important to consider the following:

- Unnecessary modifications in the "entrance area" are to be avoided
- Changes in form and volume of the ear canal are to be avoided, acting only in those portions that do not allow a satisfactory surgical approach
- The anterior tympanomeatal angle should, if possible, not be modified

MECHANO-ACOUSTICAL CHANGES DUE TO RECONSTRUCTION OF THE TYMPANIC MEMBRANE

While closure of perforation in tympanoplasty can be achieved in 85–90% of cases, normal hearing (gap of 10 dB or less) is achieved only in 43–80%.[12-16]

This difference between morphologic and functional success reflects that we not only need to achieve closure, but also recovery of functionality (acoustical properties) of the membrane.

Tympanic membrane reconstruction pretends to achieve three objectives:

1. Improve hearing
2. Prevent future infections
3. Isolate the middle ear cavity

The purpose of a myringoplasty is to obtain a membrane with functional properties similar to the natural membrane (Figures 8A and B). Many deficits in achieving closure within 10 dB are due to failures in reparative techniques.

The reconstruction of a central perforation (Figure 9) achieves a neomembrane that has the external (ectodermal) and internal (endodermal) epithelial layers, and not the middle (mesodermal) layer because it does not regenerate. Therefore, the pars tensa will not have the collagen fibers that in normal physiologic conditions has both radial (external) and circular (internal) layers as well as parabolic or connection fibers (Figure 10). The mechanical function of a tympanic membrane that is reconstructed is not comparable to the natural membrane. The thickness of 30–90 μm is generally surpassed and the disruption of fibers causes a loss of the conical shape with an angulation of 120° (Figure 11). The convexity at the umbo causes a special tension in the radial fibers, which in turn cause a stronger force over the umbomalleus handle area than in the rest of the membrane (Figure 12). That is to say, the lack of capacity of completely recovering the normal structure does not allow a perfect recovery of the efficiency of the natural membrane (Figure 12).

The pars flaccida of the tympanic membrane has elastic fibers that are at random and not seemingly oriented to a mechanical function nor possess a special strength to tolerate pressure forces. They seemingly allow a predisposition to the development of attical retraction pockets, pathological entities that put the surgeon in a difficult position either to operate or to observe. The poor mechanical function of the pars flaccida is compensated by other duties. The Schwann cells and axons of this area are considered some sort of mechanoreceptors[17,18] that can constitute a reflex arch (Figure 13) that stimulates tubary function in cases of low pressure in the tympanic cavity.[19]

If the structure of the tympanic membrane is considered together with the energy transfer at the malleus (Figure 14), and the articular and muscular organization of the ossicular chain, we will understand that the malleus does not vibrate in a fixed axis of rotation (Figure 15), and that its movement can change in all directions with movements of rotation and translation.

While it is impossible to re-establish all these and other functions with a myringoplasty, a normal hearing is still achieved

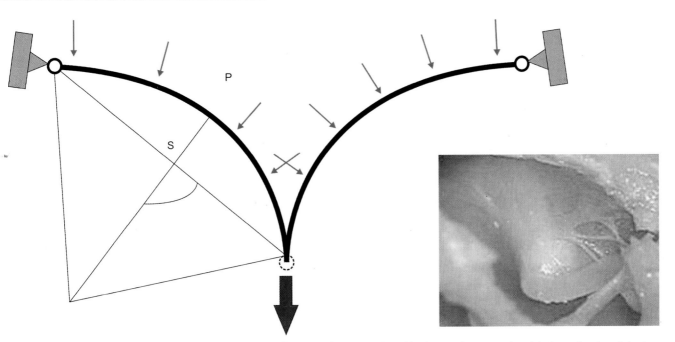

Figure 12 The tympanic membrane is convex to the outside. Small pressure changes originated by the sound waves reach mainly the malleus handle/umbo

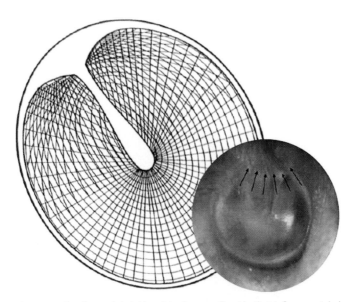

Figure 13 A reflex arch is initiated in the pars flaccida that influences tubal opening

between 43% and 80% of cases. This suggests the existence of compensatory mechanisms post surgery.

The mechano-acoustic properties of a repaired membrane depend on:

- The properties of the material that is used as a graft (size, mass, rigidity, etc.)

- The technique employed in the reconstruction (position of the graft, position in relationship to the malleus handle and tympanic frame)

There are different basal conditions for different elasticity properties of the natural structures compared to the grafting materials used for reconstruction.[9]

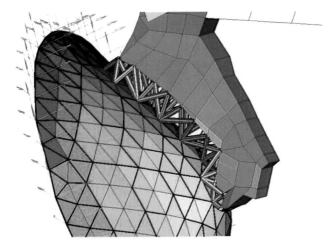

Figure 14 The strong fibrous union between the tympanic membrane and the malleus handle is essential for energy transfer between both structures

Pars tensa .... 3.3x107 N/m²
Pars flaccida .... 1.1x107 N/m²
Temporal fascia ....1.5x107 N/m²
Perichondrium ....2.0x107 N/m²
Conchal cartilage ....0.6x107 N/m²
Tragal cartilage ....0.3x107 N/m²

Grafting Materials and Their Use

Temporal fascia, perichondrium and cartilage are the most frequently used grafting materials.

Fascia and perichondrium have the advantage that their acoustical properties are similar to those of a normal membrane. The disadvantage is that their stability is worse than that of other materials.

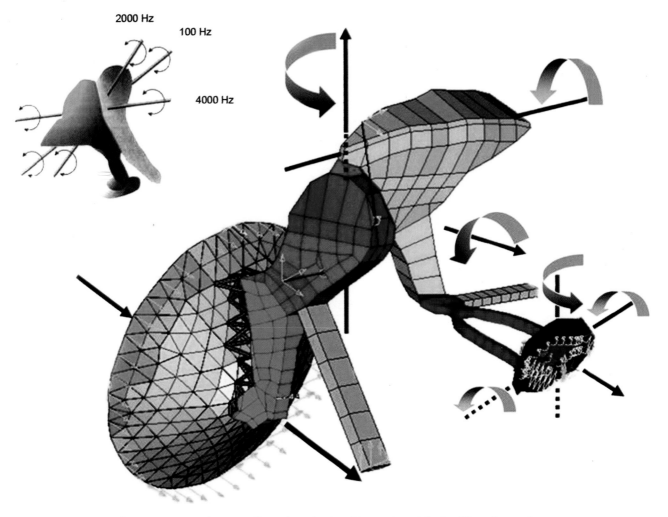

Figure 15 Rotation axis of the tympano-ossicular system. Above: classic drawing of the rotation axis for the different frequencies

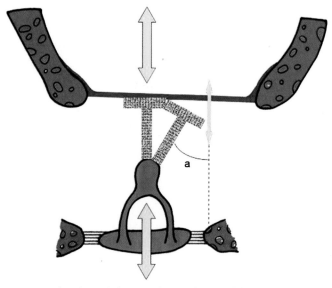

Figure 27 When the angle between the prostheses and the transmission axis is smaller, the system is more stable and efficient

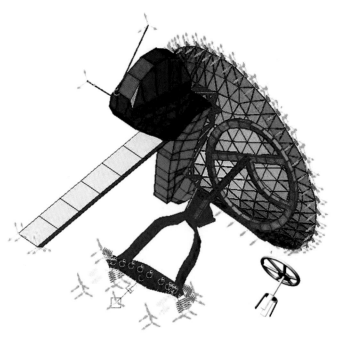

Figure 28 Securing the PORP to the head of the stapes with a clip, gives more stability

since it has a greater chance of being trapped and moved by retracting scar tissue and has a greater chance of leaning on the bony tympanic framework.

Weight of the prostheses: Weight has little influence in the modification of the mechano-acoustical factors in tympanoplasties (Figure 30).

In our computerized 3D model, the detriment is only 4dB when we multiply the weight of the prostheses by 8, and it is only 10 dB and only in high frequencies if the weight is increased 16 times.

The total weight of the ossicular chain is 56 mg. The weight of a titanium prosthesis (Kurz) is 4 mg and a gold prosthesis

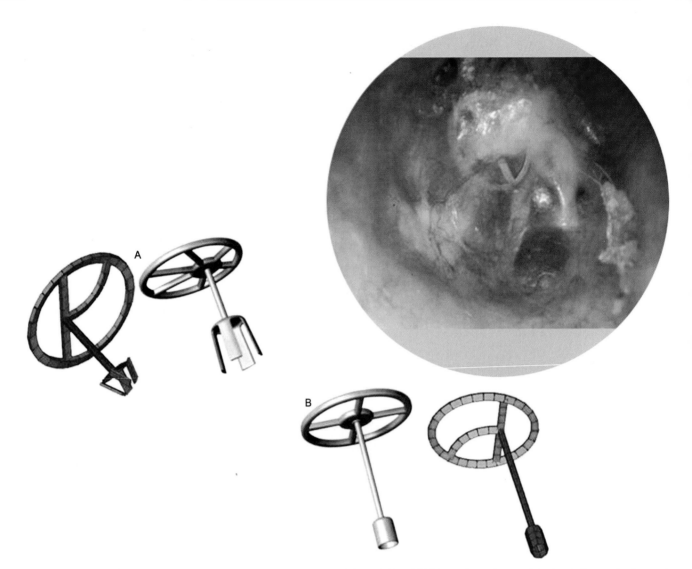

Figure 29 Larger heads have advantages and disadvantages (see text). Modeling TORP and PORP prostheses. Image of the head of a prosthesis seen by transparency

(Kurz) is 42 mg. Even if the difference is significant, the practical surgical result is the same.

Elastic coefficient and vibratory properties of the prostheses: Experimentally (simulated 3D), a more rigid prostheses has no clinical significance (Figure 31).[35-38]

Contact between the prostheses and the tympanic membrane, or the malleus handle:

- The contact is safe only when the length of the prostheses is adequate (Figure 32)
- The prostheses must be slightly lengthy so that its interposition has tightness when it is placed in between the chain remnants. By doing this there is:

- Less possibility of displacement by scar tissue
- Less displacement secondary to sudden pressure changes (nose blowing displaces the tympanic membrane 1 mm)
- A better contact of the prostheses with head of the stapes or stapes footplate

However, the length of the prostheses must not be too much because it can cause an excessive tension in the chain. In addition, too much footplate displacement elongates the fibers of Rudinger's ligament (Figure 33). Excessive tension by a prostheses can cause a loss up to 40 dB in the high frequencies.

A prostheses that is too long, can penetrate the vestibule and harm the saccule and utricle (Figure 34).

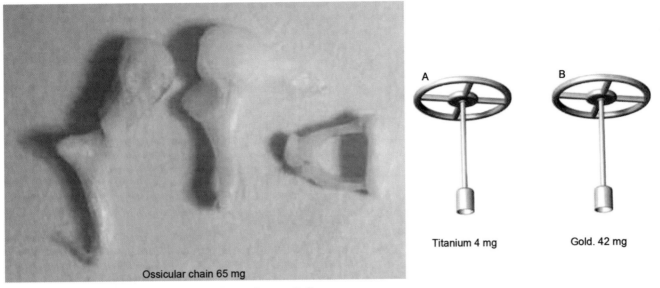

Figure 30 The weight of the prostheses has very little or no functional influence

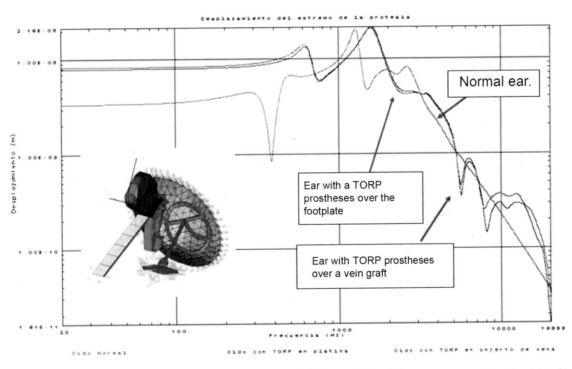

Figure 31 The rigidity of a prosthesis does not have clinical bearing. 3D FE shows a similar displacement response when placed directly over the footplate or over an open window covered by a vein graft, even if both elements have a different impedance

All these criteria are important in order to achieve stability of the reconstructed ossicular chain and in trying to avoid extrusion or displacement that would result in a loss of functional gain (Figures 35A to C).

MALLEOVESTIBULOPEXY

Theoretically, is the most stable system. The difficult part is to obtain a satisfactory prostheses design. The malleus handle

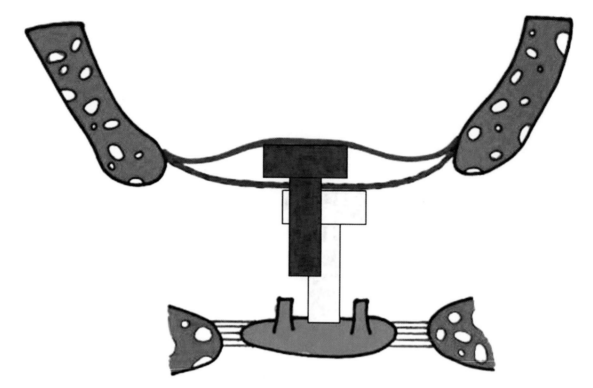

Figure 32 A short prostheses has poor stability

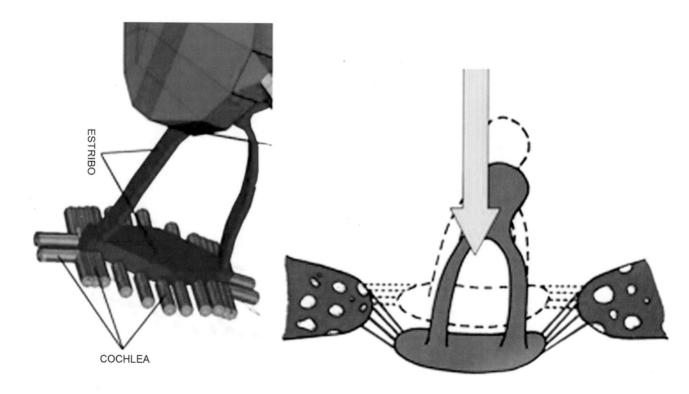

ESTRIBO

COCHLEA

Figure 33 An excessively large prosthesis can distend the fibers of the annular ligament and can even fix the system

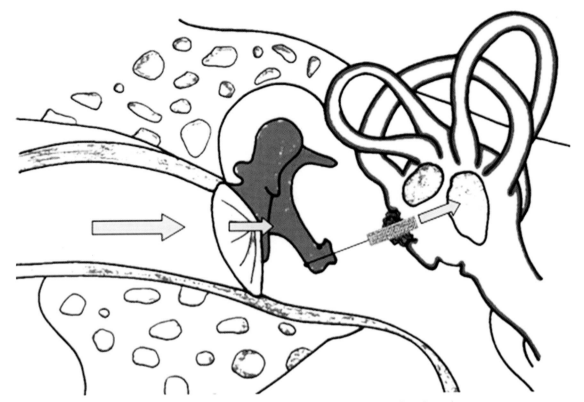

Figure 34 The distal end of the prostheses can penetrate the vestibule and damage the utricle and saccule

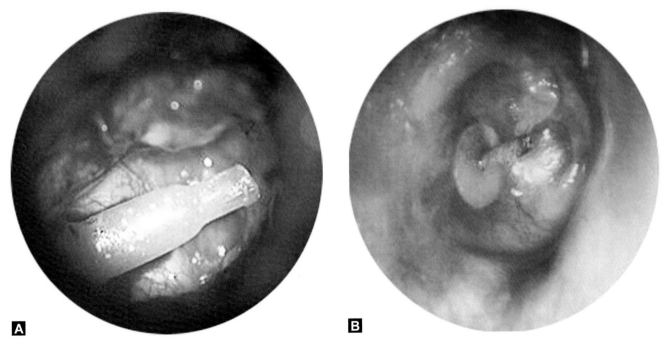

Figures 35A and B

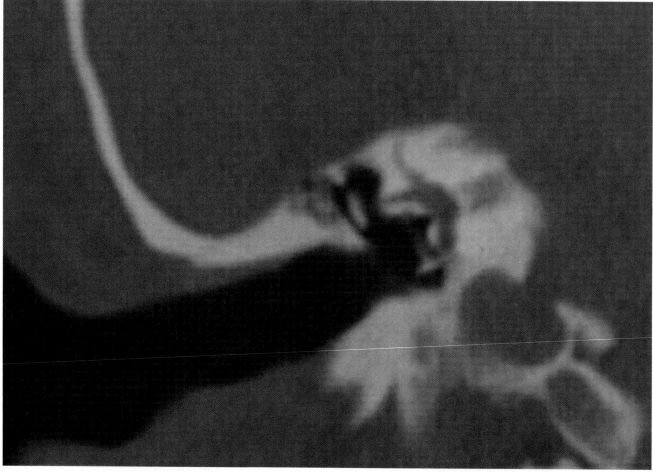

Figure 35C

Figures 35A to C Adequate criteria minimize possibilities of disarticulation or extrusion. (A and B) CT of a prosthesis laying over the promontory; (C) Prostheses extruding through the tympanic membrane

is eccentric with respect to the oval window, therefore, some angulations have to be developed. We have modified fluoroplastic prostheses and have obtained satisfactory results. Fixing the prostheses to the malleus handle requires separating the handle from the tympanic membrane and this deteriorates the area of contact between the membrane and the malleus (Figures 36 to 38).

The ostrich has a solid attachment of a columella to the tympanic membrane with three arms, and has only one muscle (since there is only one ossicle) and has no joints. This system is similar to malleovestibulopexy. Based on this observation, we developed a prostheses that optimizes these mechano-acoustical conditions and has a soft contact with the malleus handle. We modeled it through our 3D method of finite elements (3D FE) and verified its efficiency in a middle ear artificial model that they developed [Figures 39(A to C) to 41].

Practical Suggestions

Considerations for ossicular chain reconstruction are as follows:

- The selection of a good prostheses
- Alignment has to be efficient
- Proximal and distal ends of the prostheses must be adjusted adequately

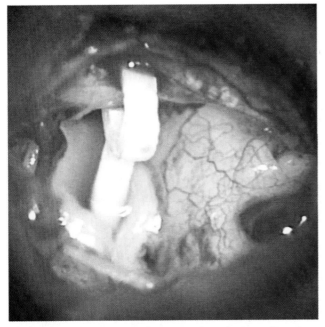
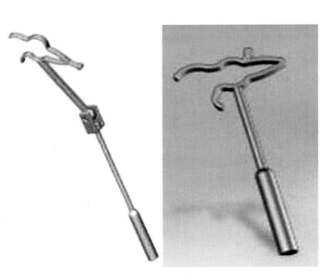

Figure 36 For malleovestibulopexy we use a fluoroplastic prostheses (see text)

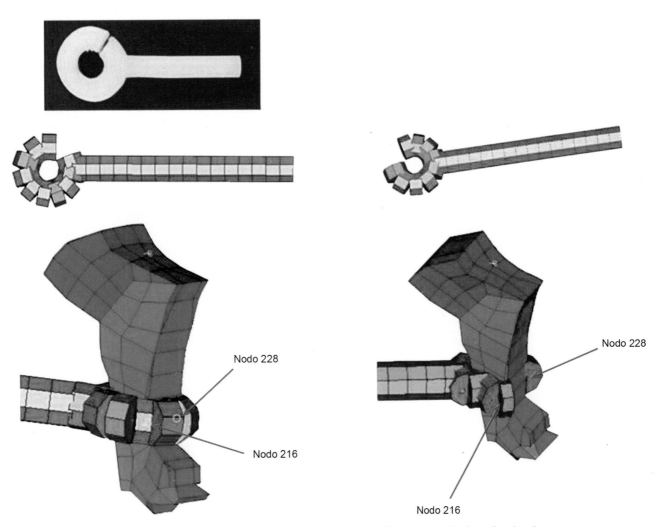

Nodo 228

Nodo 216

Nodo 228

Nodo 216

Figure 37 Malleovestibulopexy. Modeling of a fluoroplastic prostheses that has been modified and placed in the malleus handle

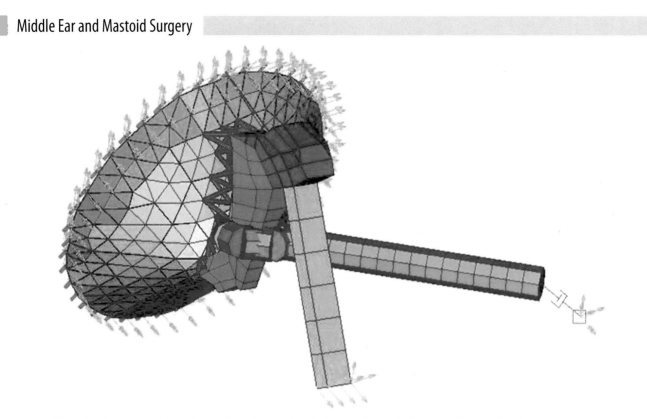

Figure 38 The junction of the malleus and membrane is altered when a malleovestibulopexy prostheses is placed

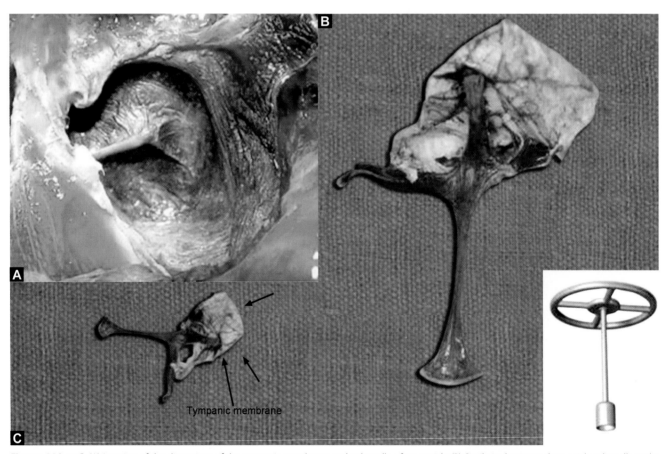

Figures 39A to C (A) Imaging of the dissections of the tympanic membrane and columella of an ostrich; (B) Similarity between the ostrich columella and a TORP; (C) Tympano-ossicular system of the ostrich (in mm)[43]

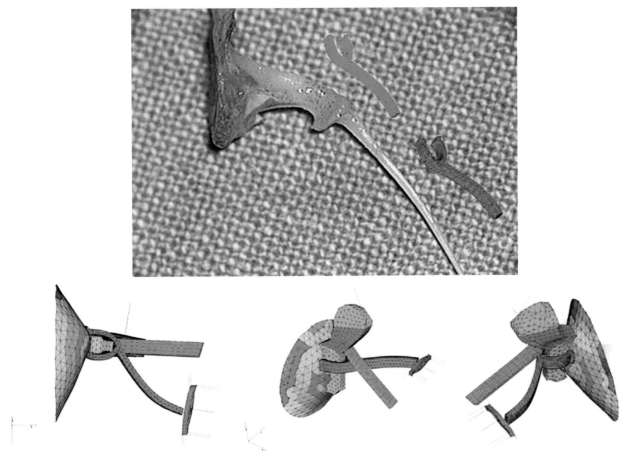

Figure 40 Design of a prosthesis. It attaches to the malleus like a crutch without having to dissect the malleus handle

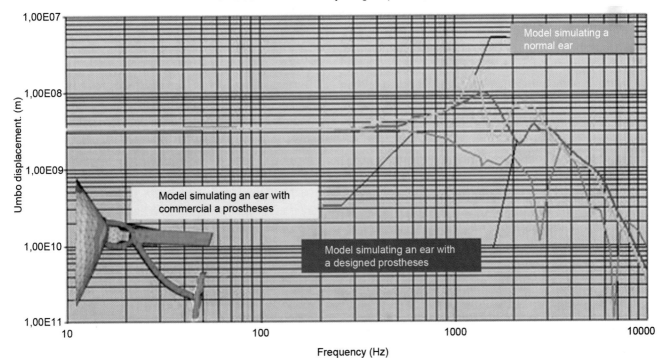

Curves of a simulated normal ear versus a simulated ear with a commercial prostheses and a simulated ear with a newly designed prostheses

Figure 41 3D FE validation. Comparison between a normal ear, the behavior of a conventional prosthesis and the prostheses designed by us

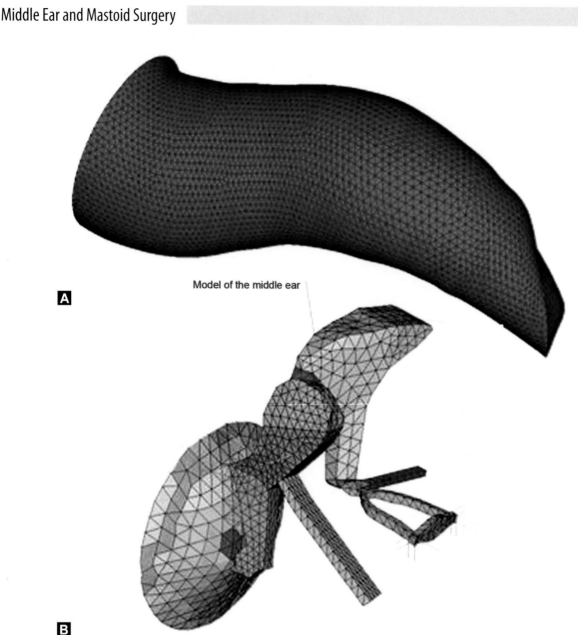

Model of the middle ear

A

B

Figures 42A and B 3D FE model of EAC and of the complete middle ear

- Contact with the tympanic (bony) frame is to be avoided
- Stability has to be achieved in order to avoid extrusion or displacement
- Depending on the case one has to choose either PORP, TORP, or malleovestibulopexy
- The annular ligament of the oval window must be mobile
- A prosthesis over a graft in an open footplate has a higher chance for major complications

We end this chapter calling your attention to the fact that it is very difficult to show functional results following middle ear surgery. Middle ear pathology frequently associate with bone conduction loss (sensorineural) in hearing

tests,[39] and this also occurs following tympanoplasy and stapedectomy.[40]

Most of the criteria described in this chapter have been confirmed in our 3D simulator. Following the development of our experimental middle ear,[41] we developed the experimental external auditory canal (Figures 42A and B); the model that couples both of them (Figure 43) and the model of overall system (Figure 44).

These models (Figures 45 and 46) are useful instruments for the study of middle ear physiology and of its function when modifications are introduced simulating tympanoplasty (Figures 47 and 48).

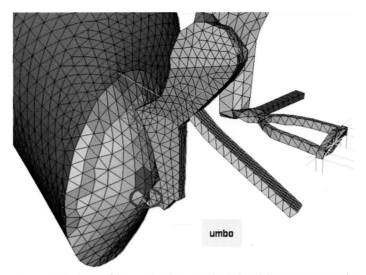

Figure 43 Modeling of the coupling between the EAC and the tympano-ossicular system

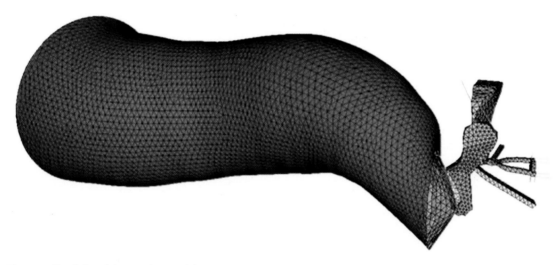

Figure 44 Simulation of the complete model

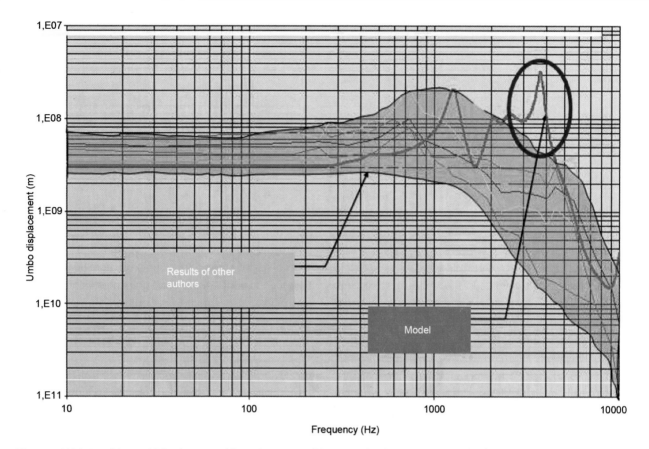

Figure 45 Validation of the model. Displacement of the umbo in our model compared to the experimental result of other authors. In gray are the results of other authors, in red; our model

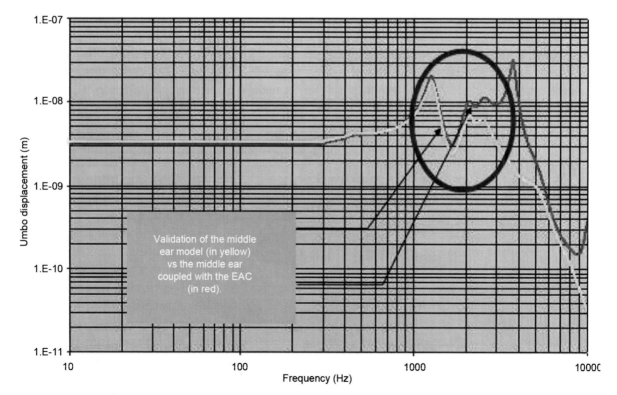

Figure 46 Validation of the middle ear model vs the middle ear coupled with the EAC. The differences that can be seen between 2 kHz and 5 kHz are due to the effect of the first resonance of the EAC

5.2.4A (III)

The Use of Cartilage in Tympanoplasty

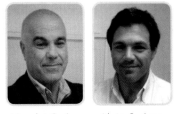

Hamlet Suárez,   Alejo Suárez

INTRODUCTION

The term "tympanoplasty" implies the concept of reconstruction of the middle ear with the purpose of re-establishing continuity of the structures involved in sound transmission to the inner ear that have been involved in a pathological process.

This involves tympanic membrane and ossicular chain reconstruction considering principles that include the resolution of pathology as well as functional sound transmission.

Until the 60s, the concept of functional reconstruction that prevailed were established by Wullstein and Zollner,[1,2] but soon thereafter other authors, such as C Janssen[3] started using autologous materials, such as perichondrium, fascia and the patient's own cartilage. In the following years synthetic materials started appearing to be used in reconstruction of the ossicular chain with the purpose of re-establishing functionality of the middle ear.

In this section we will describe some aspects of interest in the use of cartilage in reconstructive procedures of the middle ear, procedures that we perform in our medical practice.

Many forms of chronic otitis media can present with tympanic lesions. These can vary from simpler inflammatory reactions, such as, those in mucoid otitis to severe forms, such as, those of adhesive otitis with atelectasis of the tympanic membrane with aggression to the ossicular chain and/or the development of cholesteatoma, which generally evolves with phenomena of osteolysis.

Surgery is in these cases a therapeutic intervention oriented toward eradicating the underlying disease as well as to reconstruct the tympanic membrane. The use of different grafting materials, such as temporal muscle fascia and perichondrium has been described, however, not infrequently when there is tubal dysfunction with the presence of atelectasis; these materials tend to fail and re-perforations occur. This is crucial when there is an associated alteration of tubal function, where in the tensional intratympanic changes end up with a re-perforation of the grafted membrane. For this reason the use of auricular cartilage was proposed in order to strengthen the membrane and protect it from the tensional

changes occurring within the middle ear cavity, and at the same time protect it from the development of retraction pockets and secondary atelectasia.[3-6]

CHARACTERISTICS OF THE AURICULAR CARTILAGE

It is an elastic cartilage which like the other types of cartilage (hyaline, articular, fibrous), is a variety of connective tissue and the main supporting element of bone.

It is constituted by two main cells: chondroblasts (young cells) and chondrocytes (mature cells), a matrix with elastic and collagen fibers and ground substance (glycoproteins). It is covered by perichondrium which has two layers; an external constituted by collagen fibers and fibroblasts and an internal with undifferentiated mesenchymal cells. The nutrition of the cartilage comes from the perichondrial vessels; however, blood vessels do not penetrate the cartilage itself (nutrients diffuse).

The elastic auricular cartilage is characterized by abundant elastic fibers which give it elasticity and consistency (Figures 1A and B).

The characteristics, in terms of thickness and position of the cartilage to be placed, have been measured with optoelectronic holography with laser.[7]

Indications

Although some authors indicate the universal use of cartilage in all cases for tympanic membrane repair, the formal indications that we use are as follows:

1. *Recurrent tympanic membrane perforations:* In many instances the otologic surgeon has to repair a perforated membrane that has recurred after many previous surgical attempts. In general, this type of failures are secondary to tubal dysfunction related to chronic rhinosinusitic processes that can be clinically evident or not that evident. This implies that any surgical repair (in addition to treating the nasal and sinus problem) will require a mechanism that provides a stronger support in order to resist the tensional changes of a middle ear cavity with poor tubal function. Cartilage has shown to be a good option in these cases, providing definite closures.[3-6]

2. *Total tympanic membrane perforations:* When the tympanic lesion implies a complete or almost complete destruction of the membrane the search for supporting material such as cartilage becomes essential.

   Frequently, the annulus margin is minimal and this does not allow adequate positioning of a temporal muscle fascia, and the chances of graft retraction, reabsorption and re-perforation are high. Therefore, placing cartilage that will allow separation of the fascia from the promontory is essential (Figure 2).

   Palisade technique or placing a wide piece of cartilage can be used. Bernal Sprekelsen et al.[8] represent one of the groups that have proposed this technique of placing cartilage in the form of a palisade in cases with and without posterior canal wall. They have used it even in some cases of cholesteatoma with a 98.3% of definite closure with recurrence of cholesteatoma in 2.2% of patients. The gap closure was of 50%.

   On occasions when there are rigidities of the chain with fibrosis and incudo-malleal autolysis, placing the cartilage over the incudostapedial joint will allow sound transmission from the new tympanic membrane to the stapes. On other occasions when there is significant lysis or rigidity of the ossicular chain, it is best to use a prosthesis of synthetic material.[8]

3. *Chronic otitis media with severe atelectasis of the tympanic membrane:* In some chronic inflammatory processes of the middle ear the tympanic membrane retracts without having a perforation. The membrane looses its middle layer and becomes a bimeric membrane that is adherent to the ossicular chain, and oval and round windows. This causes an auditory deficit and at times, with interruption of the functional integrity of the ossicular chain, an added risk of developing a secondary cholesteatoma.

   Aidonis et al.[9] published a report of 62 patients with atelectasis with reconstruction of the membrane and used auricular cartilage shaped like a shield. They obtained significant improvements in audiometric thresholds, and absence of recurrence of pathology and re-perforations. In these cases, a tympanoplasty with conventional techniques, as compared to the use of cartilage, has a high risk of failure because of the underlying tubal dysfunction.

   If possible, the bimeric membrane that is adherent to the promontory and ossicular chain is removed in block. More often than not, this is not possible because it usually breaks down (since there is no fibrous layer) and it has to be removed piece by piece.

   Placement of cartilage is done following this "de-epithelialization", making sure that the ossicular chain is intact and that there is no residual cholesteatoma under the cartilage (Figure 3).

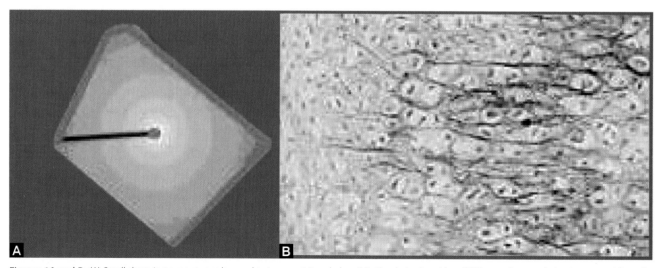

Figures 1A and B (A) Small sharp instruments can be used to transport it and place it in the desired position; (B) The cartilage graft that is removed from the auricular tragus or the pinna must be handled with care in order to avoid structural alterations of its elastic structure

5.2.4A (IV)
Harvesting of Cartilage and Perichondrium

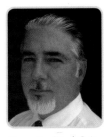

Ernesto Ried G Jr

GRAFTING MATERIALS IN OTOLOGIC SURGERY

The most used grafting materials in all countries are: temporalis muscle fascia, cartilage and perichondrium. The great majority of these grafts are used for sequelae of chronic otitis media. The additional use of cartilage has been preferred in cases of Eustachian tube dysfunction, retraction pockets, atelectasis and attical cholesteatomas, as well as in revision surgery. Cartilage is also used in cases in which partial or total ossicular prostheses are placed in order to increase the surface that is in contact with the overlying tympanic membrane or graft.

Obtaining Tragal Cartilage

Tragal cartilage is a structure that is easy to obtain and easy to work with. It has an adequate size and a curvature that accommodates quite well to the tympanic membrane. If it is not available in revision surgery, it can be easily obtained with a postauricular incision in children and older adults as well.

The free border of the tragus is palpated and local anesthetic solution with epinephrine is injected (Figures 1A and B). This is done prior to working in the ear canal. Injection should not be deep in order to avoid injecting the plane between cartilage and perichondrium. Infiltration must be placed in the subcutaneous tissue and the surgeon must wait for a few minutes for the vasoconstrictor to have an effect. Multiple puncture sites must be avoided.

The incision can be done in the free border or slightly towards the dorsal aspect of the tragus. This skin incision can be done with a 15 or 11 scalpel blade from the sides toward the center. The anterior border is grasped with a double hook and the assistant pulls it upwards. This allows the tragal cartilage and the ear canal to be aligned. With blunt dissection, the assistant suctions in between the scissor blades, while the surgeon helps himself with Adson forceps in order to improve vision of the operative field. The incision can also be done 4 or 5 mm posterior (dorsal) to the free border, but there is a risk of falling directly over the cartilage and harming it. The cartilage is identified and exposed with blunt scissors without touching the perichondrium (Figure 2).

The graft is obtained once the cartilage is clearly exposed. For use in smaller perforations or in stapedectomy, posterior perichondrium will suffice (Figures 3A to D). Cartilage with perichondrium can also be obtained. Four or five millimeters of the free border of the tragus should be left in place in order to avoid a cosmetic defect; however, perichondrium can be obtained up to 1 mm from the free border without influencing stability. The tragal cartilage presents a perichondrium that is adherent to the preauricular muscles. Therefore, its removal can cause a small amount of bleeding. It is useful to free all adherences of tragus to cartilage of the ear canal priorly at the level of the incisura of Santorini. The muscle fibers must be sectioned sharply without traction (Figures 4A and B).

This cartilage must be kept in saline until work under the microscope is performed. Thinning is done with a new scalpel blade from the center toward the borders (Figure 5). This allows that the graft acquires a curvature that adapts better to the perforation (Figure 6). A small piece of cartilage can be left attached to a larger piece of perichondrium. This can be used in lateral or small to medium perforations and the cartilage can be placed medial to the tympanic membrane covering remnants or ossicles in type II or III tympanoplasties.

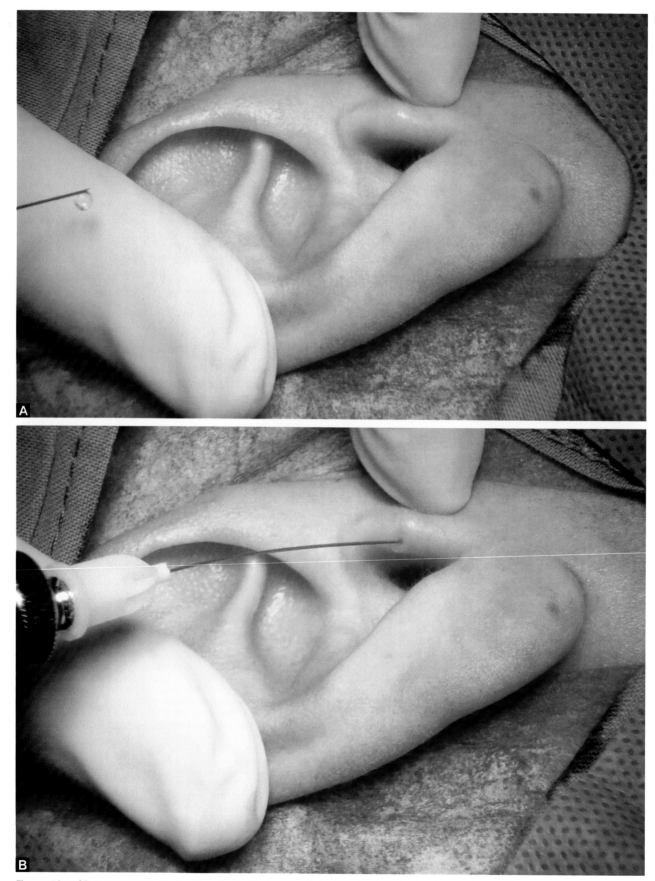

Figures 1A and B Tragal cartilage obtained by palpating the tragus and injecting a local anesthetic solution with epinephrine

Cartilage of the External Auditory Canal

It is medial to the tragal cartilage. It is smaller and has a triangular shape with a superior and two inferior "roots". Of these two, one goes toward the auricular concha and the other toward the external auditory canal. It is not commonly used since it is smaller than the tragus. It is more firm, thicker and its perichondrium is firmly attached. When there is a need of cartilage, it can be removed simultaneously with the tragal cartilage. It should be removed prior to the tragal cartilage since it has no tight muscular adherences and bleeds minimally; therefore the operative field remains cleaner.

The posterior side should be separated first and then through the Santorini incisure, the anterior side should be separated until reaching the beginning of the osseous external auditory canal. Once it is free in both sides, it is held firmly with Adson forceps, and is retracted superiorly and both inferior "roots" are sectioned. Then it is pulled inferiorly so to section the superior root. Its removal is not complex and leaves a surgical field that rarely requires the use of cautery. The graft can be "carved" or thinned under the microscope according to need.

Cartilage from the Auricular Concha

This graft is a good option for patients who have had surgery and tragal cartilage is not available. It can be obtained directly from the auricular concha with an incision in the posterior border from the antitragus to the root of the helix. Infiltration is done previously with an anesthetic and with epinephrine.

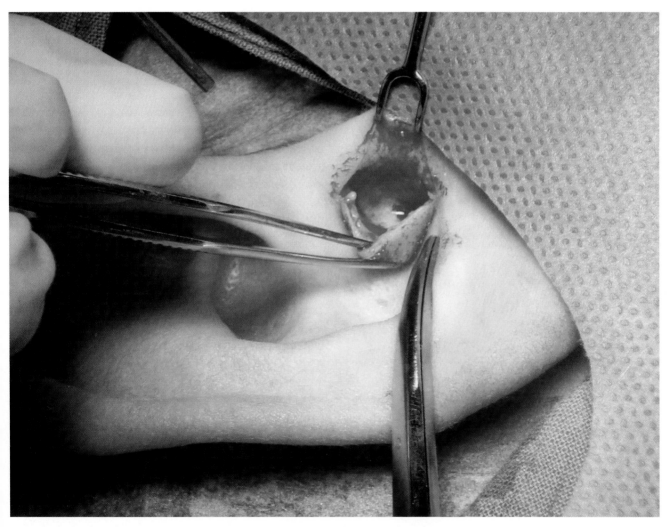

Figure 2 Cartilage identified and exposed with blunt scissors without touching the perichondrium

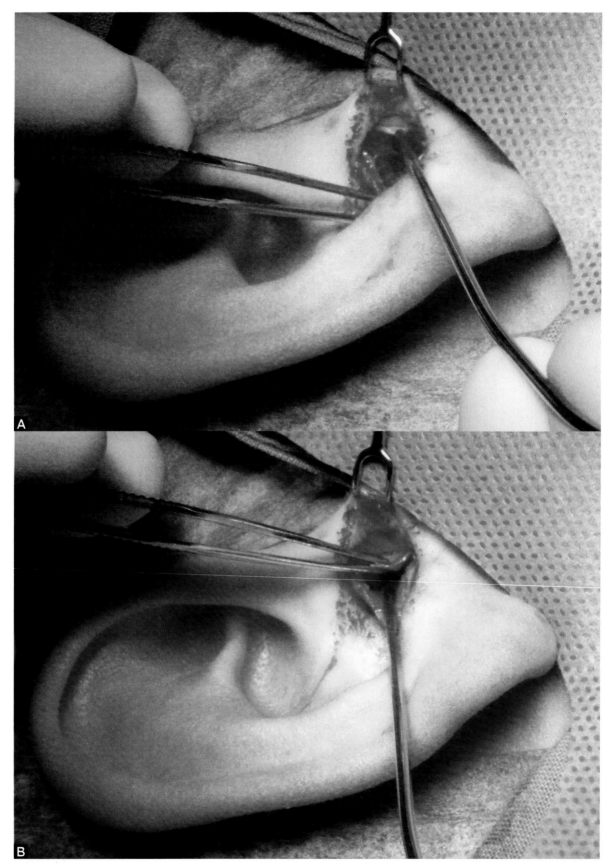

Figures 3A and B

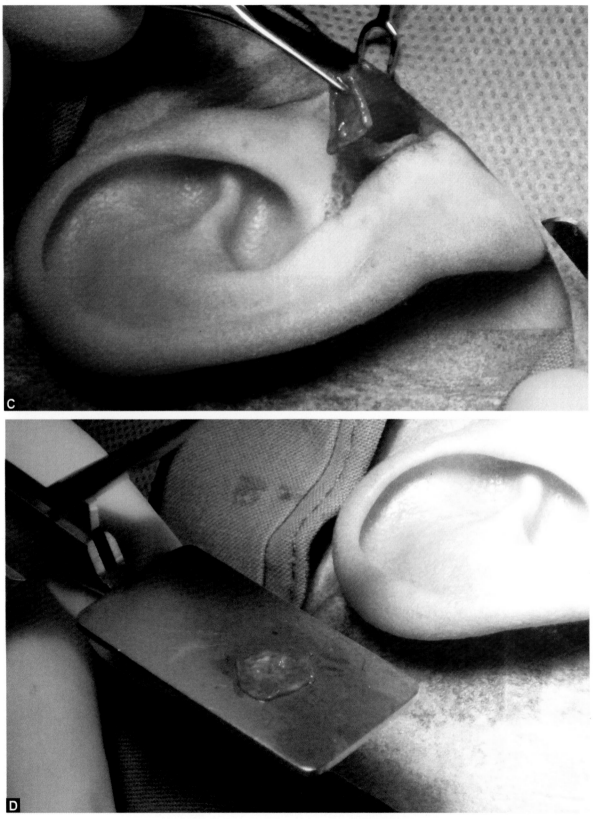

Figures 3C and D

Figures 3A to D The graft is obtained once the cartilage is clearly exposed. For use in smaller perforations or in stapedectomy, posterior perichondrium will suffice

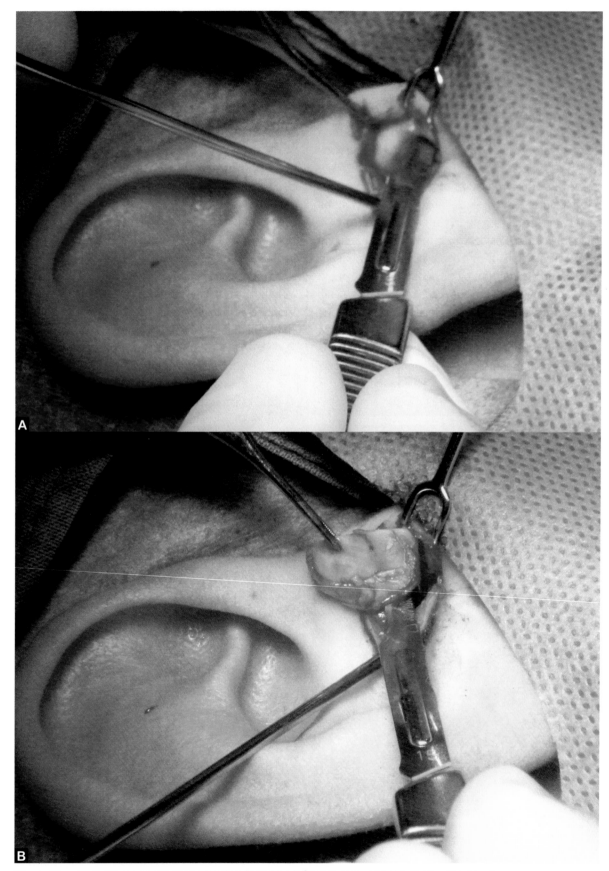

Figures 4A and B Cartilage presenting with a perichondrium; muscle fibers must be sectioned sharply without traction

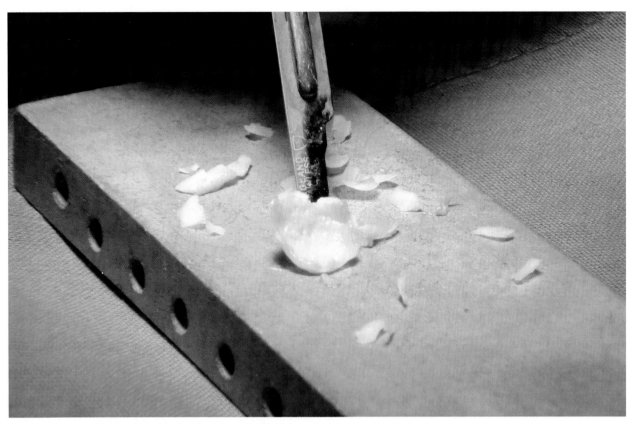

Figure 5 Thinning of the cartilage is done with a new scalpel blade from the center towards the borders

The skin incision is done until the free border of the cartilage is reached. The cartilage is sectioned and a blunt dissection is done in its medial surface. Hemostasis is done with bipolar cautery. Closure is done in one plane and compression is done with a gauze. The cartilage can also be obtained through a postauricular incision. In this case, cartilage work should be done palpating the anterior surface with the index finger in order to avoid damaging the conchal skin.

This cartilage is stiffer and its lateral surface adapts quite well to the size and curvature of the tympanic membrane. It must be prepared very carefully under the microscope because it breaks quite easily if the perichondrium of one of its surfaces is removed. It is better to thin it with a new scalpel blade with gradual removal of thin pieces until reaching the desired size and thickness. It can be used in large tympanic membrane perforations, closure of cavities and reconstruction of posterior wall or attic defects. The drawback of this graft is that obtaining it requires more work and closure is more uncomfortable. Moreover, in elderly patients this cartilage can be calcified and it is hard to thin it.

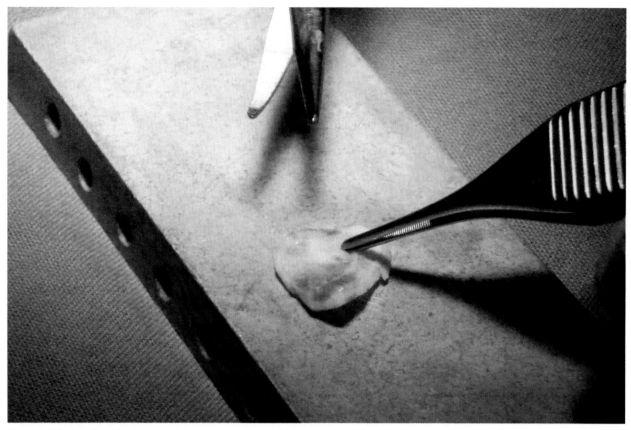

Figure 6 Thinning allows the graft to acquire a curvature that adapts better to the perforation

5.2.4B

Onlay Tympanoplasty Techniques

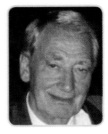

Mirko Tos

INTRODUCTION

Onlay myringoplasty denotes placement of the fascia graft (Ørtegren 1964) or of the perichondrium graft onto the denuded lamina propria of the perforated eardrum, in contrast to the underlay myringoplasty, where the fascia or perichondrium graft is placed under the perforated lamina propria. Onlay myringoplasty was started in the fifties, slightly before, than the underlay myringoplasty. Wullstein (1952, 1963, 1968), Zöllner (1954, 1957, 1959).

ONLAY MYRINGOPLASTY WITH SKIN GRAFTS

Before the onlay placement of the fascia or of the perichondrium onto the denuded lamina propria "the pedicled ear canal skin graft" was used by Zöllner (1954) and Frenckner (1955), for a period of two years. It was soon replaced by Wullstein's "free split-skin grafts." The split-skin graft, harvested from the posterior auricular skin, includes only two-thirds or three quarters of the thickness. "Thin meatal skin" was used and popularized by Plester (1960, 1963, 1989) as free full thickness graft, and used it commonly during the sixties.

ONLAY MYRINGOPLASTY WITH FASCIA OR PERICHONDRIUM

In relation to the management of the keratinized squamous epithelium of the eardrum remnant, and of the fibrous annulus, the onlay techniques are subdivided in:

• Removal of the epithelium from the eardrum remnant (Figure 1) and eventually from the fibrous annulus, without covering of the denuded graft. The denuded lamina propria will be "gradually epithelialized" from the border of the ear canal skin. This method has a risk that the perforation will not be closed completely; therefore I will not recommend it.

• Elevation and outward dissection of the epithelium of the eardrum remnant, followed by covering of the denuded eardrum and the perforation with the fascia or the perichondrium. Finally, the epithelial flaps are replaced (Figure 2).

• Sandwich techniques, with complete removal the eardrum-remnant epithelium and ear canal skin, placement of the fascia on the denuded fibrous annulus, and covering the fascia with ear canal skin.

ONLAY MYRINGOPLASTY IN VARIOUS PERFORATIONS

In the early period of myringoplasty, in the early fifties, the split-skin grafts and the ear canal skin grafts, were used as onlay techniques, but soon, as underlay techniques with fascia or perichondrium were used.

In my *Manual of Middle Ear Surgery volume 1* (Tos 1993) perforations of pars tensa were divided in anterior, inferior, posterior, subtotal and total perforation. This nomenclature is to be used here.

Each of the perforations has some differences and onlay closures of the different perforations will be described here.

Anterior Perforation

Onlay technique is in my opinion the most rewarding technique for the anterior perforation, especially because it is easier and safer than the underlay technique. Anterior perforation can be closed by the onlay technique in different methods:

• Technique with total removal of the epithelium: edge of the perforation is in all methods cleaned for squamous epithelium. Incision of the epithelium is made along the posterior border of the malleus handle, along the anterosuperior border of the eardrum and along the anteroinferior part of

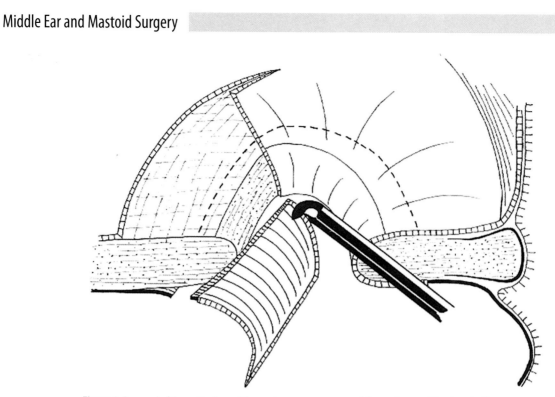

Figure 1 Removal of the epithelium of the eardrum remnant around the perforation. The denuded lamina propria and the perforation will be gradually epithelialized (Tos 1993)

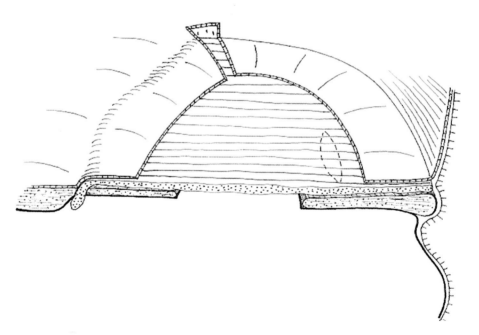

Figure 2 Final situation of cleaning the edge of the perforation, elevation of the epithelium flaps, placement of the fascia graft onto the denuded eardrum, and replacement of the elevated epithelial flaps (Tos 1993)

the eardrum. Finally an incision is made in the ear canal skin 1 mm lateral to the annulus. The epithelium is elevated and removed, and the fascia covers the denuded area (Figure 3).

- *Epithelial flap technique:* Epithelium is removed from the edge of the perforation. An anterior incision of the ear

canal skin is made 1 mm lateral to the anterior fibrous annulus. The skin flap is cut at 9 o`clock position and an anterosuperior epithelial flap is elevated, exposing the superior part of the malleus handle. Epithelium from the anteroinferior part of the eardrum is removed (Figure 4).

The fascia is placed onto the denuded area of the eardrum, onto the superior part of the malleus handle and onto the ear canal bone. The superior skin flap will be replaced and fixated by gelfoam balls.

- *Elevation of the anterior ear canal skin flap together with the epithelium around the perforation* (Figure 5): The anterior meatal skin flap is elevated together with the epithelium around the perforation including the malleus handle. The fascia graft is placed onto the denuded eardrum and the epithelium, with the ear canal skin is replaced and covered with the gelfoam balls.

- *Outward elevation of the anterior ear canal skin flap, together with the epithelium surrounding the anterior perforation* (Figure 6): A bulged anterior ear canal bone can easily be drilled away and the denuded anterior lamina propria will be covered with the fascia or with perichondrium.

Here only the basic methods are described, in the literature some small variations will be found.

In my opinion, onlay closure of the anterior perforation is the easiest and safest procedure. Placement of the fascia onto the denuded lamina propria is easy and safe. Underlay placement of the fascia need a support under the eardrum, such a support is usually gelfoam.

Inferior Perforation

The inferior perforation of various sites is easily and safely closed in onlay techniques. The surgeon can in all approaches; the transcanal, endaural and retroauricular approach easy close an inferior perforation. Some onlay methods of myringoplasty caused by simple chronic otitis media without cholesteatoma will be described below.

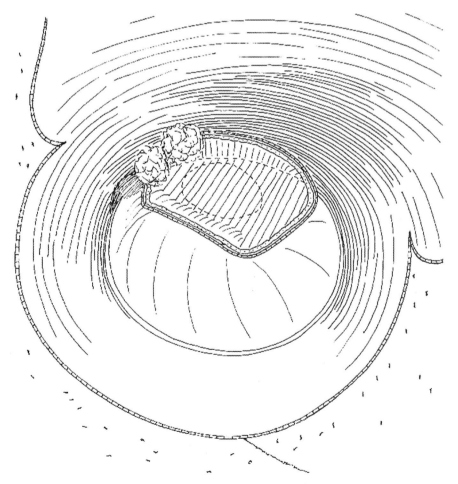

Figure 3 Onlay technique with removal of the epithelium around the anterior perforation. Edge of the perforation is cleaned for squamous epithelium, and four incisions of the epithelium are made: one along the posterior edge of the malleus handle, one along the anterosuperior, one along the anteroinferior and one is anterior skin incision of the ear canal. Fascia covers the denuded part of the eardrum, malleus handle and the bony annulus (Tos 1993).

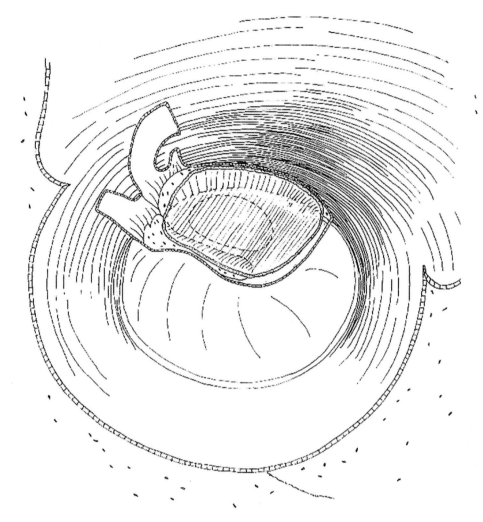

Figure 4 The superior two epithelium flaps are elevated, the epithelium around the inferior half of the anterior perforation is removed. The denuded eardrum with the anterior fibrous and bony annulus will be covered by the fascia graft (Tos 1993)

- *Elevation of the epithelium around the small perforation:* Denuded lamina propria and the perforation are covered with the fascia or the perichondrium and finally the elevated epithelium is replaced and covers the perforation. Such simple method is used for small perforations.
- *Superior onlay epithelium flap technique in a large inferior perforation:* Incision of the ear canal skin 1 mm lateral to the fibrous annulus, from the 9 o'clock to the 3 o'clock position is performed. The elevated skin and the epithelium are removed. Superiorly, the epithelium is elevated. A fascia covers the denuded eardrum, fibrous annulus and the denuded ear canal bone (Figure 7). Finally, the superior epithelium flaps are replaced.

- *Outward elevation of the epithelium and partly of the ear canal skin in a large inferior perforation* (Figure 8): Three radial incisions at 3, 6, and 9 positions are performed and the three epithelium flaps with some ear canal skin are elevated. Fascia is placed onto the denuded lamina propria and the elevated epithelium and skin flaps are replaced.
- *Onlay epithelial flap technique with a large tympanomeatal flap:* An incision is made from the 9 o'clock to the 3-o'clock position 5 mm lateral to the fibrous annulus and the skin flap with the epithelium of the eardrum is elevated. Fascia is placed onto the denuded eardrum (Figure 9) and the perforation. The skin flap with the epithelium flap will be replaced.

5.2.4C(V)
The Yo-Yo Technique for Small Central Perforations

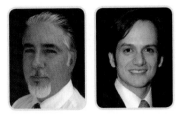

Ernesto Ried G, Nicolás Albertz

INTRODUCTION

Myringoplasty is a surgical method that is used to re-establish the integrity of the tympanic membrane in cases of small or mid-sized perforations without associated compromise of the ossicular chain. These perforations are usually secondary to trauma or otitis media.[1,2] It was introduced by Berthold and corresponds to a Type I tympanoplasty in the Wullstein classification.[3] Its purposes are to close the perforation and restore normal hearing.

Myringoplasty with a compound cartilage-perichondrium graft offers the advantage of providing a higher resistance of the repaired tympanic membrane. In addition, cartilage is irrigated by diffusion and does not need neovascularization in order to survive in early stages.[4] Compound grafts can be used with different techniques (lateral, medial or lateromedial) and the graft can be designed in different shapes, such as island, butterfly, ring, palisade, etc.[5]

In order to obtain optimal stability and resistance we have developed an approach which we have termed the yo-yo technique, which is described to follow.

SURGICAL TECHNIQUE

Under general anesthesia or using local anesthesia with sedation, tragal cartilage is obtained with perichondrium in both sides (Figure 1). The perforation is visualized by a transcanal approach (Figure 2), doing a canalplasty as needed and radial epithelial flaps are developed from the borders until obtaining a satisfactory fibrous layer that can "receive" a graft. A composite "yo-yo" graft is then carved (Figure 3). The cartilage is cut of a size that is slightly larger than the perforation. The thicker perichondrium of the anterior tragus is removed (Figure 4),

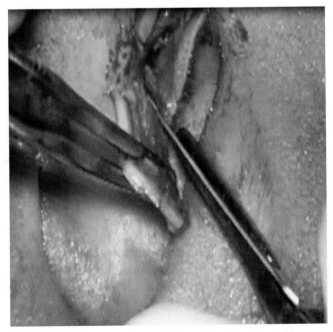

Figure 1 Tragal cartilage is obtained with perichondrium in both sides

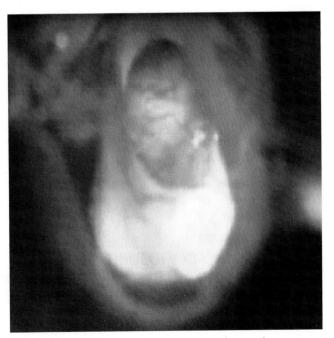

Figure 2 The perforation is visualized by a transcanal approach

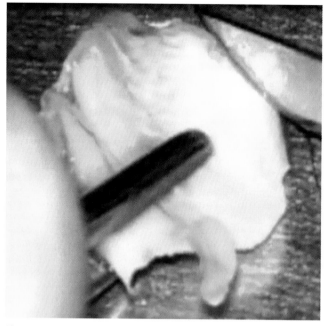

Figure 3 A composite "yo-yo" graft is then carved

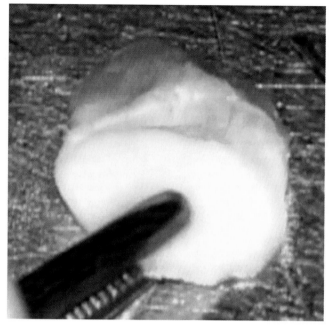

Figure 4 The thicker perichondrium of the anterior tragus is removed

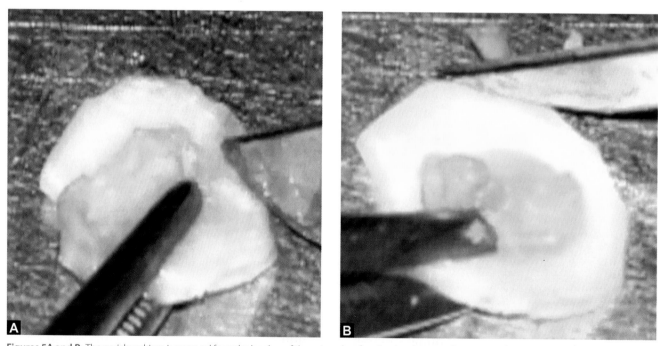

Figures 5A and B The perichondrium is removed from the borders of the external surface leaving the central portion in place. The size of the central portion is of the same size or slightly smaller than the perforation

leaving the posterior perichondrium for the external or lateral side of the perforation. The perichondrium is removed from the borders of the external surface leaving the central portion in place. The size of the central portion is of the same size or slightly smaller than the perforation (Figures 5A and B). The edges of the cartilage are thinned and so is the center but to a lesser degree. This improves sound conduction and the graft acquires a curvature which adapts quite well to the shape of the tympanic membrane, leaving a cartilaginous cover of a size that is slightly larger than the perforation.

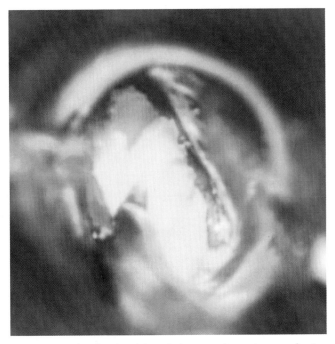

Figure 6 Carved graft is placed through the tympanic membrane perforation just as a button through a buttonhole, with the cartilage placed medial to the tympanic membrane

Once the graft is carved, it is placed through the tympanic membrane perforation just as a button through a buttonhole, with the cartilage placed medial to the tympanic membrane (Figure 6). The perichondrium that was left in place in the lateral surface of the graft is extended over the lateral surface of the tympanic membrane, over the de-epithelized fibrous layer (Figures 7A and B). The epithelial flaps are repositioned over the perichondrium and small pieces of gelfoam® are placed over the surface of the tympanic membrane. Gelfoam® is not used in the middle ear.

CONCLUSION

Over the years, this yo-yo technique has become very useful since it is easy to perform and provides excellent anatomic and functional results (Figure 8). The oversized cartilaginous medial portion of the graft provides stability and integrates very well to the tympanic membrane structure. These results have been satisfactory in both children and in adults, for small or mid-size central perforations regardless of their location.

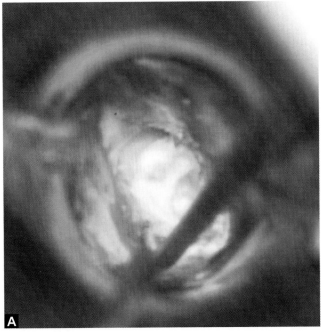

Figures 7A and B Perichondrium is extended over the lateral surface of the tympanic membrane, over the de-epithelized fibrous layer

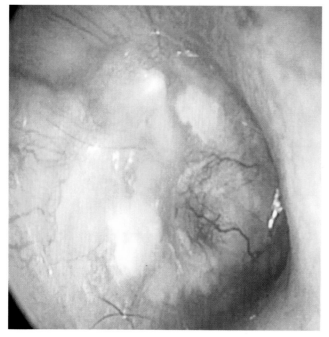

Figure 8 Yo-yo technique provides excellent anatomic and functional results

REFERENCES

1. Paparella MM, Shea D, Meyerhoff WL, et al. Silent otitis media. Laryngoscope. 1980;90(7 Pt 1):1089-98.

2. Goycoolea MV, Paparella MM, Juhn SK, et al. Otitis media with perforation of the tympanic membrane: a longitudinal experimental study. Laryngoscope. 1980;90(12):2037-45.

3. Wullstein H. Theory and practice of tympanoplasty. Laryngoscope. 1956;66(8):1076-93.

4. Altuna X, Navarro JJ, Martinez Z, et al. [Island cartilage myringoplasty. Anatomical and functional results in 122 cases]. Acta Otorrinolaringol Esp. 2010;61(2):100-5.

5. Tos M. Cartilage tympanoplasty methods: proposal of a classification. Otolaryngol Head Neck Surg. 2008;139(6):747-58.

5.2.4D
Pertinent Histopathology

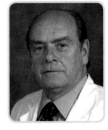

Marcos Goycoolea

Chronic otitis media with perforation of the tympanic membrane. The lower magnification (Figure 1) shows the three layers of the tympanic membrane: (1) the outer epithelium (stratified squamous epithelium), continuous with that of the external ear canal; (2) the middle ear connective tissue layer, continuous with both the connective tissue layer of the external ear canal and middle ear; and (3) the inner mucosal layer, continuous with that of the middle ear. The higher magnifications (Figures 2A and B) clearly show the in-growth of outer stratified squamous epithelium (arrows). This epithelium is removed before placement of a connective tissue graft; otherwise there will be no migration of epithelial cells over the graft. The purpose of the graft is to "replace" the lost connective tissue and to serve as a bridge for migration of epithelial cells to close the gap (perforation). These photomicrographs illustrate the concepts of perforation and grafting; they are not meant to imply or to suggest grafting a perforation during an acute episode of otitis media.

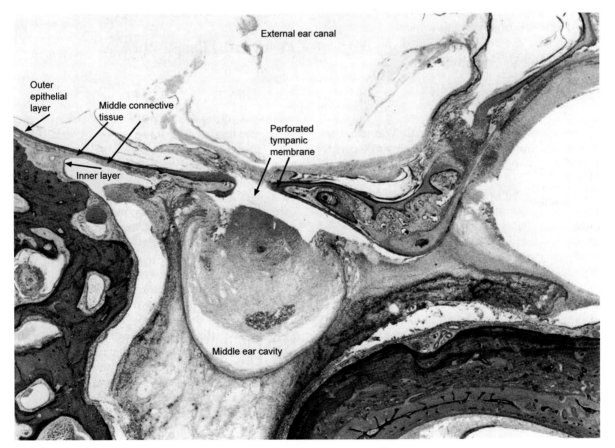

Figure 1 Chronic otitis media with perforation of the tympanic membrane. Lower magnification

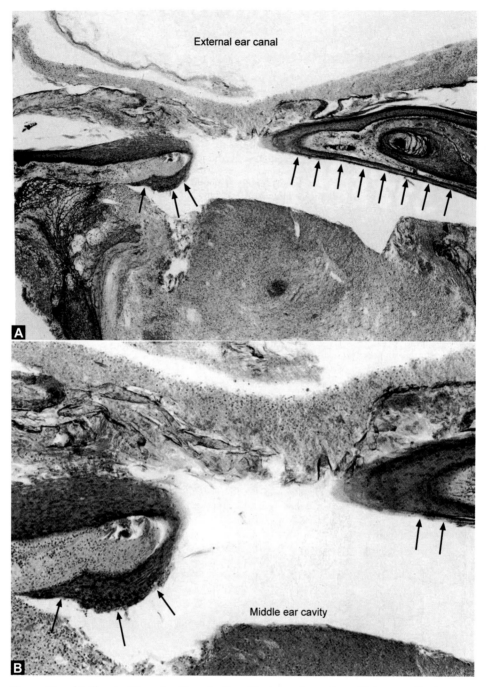

Figures 2A and B Chronic otitis media with perforation of the tympanic membrane. Higher magnification

be as good as in otosclerosis. However, it is essential to do this stapedectomy in a "dry ear" and as a single procedure. It should not be performed in conjunction with a tympanoplasty because of a high-risk of sensory hearing loss. If a tympanoplasty is performed, the stapedectomy is delayed. Careful staging is crucial.

Fractures of the crura are treated with a piston prosthesis from the incus to the oval window, unless the fracture is the rare one that allows a crurotomy. Again, these procedures are done in a "dry ear". In cases of fractured crura and footplate, it is safer to remove the footplate and use connective tissue to seal the window. (Wire connective tissue prosthesis is preferred but it is not essential.) An alternative in fractured crura and intact mobile footplate is the use of an inverted allograft stapes or the use of a short prosthesis (Figures 15A and B).

Combined Ossicular Problems

Repairs become more troublesome if the malleus handle or stapes (or both) are absent. This means that the prosthesis must be supported by the grafted tympanic membrane, which carries a higher risk of failure, or a longer prosthesis must be used from the tympanic membrane to the oval window.

Fixation of the head of the malleus associated with a fixed stapes footplate has been shown to be repaired with a malleus-to-oval-window wire connective tissue prosthesis. While this is a good alternative, it has the drawbacks of lateralization and loss of adequate conductivity. It must be remembered that whenever the stapes footplate is removed, a fistula of the oval window is a potential complication. Regardless of the graft or prosthesis, an adequate seal is essential. Alternatives include the use of a TORP, a TORP-shaped cortical bone ossicle, cartilage, or ceramic prosthesis, or a sculptured ossicle.

In cases of fixation of the ossicular chain by tympanosclerosis, the first stage implies mobilization, completion of the malleus, disarticulation of the incus, and so on. This prepares for a second procedure in which the stapedectomy is done. Surgical repair involves the alternatives described below.

When both the malleus and incus are absent (usually seen in chronic otitis media cases, and not uncommonly in tympanomastoidectomy procedures), or when both ossicles are a single, congenital, nonfunctional "mass", the alternatives are a classic Type III tympanoplasty or use of a short prosthesis or graft (described above), if the stapes is intact and mobile. If the stapes is fixed or damaged, a long prosthesis (tympanic membrane to footplate or oval window graft) is necessary.

If the malleus is absent and there is an intact and mobile stapes, a short prosthesis is used. However, a long prosthesis is indicated if the stapes is damaged (Figure 16).

In cases of tympanomastoidectomy, the concept of space becomes relevant in terms of reconstruction. At this point and with this type of disease, an intact-bridge tympanomastoidec-

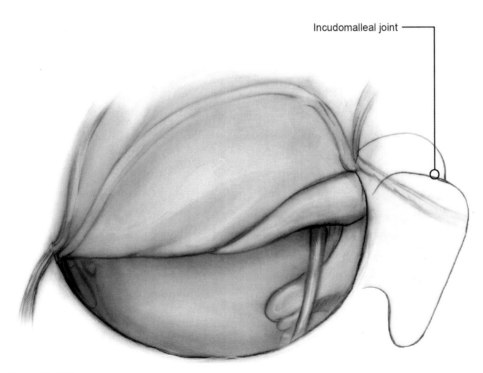

Incudomalleal joint

Figure 1A Malleus

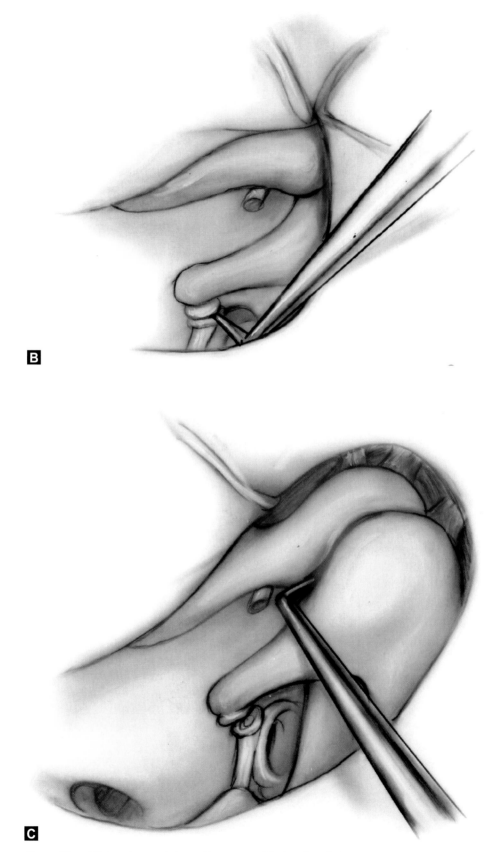

Figures 1B and C An atticotomy is done with exposure of the incudomalleal joint

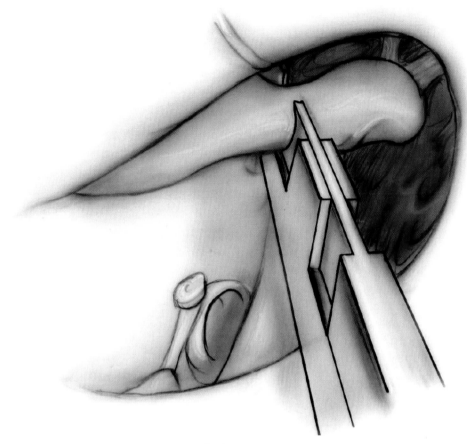

Figure 2 The head of the malleus is amputated with a nipper

Graft

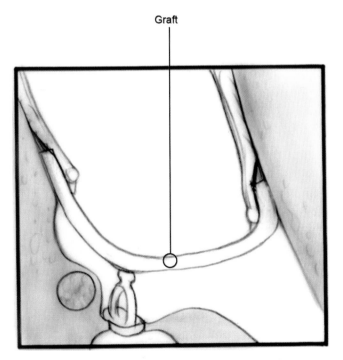

Figure 3 Laying the tympanic membrane over the head of the stapes (Classic Type III tympanoplasty)

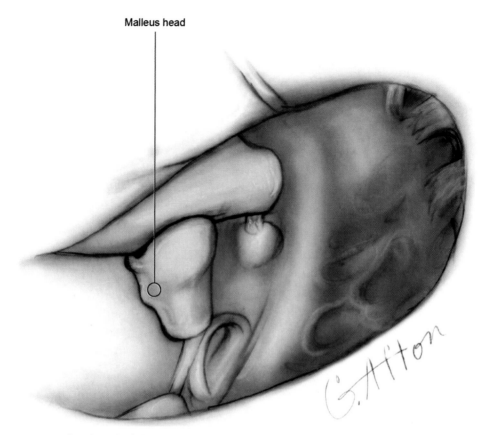

Malleus head

Figure 4 Malleus shaped to fit between the head of stapes

tomy makes good sense (if needed, of course; if possible, an intact-wall procedure is preferred).

As mentioned earlier, a critical factor is the presence or absence of the malleus handle. An equally important factor (sometimes overlooked) is the presence or absence of a mobile footplate. For practical purposes, the use of a TORP will be described, followed by other alternatives.

Placement of a TORP

Two points of contact are crucial. The usual tendency is to think in terms of extrusion and forget the distal end of the TORP (over the footplate or oval window graft).

The TORP is cut to the necessary length. This may be 3.5 mm for an open cavity, 4 mm if the malleus handle is present, or 5 mm if it is absent.

A thin, but large piece of cartilage is placed over the TORP (beneath the malleus or tympanic membrane graft) to provide protection from extrusion (some surgeons suture it to the TORP). If there is a footplate or membrane, the TORP is placed over it and is supported with abundant Gelfoam® to secure it in position. A TORP with a peg can be used to provide more stability at the footplate and prevent slipping (Figures 17A and B). Once the TORP is placed, it should impart some tension to the tympanic membrane. A TORP-shaped piece of cartilage or cortical bone can be used, as well. A small piece of Silastic can be placed, surrounding the prosthesis at the oval window area, in order to prevent adhesions (Figure 18). A ceramic TORP can also be used (Figure 19), as well as a sculptured cartilage (Figures 20A and B). The latter should be flattened toward the tympanic membrane in order to provide a smooth and wide contact. If the malleus handle is present, drilling a groove in the TORP provides better stability. Titanium prostheses work quite well and can be trimmed to size, ending up as stable prosthesis with the additional capability of tissue in-growth. Whenever a long prosthesis (TORP type) is placed over an oval window without a footplate, there is a possibility of a fistula and good seal is needed. If there is a potential for retraction (for example, Eustachian tube dysfunction), these prostheses may lead to fistulization by sliding into the oval window.

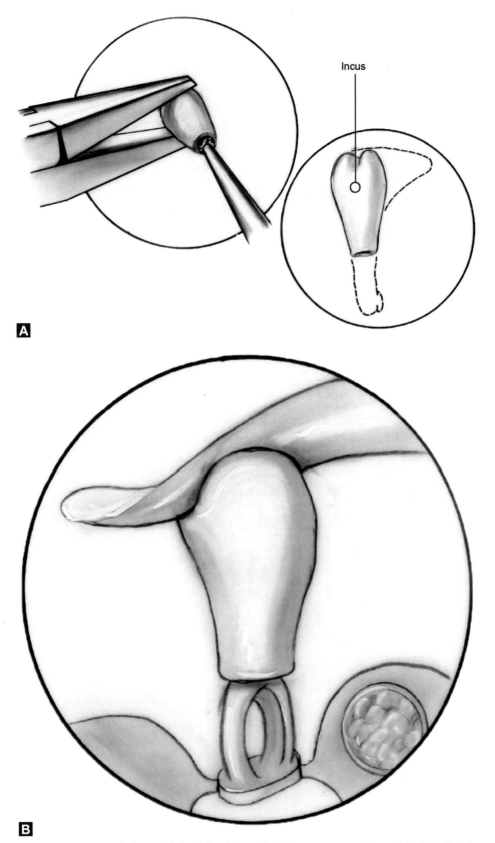

A

B

Figures 5A and B Acetabulum is drilled and then followed by drilling a groove over the remaining body for fitting under the malleus handle

Cortical bone

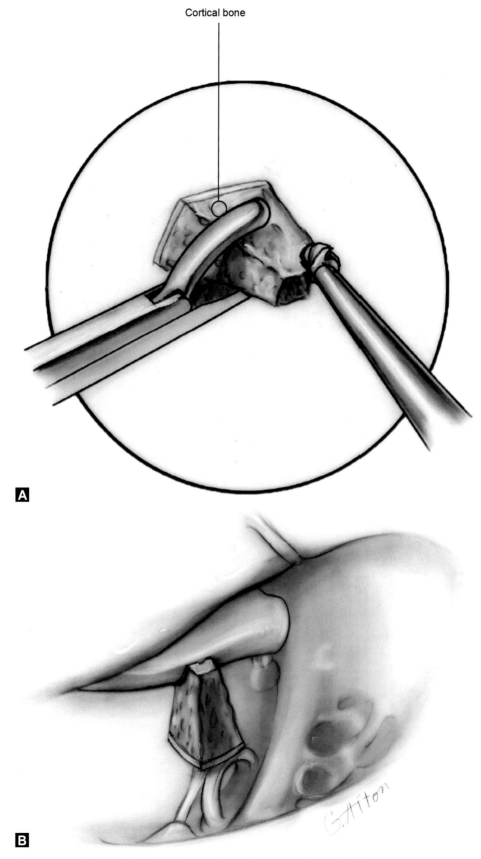

A

B

Figures 6A and B Graft is shaped similar to a sculptured incus or malleus head, drilled, creating a concave hole to fit under the malleus handle

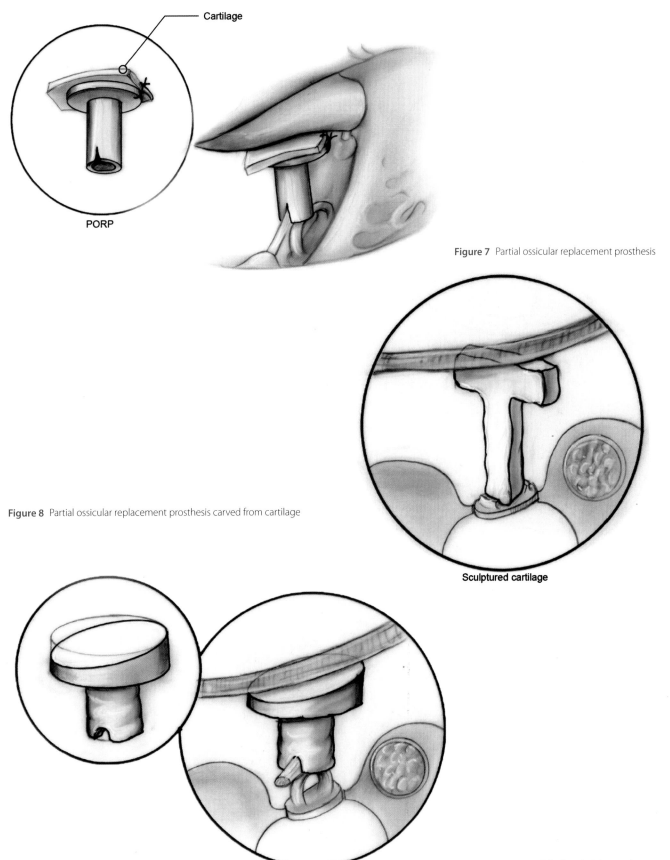

Cartilage

PORP

Figure 7 Partial ossicular replacement prosthesis

Figure 8 Partial ossicular replacement prosthesis carved from cartilage

Sculptured cartilage

Cartilage PORP

Figure 9 Trimming of the head of the cartilage to fit the angled position of the membrane

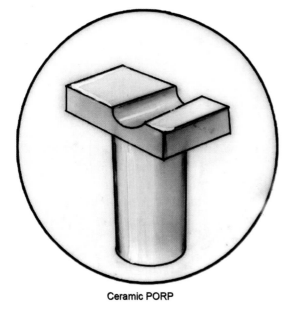

Ceramic PORP

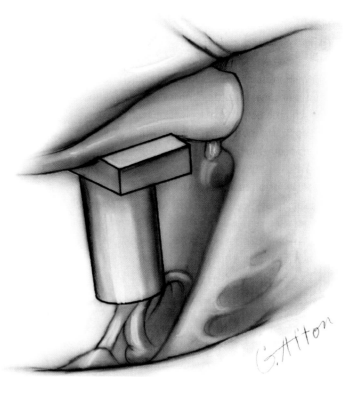

Figure 10 Ceramic partial ossicular replacement prosthesis

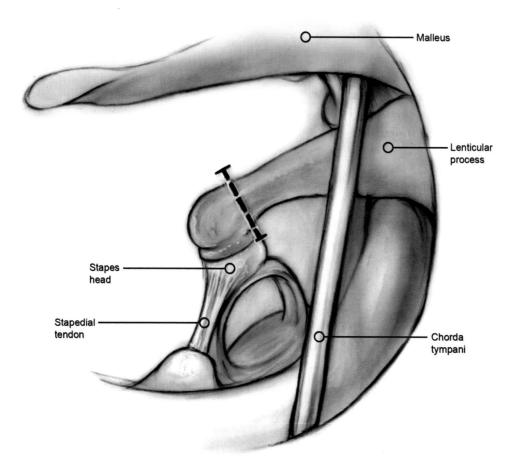

Malleus

Lenticular
process

Stapes
head

Stapedial
tendon

Chorda
tympani

Figure 11 Incus

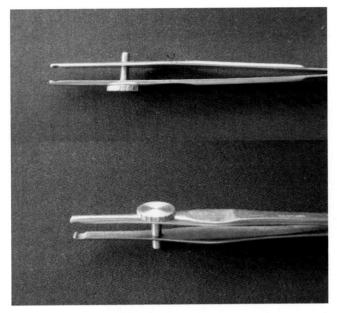

Figure 2 Forceps with an adjustment screw to maintain a stable ossicle while drilling it with diamond microburrs
(*Source:* Original design by James Sheehy)

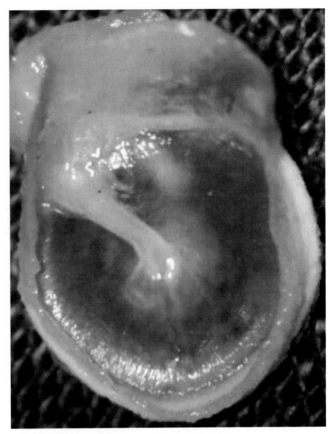

Figure 3 Tympano-ossicular homograft (tympanic membrane, malleus, incus in one piece) of high quality (produced in the ear bank of the Otological Foundation of Venezuela)

hydroxyapatite or titanium allow better adaptability and coupling with better functional results.

Biophysical Factors that Influence Ossicular Reconstruction

Regardless of the material that is used, the surgeon should have a thorough knowledge of the biophysical factors that can influence reconstruction. These factors are: mass, friction, rigidity, coupling, alignment and length.

Mass: Experimental analysis in middle ear models[10] has demonstrated that a moderate increase in mass in the substitution mechanism of the ossicular chain has no significance in sound transmission. An increase in 5 mg in the stapes mass (over the capitulum) causes a loss of 13 to 15 dB in high frequencies.

Friction: Friction of the prostheses with neighboring structures of the middle ear must be avoided, especially with the scutum (lateral wall of the attic) in order to avoid fixations or adherence formation that could reduce the vibration capacity of the prostheses.

Rigidity: When the middle ear mucosa is intact, adherences and scarring that compromise prostheses mobility are avoided.

Coupling: It is not always easy to obtain a stable coupling between the two extremes of the substitution mechanism because a firm union of the prostheses to the stapes footplate is difficult because of the lack of connective tissue and scarring at this point of contact (stapes footplate). Also, the contact with the neotympanum requires a contact surface of at least 3 to 4 mm for the coupling to be efficient.[11,12]

CONCLUSION

The reposition of autologous ossicles (when they are free of pathology) is a valid and current surgical alternative that can lead to acceptable functional results. Unfortunately, the use of

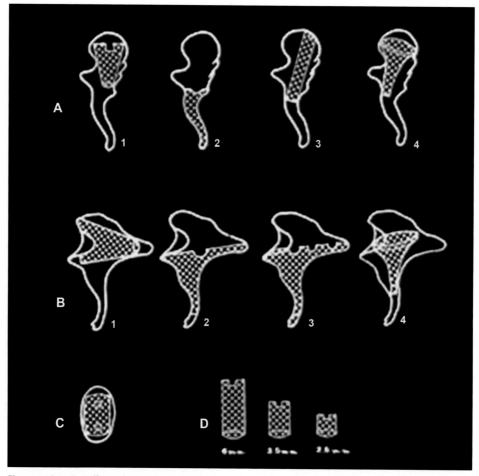

Figures 4A to D Different forms of ossicular homografts that have been carefully carved in multiple forms in order to be useful for any type of ossicular reconstruction. Preserved in Cilait (mercurial solution). (A) Malleus; (B) Incus; (C) Stapes; (D) Cortical mastoid bony columns

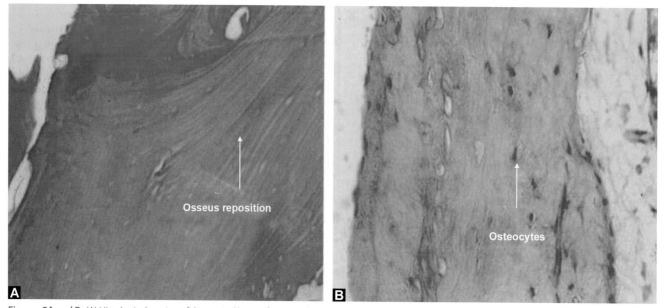

Figures 5A and B (A) Histological section of the cortical bone of an incus homograft removed from a patient 10 years after having been implanted in his middle ear. The laminar structure of bone is well preserved and there are no signs of resorption; (B) Section of the same incus where some osteocytes can be observed with well defined nuclei (original magnification 400 X; hematoxylin-eosin)

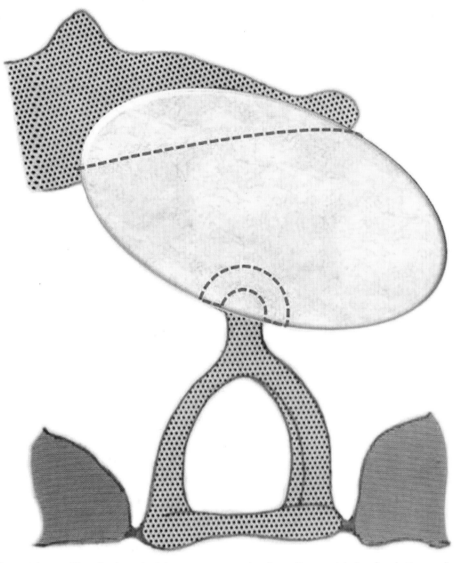

Figure 6 Interposition of an incus body between stapes and malleus with an acetabulum for a better coupling with the stapes head

these bones of the patient himself/herself is limited because they are frequently damaged by the pathological process which can render them useless.

The use of ossicular homografts obtained from fresh temporal bones was a very successful approach and had good results between the 60s and 90s. Later their use became limited because of the nondemonstrated belief that they could be contaminated by emerging viral processes. At present, they have been substituted by alloplastic prostheses.

In our days, alloplastic prostheses of hydroxyapatite and titanium constitute the prostheses of choice in auditory functional reconstruction.

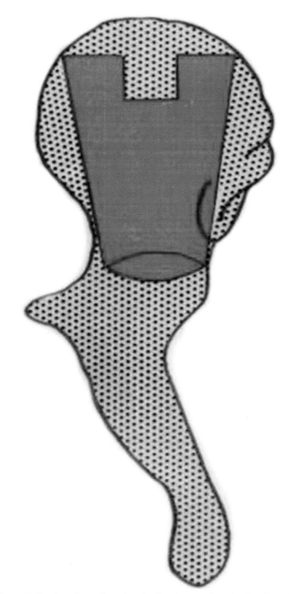

Figure 7 Carving of a malleus head with a low cut for adapting it to the malleus head and an acetabular surface to maintain it over the stapes capitulum

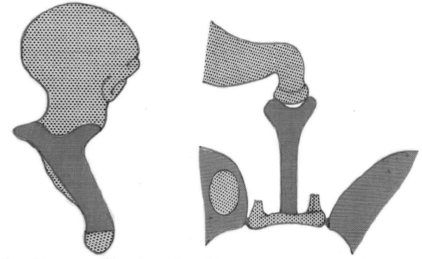

Figure 8 Long process of the malleus and its possible use

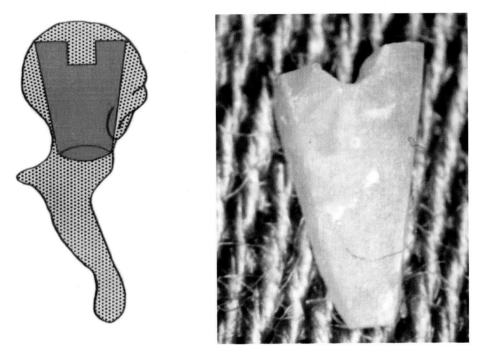

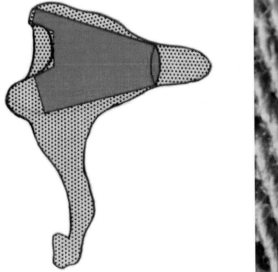

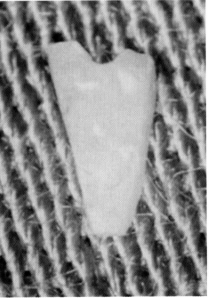

Figure 9 Osseous piece for interposition that was carved from a malleus head

Figure 10 Piece that is similar to Figure 9 but carved from an incus body

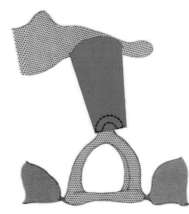

Figure 11 Interposition of the carved osseous pieces of Figures 8 and 9 between the capitulum of the stapes (head) and the long process of the malleus

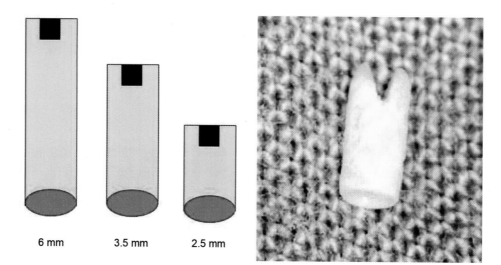

6 mm   3.5 mm   2.5 mm

Figure 12 Osseous columns made from mastoid cortex and molded to different sizes used for ossicular reconstruction

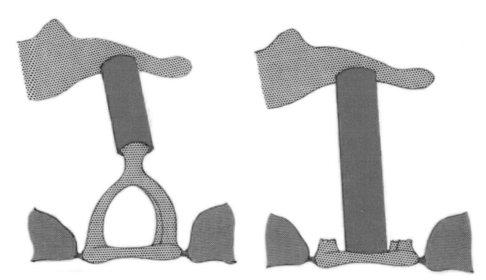

Figure 13 Different possibilities of ossicular reconstruction with bony columns carved according to need

and the crus of the helix. It is started at the level of the bony-cartilaginous junction and continued laterally for 5 to 10 mm, finishing just outside the EAC.

The temporalis muscle is identified at the superior edge of the EAC, and 3–4 mm of superficial temporalis fascia is harvested in case it will be necessary. The remainder of the soft tissues are separated from the bone using a small periosteal elevator until the underlying bone superior to the EAC is revealed.

Two two-armed retractors are placed at the osteo-cartilagenous junction, perpendicular to each other, to enlarge the EAC to approximately twice the original diameter. The retractor that is placed in the anteroposterior plane is placed with one arm inside the endaural incision and one on the canal skin.

Tympanomeatal Flap (Figures 1A to C)

Two incisions are performed from the medial end of the endaural incision. One is directed posteroinferiorly and then is directed towards the tympanic membrane, reaching the annulus between the middle and inferior-thirds of the posterior annulus (7 o'clock).

The second incision is directed in an anterior direction, until it reaches the tympanic membrane beyond the level of the lateral process of the malleus (1 o'clock).

The flap is elevated using round knife and microsraspatory. Any bony canal wall drilling is performed before accessing the middle ear to improve access.

Elevation of the tympanic membrane is started at the level of the posterior tympanic spine, superiorly to the chorda tympani nerve, which is found in an acute angle when dissecting in a superior to inferior direction. This direction of dissection is safer for the nerve and annulus. The complete pars flaccida is elevated until the neck, lateral process of the malleus and anterior tympanic spine are identified. Then, the dissection is carried out slightly inferiorly to the chorda, and the posterior annulus is elevated.

Exposure of the Malleus Handle (Figure 2)

The first millimeter of the malleus handle must be released from the tympanic membrane.

Excessive exposure of the malleus handle must be avoided, to maintain connection of the malleus to the tympanic membrane.

Exposure of the Oval Window (Figure 3)

In most cases, the posterosuperior edge of the tympanic rim occludes the oval window. A curette is used to remove this bone until the pyramidal process is seen.

Care is taken to avoid injury to the chorda tympani nerve.

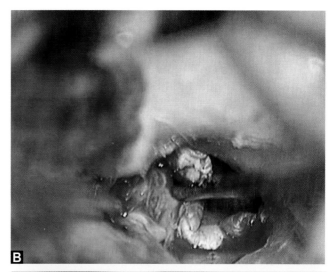

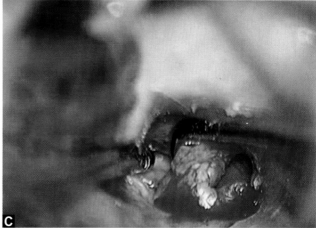

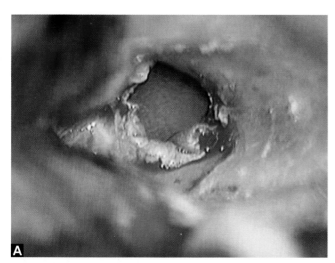

Figures 1A to C Left ear. Tympanomeatal flap

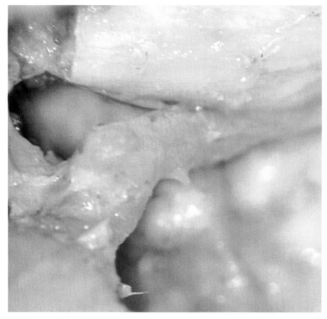

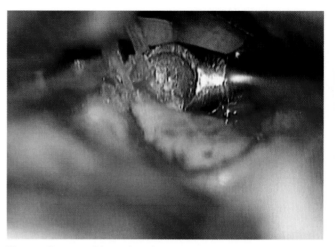

Figure 3 Exposure of the oval window

Figure 2 Exposure of the malleus handle

Adequate exposure from the short process of the malleus to the pyramidal process must be achieved in order to safely perform further surgical steps.

Ossicular mobility requires careful assessment with a 45° hook. Accurate assessment of malleus and incus mobility may require incudo-stapedial joint division. Minor fixation may be difficult to detect.

When present, the damaged incus is removed at this stage.

Removal of the Malleus Head

In mallear head fixation situations, removal of the head usually creates normal malleus mobility. Further fixation may be caused by anterior mallear ligament fixation. This may be divided by scissors or drilling. Since it is attached to the malleus at the level of the anterior process, which is inferior to the malleus neck, the only possible way to liberate the malleus is to remove away the anterior mallear process, which is better performed with a drill.

Laser-Aided Removal of Stapes Arch

This step is performed only if stapes suprastructure is present.

The Argon laser is used with an angled handpiece to atraumatically remove the stapes tendon, then stapes arch.

Determination of Prosthesis Length and Preparation of the Prosthesis (Figures 4A and B)

A measuring rod is placed between the stapes footplate and the lateral process of the malleus handle, and the prosthesis length is defined.

A 0.4 x 8.5 mm shaft titanium stapes piston or more recently a specially designed prosthesis (Grace Medical) is placed on a cutting block. The length is compared to that obtained with the measuring rod, and cut accordingly.

Then, to confirm correct prosthesis length, the prosthesis is placed between the stapes footplate and the malleus handle. The specially designed prosthesis length is right if the loop of the prosthesis surpass the level of the malleus handle by 0.5 mm.

The shaft of the prosthesis may be bent to accommodate for an anteriorly situated malleus. Also, when necessary, the loop of the prosthesis may be enlarged at this stage.

Laser-Aided Stapedotomy (Figure 5)

The laser is used now to create a rosette in the middle of the footplate. The correct size is confined with a 0.4 mm measuring caliper.

Fixation of the Prosthesis (Figure 6)

The prosthesis is first laid on the malleus handle, usually inferiorly to the chorda tympani. Then it is introduced into the vestibule.

This meticulous care is essential until epithelialization occurs. If skin grafting is needed (see the discussion of Thiersch grafting), it is done six to eight weeks after the surgery. Skin coverage prevents infection of the exposed areas.

All the different approaches that have been mentioned will be discussed in this section. In addition, the alternatives (and indications) of performing mastoid obliteration and reconstruction of the posterior canal wall will be described.

The main pathological entities in chronic otitis media requiring the procedures that have been discussed are granulation tissue, cholesterol granuloma and cholesteatoma. These changes occur within the continuum of otitis media, which is quite often bilateral and deserve special consideration. Therefore, surgery on the contralateral ear and a detailed review of cholesteatoma surgery (acquired and congenital) will precede the discussions following after this.

5.2.6B
Surgery for Cholesteatoma

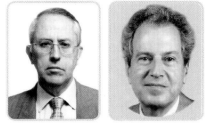

Rodrigo Posada Trujillo, Ugo Fisch

CLASSIFICATION OF CHOLESTEATOMA

- Congenital cholesteatoma
- Acquired cholesteatoma
  - Primary acquired cholesteatoma
  - Secondary acquired cholesteatoma

Congenital Cholesteatoma

It is a developmental defect consisting of a cystic epidermoid growth arising from rests of keratinizing squamous epithelium present before birth. The patients have no history of ear disease and present a normally pneumatized mastoid.

Acquired Cholesteatoma

Acquired cholesteatoma occurs after birth and is caused by invasion of the middle ear cleft by keratinizing squamous epithelium originating from the lining of the external auditory canal or from the tympanic membrane. Patients with acquired cholesteatoma usually present with a history of recurrent ear disease and with a reduced pneumatization of the mastoid. According to the condition of the tympanic membrane, acquired cholesteatoma can be divided into primary and secondary.

Primary Acquired Cholesteatoma

Primary acquired cholesteatoma develop behind an intact tympanic membrane.

Secondary Acquired Cholesteatoma

Secondary acquired cholesteatoma grow in the middle ear mostly through a marginal perforation of the tympanic membrane.

PRINCIPLE

Surgical treatment of cholesteatoma must be as radical as possible, due to the aggressiveness of its pathology, but, paying extreme care to the anatomical structures and trying to recover, at maximum, the hearing function.

There are surgical principles which must be observed and respected in order to obtain the best results over the long term.

Principles of the Zurich School

1. *Wide exposure:* To achieve a complete removal of the cholesteatoma and its associated pathology.
2. *Skeletonization:* To make the anatomical structures transparent, without having to expose them, leaving the last shell of protecting bone, at the level of the middle cranial fossa dura, sigmoid sinus, facial nerve, sinodural angle and labyrinth.
3. *Exenteration:* Removal of all infected pneumatic cells, eliminating not only the cholesteatoma but also the infected mucosa leaving no residual cholesteatoma.
4. *Exteriorization:* Shaping the cavity with a lateral diameter twice the size of the medial diameter.

The Zurich Otology and Skull Base Surgery School considers that only the mastery of surgical techniques, the most precise knowledge of surgical anatomy, the continued practice of temporal bone dissection besides appropriate instrumental, along with highly trained support staff, participating in conjunction with the surgeon, guarantee the best results.

SURGICAL TREATMENT OF ACQUIRED CHOLESTEATOMA

AIMS

- Eradication of disease
- Prevention of recurrent and retention cholesteatomas
- Formation of a dry and self-cleansing cavity
- Restoration of tympanic aeration
- Reconstruction of a sound-transformer mechanism

Closed Cavity: Principle

The principle of the intact canal wall tympanomastoidectomy (closed-cavity) is to completely remove the cholesteatoma matrix and its related pathology from the tympanic cavity and mastoid working on both sides of the preserved bony canal wall.

Closed Cavity Indications

- Good lumen of the Eustachian tube (Figure 1)
- Well-pneumatized mastoid (Figure 2)
- Limited cholesteatoma (Figures 3 and 4)
- Easy postoperative follow-up of the patient.

Open Cavity (Open Mastoido-Epitympanectomy) Principle

The open cavity technique consists in removing the posterior and superior wall of the bony external auditory canal creating a wide cavity which includes the mastoid and epitympanum.

Open cavity Indications

- Insufficient Eustachian tube function
- Sclerotic mastoid with extensive disease
- Only hearing ear
- Brain complications secondary to cholesteatoma

- Destruction of the posterosuperior canal wall
- Difficult postoperative follow-up of the patient.

CONCLUSION OF ABOVE DISCUSSION

Open cavity technique is chosen when it is impossible to radically remove the cholesteatoma matrix beyond doubt using the closed cavity technique.

CANALPLASTY

The first step is to create a vascularized meatal skin flap, which is pedicled inferiorly. The flap is elevated out from the external auditory canal and, therefore, does not interfere with the subsequent widening of the bony canal.

A large canalplasty is mandatory in all patients who undergo surgery due to chronic otitis media with cholesteatoma to avoid postoperative complications due to insufficient removal of the primary disease or insufficient reconstruction of the tympanic membrane (e.g. recurrent perforations).

Advantages

- Improved intraoperative assessment of functional status of the ossicular chain, particularly the anterior malleal ligament.
- Visualization of all edges of the perforation and even the annulus, with one position of the microscope.
- It improves the self-cleansing capacity of the canal, under the premise that canalplasty must be as uniform as possible, performed by a skillful surgeon, using diamond burr and angled hand piece.
- It is excellent for a second functional procedure.

OUTSTANDING SURGICAL STEPS

Open and Closed Cavity

Outstanding surgical steps of open and closed cavity are based on FIMF Pereira-Colombia Surgical Archive (Figures 5 to 19).

Closed Cavity

Figures 20 to 23 refer to some steps of the closed-cavity technique which are as follows:
1. Mastoidectomy
2. Epitympanectomy
3. Wide skeletonization of the middle cranial fossa dura

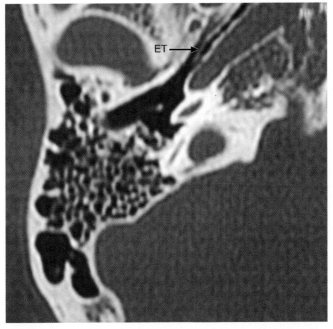

Figure 1 CT, Axial plane: good pneumatization of the mastoid with excellent Eustachian tube (ET) patency. The CT of the temporal bone is the better test good to evaluate the lumen of the Eustachian tube function. In addition, it informs about the history of the disease and guides the planning of surgery. In this case, normal pneumatization is observed as a result of the absence of a recurrent or chronic acute otitis during the first 14–18 years of life. Normal cellular mucosa is seen, as a result of good middle ear ventilation

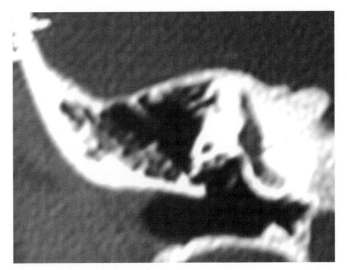

Figure 2 CAT, Coronal plane: Good pneumatization of the mastoid with excellent aeration of the tympanic cavity

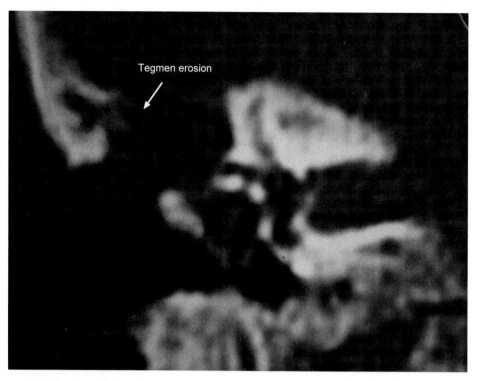

Figure 3 HRCT coronal plane, cholesteatoma in the epitympanum having induced an erosion of the Tegmen tympani and a beginning erosion of the lateral semicircular canal

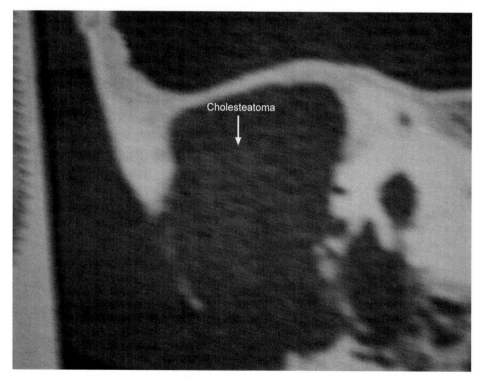

Figure 4 Coronal plane. Typical image of a cholesteatoma with sharp knife-like destruction of the affected bone

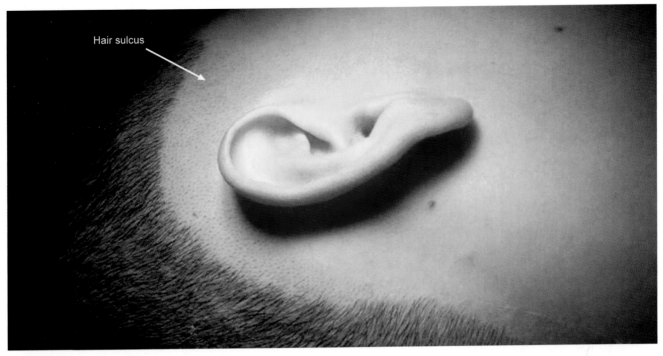

Hair sulcus

Figure 5 The hair is shaved 2 cm behind the hair sulcus

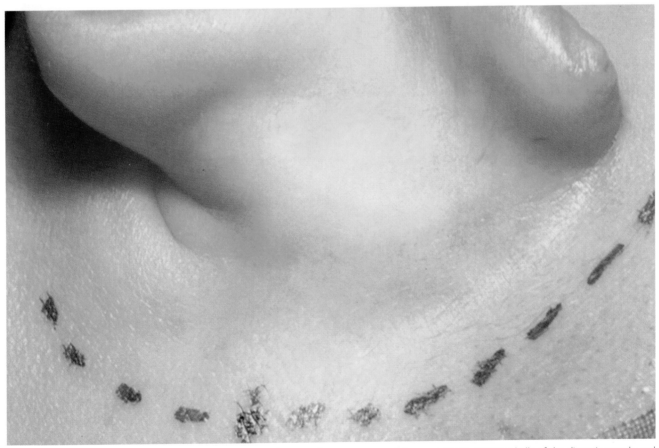

Figure 6 Retroauricular incision along the hairline (left ear), achieving a better exposure of the mastoid, the posterior belly of the digastric muscle and stylomastoid periosteum

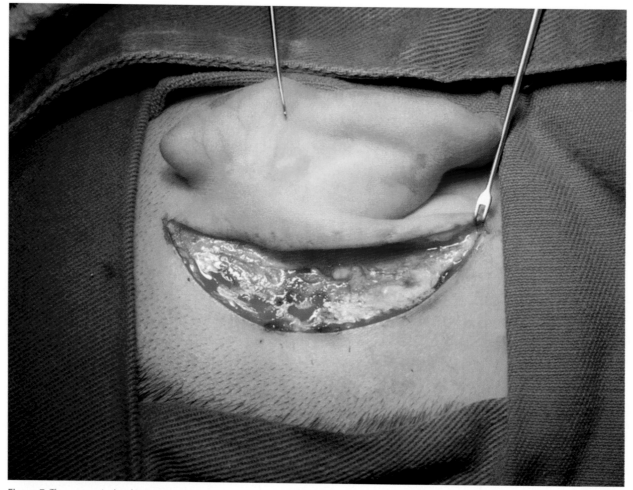

Figure 7 The retroauricular skin incision is carried out along the hairline and behind the mastoid tip. It is made only through skin, preserving the underlying fascia and periosteum

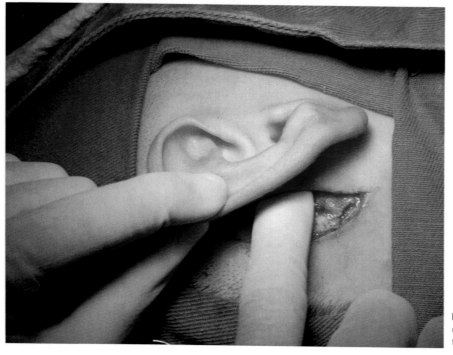

Figure 8 Creating a periosteal flap of the diameter of the index finger and matches that of the external auditory canal (EAC)

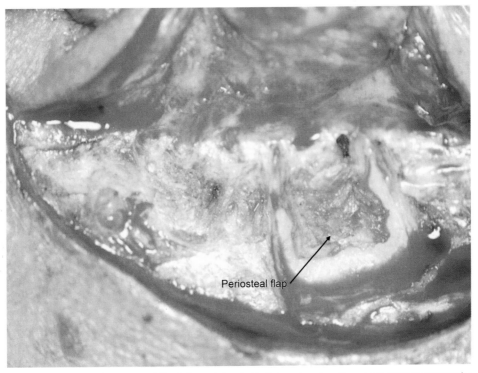

Figure 9 A retroauricular periosteal flap is formed, just behind the external auditory canal (EAC), to protect the posterior wall of the bony EAC when a closed cavity technique is being carried out

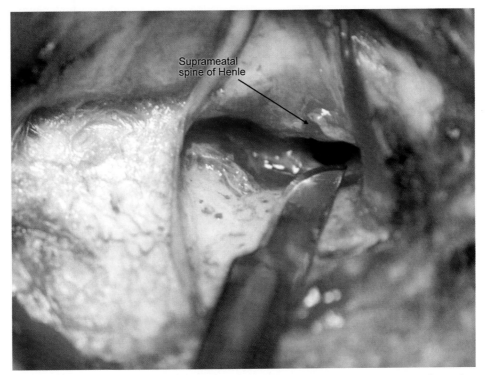

Figure 10 The posterior limb of the canal incision is carried out with a № 15 blade, remaining 2 mm deeper than the entrance of the bony external canal (right ear)

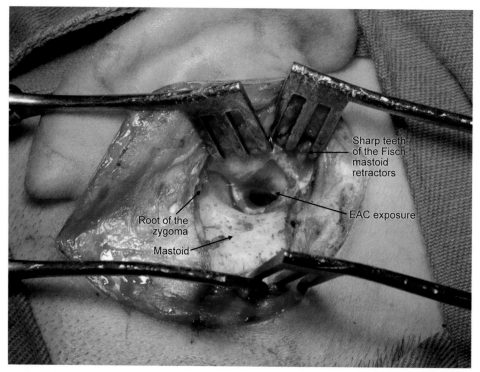

Figure 11 Placement of articulate retroauricular retractors with sharp teeth to adequately adhere to the tissues (right ear)

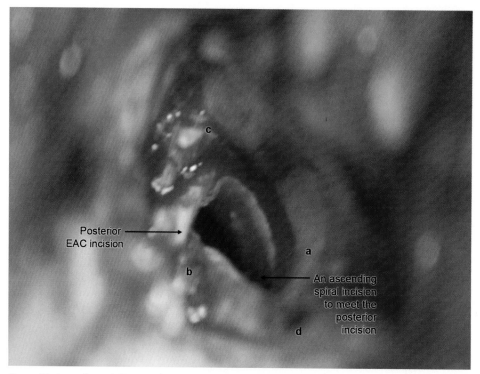

Figure 12 Ascending spiral incision from 7 in the right ear, and from 5 in the left ear to meet the posterior EAC incision. (a) Anterior wall; (b) Posterior wall; (c) Superior wall and (d) Inferior wall

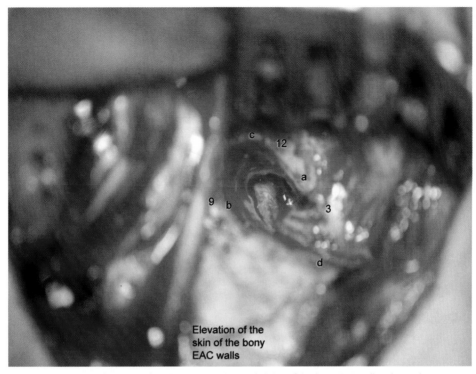

Figure 13 Elevation of the skin of the bony canal. The medial skin of the bony EAC wall is elevated, upto 2 mm above the annulus. This is done with Fisch microraspatory, designed for vertical and horizontal movements, which has a smooth and sharp end, facilitating dissection. (a) Anterior wall; (b) Posterior wall; (c) Superior wall and (d) Inferior wall

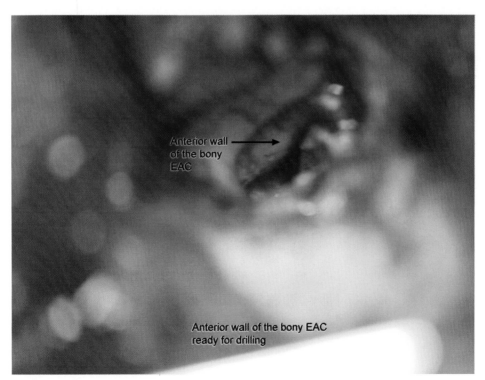

Figure 14 Exposure of the anterior wall of the bony EAC, which almost always presents bony overhangs, which are drilled to obtain a good view of the tympanic remnants

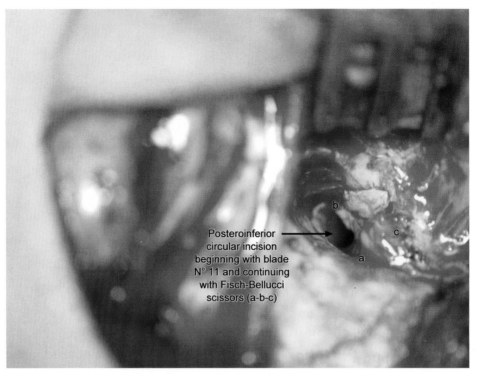

Figure 15 Posteroinferior circular incision through the skin, 2 mm above the annulus. The incision begins with blade number 11 and continues with Fisch-Bellucci tympanoplasty scissors. The real point c is 2 mm above the annulus

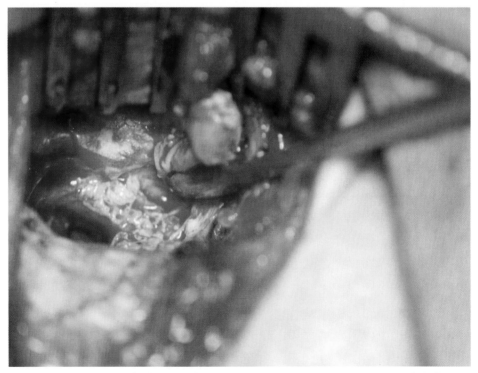

Figure 16 The inferior meatal flap has been elevated, using a key raspatory. We use two hands to lift the flap with sufficient pressure and sensitivity, in order to avoid tearing it

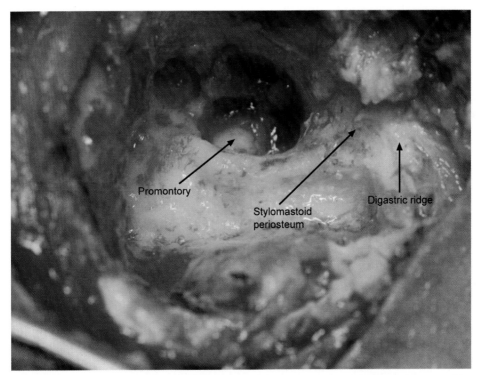

Figure 39 Lowering of facial ridge, to the level of the stylomastoid foramen, which facilitates placement of the fascial graft horizontally with better results for the auditory function. We can see the complete exenteration and exteriorization of the surgical cavity, leaving a flat cavity

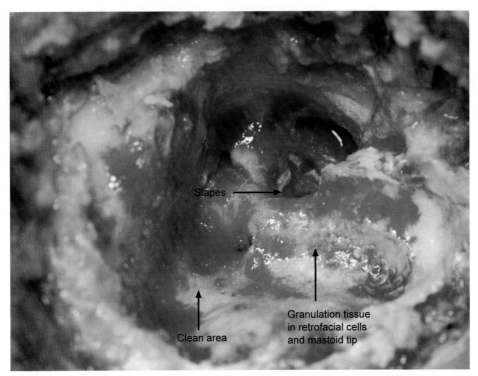

Figure 40 We can see granulation tissue in retrofacial cells and mastoid tip. Cholesteatoma surgery does not only involve the removal of the epithelium but also the removal of the granulation tissue. We must remove this pathology to avoid recurrent cholesteatoma and not to leave a wet cavity

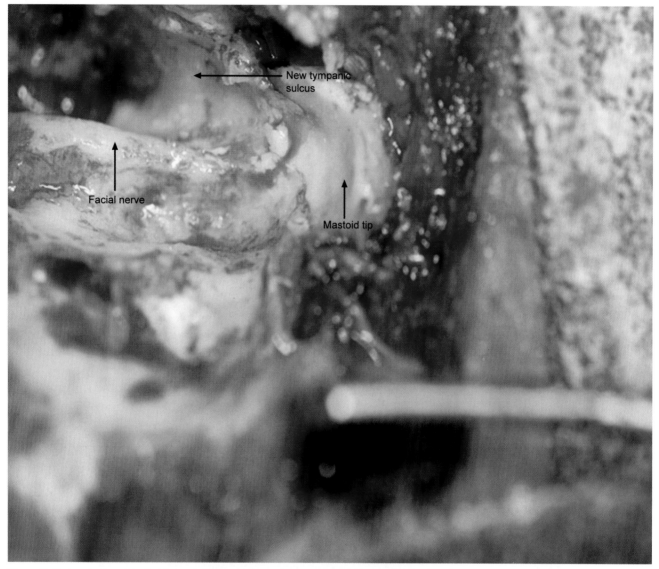

Figure 41 Skeletonization of the facial nerve with exenteration and exteriorization of the retrofacial cells, and exposure of the mastoid tip

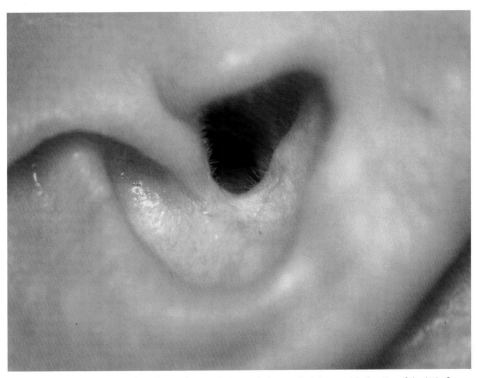

Figure 54 The typical meatoplasty has a characteristic regularly rounded shape with the size of the little finger. Take care to leave no free cartilage margins to avoid perichondritis. The small curved tympanoplasty scissors are the adequate instrument for correct dissection of the cartilage from the skin. Failure to use the curved tympanoplasty scissors will produce tearing of the skin

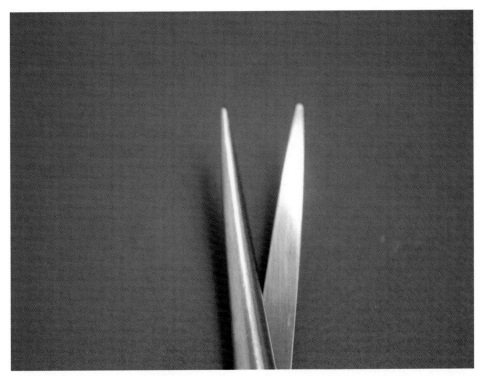

Figure 55 When carrying out the meatoplasty, you must use adequate small curved tympanoplasty scissors to separate the cartilage from the skin. Failure to use the adequate instrument will result in skin tears, since you will be unable to find the proper plane of dissection (FISCH small curved tympanoplasty scissors)

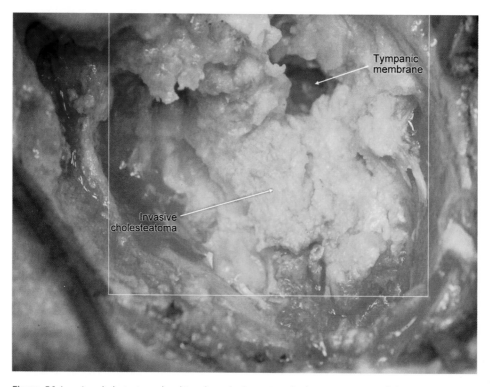

Figure 56 Invasive cholesteatoma breaking through the extremely thin outer cortex of the mastoid patient treated in a public hospital (developing country). The recommended technique in this patient was open mastoidoepitympanectomy. The cholesteatoma extended from the geniculate ganglion to the tip of the mastoid, invading the medial wall of the attic, the middle cranial fossa dura, the sinodural angle, the retrosigmoid cells, the Eustachian tube and the external auditory canal

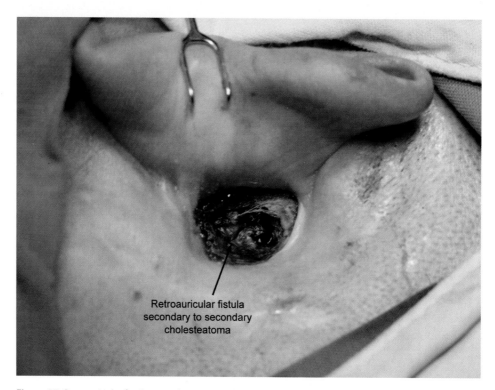

Figure 57 Retroauricular fistula secondary to secondary acquired cholesteatoma. At present, this is an unusual pathology

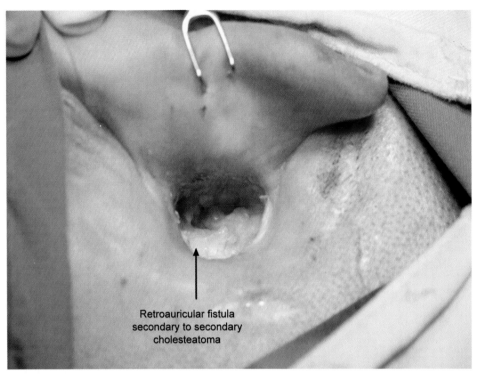

Retroauricular fistula
secondary to secondary
cholesteatoma

Figure 58 After removing the cerumen, the keratin debris of the cholesteatoma are evident. Note the scar from previous surgery performed in another medical center

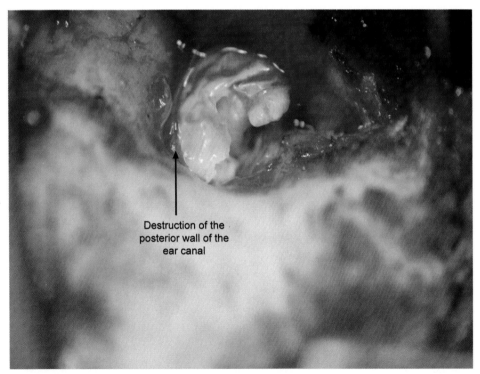

Destruction of the
posterior wall of the
ear canal

Figure 59 This case requires an open technique due to the destruction of the posterior wall of the external auditory canal and because the mastoid bone is not well pneumatized

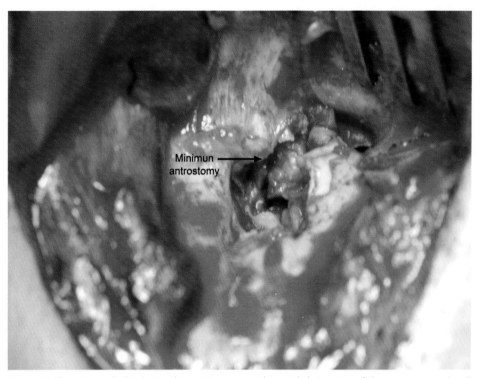

Figure 60 There is no doubt that in this revision case, with partial destruction of the posterior canal wall due to an invasive cholesteatoma in a poorly pneumatized mastoid, the indicated procedure is an open mastoidoepitympanectomy.It is not just removing the cholesteatoma matrix. The errors made in the previous surgery were: (1) Insufficient identification and skeletonization of the middle cranial fossa dura; (2) Partial destruction instead of complete removal of the posterior canal wall

RESULTS

In 1,300 cholesteatoma surgeries performed between 1981 and 2007, better results were seen with the open cavity technique.

Recurrent cholesteatoma:

10% in open cavity

25% in closed cavity

Total 13%

Most of the closed cavity had a good pneumatization.

CONCLUSION

The presented figures show that the open technique gives better results than the closed technique in cholesteatoma surgery. This is why we have performed an open cavity (mastoidoepitympanectomy) in 80% of our patients with cholesteatoma (1,040/1,300) with a recurrence rate of 10%.

We consider that the open technique is undervalued surgery. It requires on one side, a good anatomical knowledge, surgical skill and experience but offers on the other

Surprisingly the comparative analysis of temporal bones with or without TM perforation indicated that both groups were similar. When one considers granulation tissue, ossicular changes and cholesterol granuloma they were found in both groups with a difference in frequency not statistically significant. Cholesteatoma and tympanosclerosis were more frequently identified in the temporal bones with TM perforations (group II).[16] The conclusion of our study clearly shows that chronic ME inflammation may be underestimated using conventional definitions of COM.

In short, chronic otitis media has been defined under clinical and pathological criteria. Both definitions share some common aspects, but they differ deeply regarding the presence of the TM perforation. We believe that our responsibility is to shift the clinical criteria (very restrictive in our opinion) to the more encompassing and ample field of the pathological definition. Perhaps, aware of this possibility, we will investigate, understand and work more properly some ear symptoms that appear, at the first sight, obscure and unexplainable. In our opinion, to neglect these concepts is a big medical mistake. It could be interpreted as we were much more concerned about either plugging or poking holes upon the TM than actually disclosing and treating middle and inner ear pathology.

Human Clinical Studies

In the above paragraphs, we reviewed a series of studies where the *Continuum* has been consistently replicated in animal models. Strong evidences also pointing to the same direction came from elegant researches employing HTB with otitis media. For obvious reasons, the process cannot be studied longitudinally in the clinical set, since it would be ethically unacceptable to only contemplate the classic evolution of the disease from early stages of serous and mucoid effusion to the development of irreversible inflammatory pathology.

Still the ear surgeon can witness many irrefutable evidences of this march of events whenever he/she performs ME and mastoid surgery for COM. It is not rare to find during ME exploration a myriad of different pathologies dwelling the same ear: cholesteatoma in the attic and antrum; cholesterol granuloma in the tip of the mastoid and the oval and round window niches; granulation tissue over the posterosuperior quadrant and promontory; thick mucoid fluid in the protympanum and tympanic orifice of the Eustachian tube and tympanosclerosis patches all over the TM not rarely involving and fixating the ossicular chain and the cochleariform process (Figure 1).

These findings not only have confirmed that the otitis media inflammation/infection complex is very dynamic but also led to the development of new surgical techniques, especially conceived to treat this ongoing process. The prototype of these techniques is the flexible tympanomastoidectomy approach which was described in detail by Costa et al.[20] The so-called flexible approach consists in is a stepwise technique designed to explore methodically and systematically all the contents of the ME cleft and in the process to disclose, confirms and treats the disease encountered. We strongly believe that this flexible approach can be best defined as a true pathology-guided, pathogenesis-oriented surgery for the ME.

Besides the unequivocal findings during chronic ear surgery we have pursued other practical alternatives to study the *Continuum* in a human model.

For such we decided to investigate transversally the ME status of a series of patients with cleft palate.[21] The rationale behind the study was the well known fact that these patients have a chronic ET dysfunction which is not completely corrected by palate reconstruction. As a consequence, the occurrence of ME pathologies among patients with cleft lip and palate or cleft palate only is extremely high.[22,23] In this population, almost as a rule, there is an anomalous insertion of the elevator and tensor *veli palatine* muscles into the posterior margins of the hard palate. Besides, there is also muscular hypoplasia, which may cause ET dysfunction.[24-26] As pointed out before, ET tube malfunction, when persistent, may cause a negative pressure in the tympanic cavity, with the resulting transudation of fluid from the intravascular to the interstitial space, and from there to the lumen of the ME.[27] This is one of the initial landmarks of the pathogenesis of otitis media.[11,28] From this point, the sub-epithelium (and later the epithelium) reacts to the adverse situation, and there is the set-up of histological alterations that may become irreversible inside the ME, and that will define the next pathologic process.[11,28]

The goal of our study was to describe the pattern of ME alterations in 180 patients with cleft of lip and palate or isolated cleft palate followed at a university hospital in the South of Brazil with no previous otologic interventions.

Effusions in the ME were present bilaterally in 65 patients (37.6%), and unilaterally in 15 patients. Cholesteatomatous chronic otitis media (CCOM) was seen in 11 patients (6.4%) and in two patients it was bilateral. Noncholesteatomatous chronic otitis media [(NCCOM) (without cholesteatoma)] was observed in 9 patients (two of them bilaterally).

When considering the type of abnormality, patients were divided into three main groups taking into account the main finding: (1) effusion; (2) moderate/severe retractions and (3) chronic otitis media with or without cholesteatoma. Sixty-seven patients (38.2%) presented ME effusions as the main

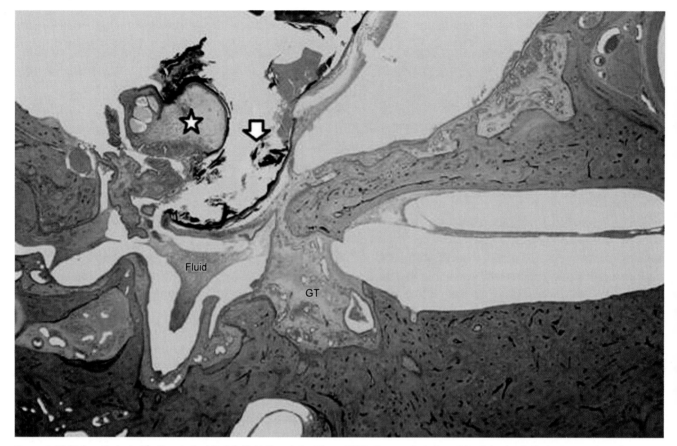

Figure 1 Multiple pathological findings in the ME cleft: Fluid; Granulation Tissue (GT) in the round window niche; Polyp (star); Cholesteatoma (arrow)

problem, 24 patients (13.3%) presented with moderate to severe retraction as the main problem and 18 patients (10%) presented with chronic otitis media with or without cholesteatoma.

There was a statistically significant association between age and the occurrence of cholesteatoma. The higher the age, the higher the prevalence of the disease (Chi-square linear trend, P = 0.008). The distribution of NCCOM among different age ranges has also shown a linear association. The higher the age, the higher the prevalence of this condition (P = 0.003). Increasing age has also correlated with the presence of retraction pockets on the TM (P < 0.0001).

The presence of ME effusions exhibited a linear association with age. Older patients tended to a lower prevalence of effusions (P < 0.0001). Figure 2 shows the linear trends in the distribution of the pathologies found: effusions, moderate/severe retractions, CCOM and NCCOM.

In conclusion the ME findings of a group of patients with theoretically known ET dysfunction supported the concept of the *Continuum:* across younger age ranges, there is the predominance of ME effusions, whereas in the older patients the prevalence of retractions and chronic otitis media are predominant. Underlined the obvious limitations of our study, we firmly believe that the progression of the severity of the ME findings in the cleft palate population through the years is in close analogy with the findings derived from may well designed longitudinal animal studies.

THE CONTRALATERAL EAR IN COM

It is curious to notice that even after such massive evidences, the *Continuum* theory is not so much explored by those who dedicate their best efforts to study COM pathogenesis and natural history. May be one of the reasons for such paradox is due to the extreme concern of the clinicians in unveiling the secrets of two groups of conditions: (1) otitis media with effusion (OME); and (2) cholesteatomas. These studies have effectively shed light to a number of questions related to the ethiopathogenesis, diagnosis and treatment of these conditions. Notwithstanding, few studies try to establish the right connections existing between these two extremes that, when separately analyzed, seems to follow parallel natural histories. A tacit example of this absurd disconnection is the joint docu-

according to the tested frequencies: low frequencies (500 and 1000 Hz); high (2000, 3000 and 4000 Hz).

We have compared with the Kruskal-Wallis test the mean ABG and the mean ABG for low and high frequencies in the CLE among the four groups and no differences were found (P = 0,567).

On the other hand when we analyzed all CLE for the occurrence of ABG of any magnitude, we found that they were present in almost 30% of the ears (135 CLE or 29.10% with ABG > 14 dBHL). There were no statistically significant differences (P = 0,940) when we compared through the chi-squared test the prevalence of the ABG among the four studied groups (30.3% NCCOM; 22.4% pars flaccida cholesteatomas; 29.4% pars tensa cholesteatomas; 34.4% open cholesteatomas).

The conclusions of the functional study are closely related to the histological and clinical ones, i.e. at least one-third of the CLE of patients with COM have a major disturbance in the tympano-ossicular system possibly related to inflammatory conditions.

The Bonus Study

Tympanic membrane perforations are the trademark of NCCOM. Their size and location are of paramount importance when surgery is planned and are also key determinants for graft-taking rates.[35] Despite the plethora of new technologies available, the dimensions and location of TM perforations and tympanosclerosis plaques have subjectively been estimated in terms of how they affected the geometry of the four quadrants since there is a lack of a specific tools that could provide such information.

A careful evaluation of the different aspects of the ME environment especially the integrity of its lateral wall (the TM) and the limitations inherent to the unaided human visual judgment of measurement-related aspects has pointed to the need of developing an alternative method to more precisely quantify these findings.

This led to the creation of the Cyclops Auris Project, which aimed at the development of quantitative computational methodologies to assess the spatial relationships between affected tympanic areas and surrounding tissue through the analysis of stored digital video-otoendoscopy.

The Cyclops Auris system was developed specifically as a standalone software tool to be used in the clinical routine for the quantitative analysis of the extension of TM pathologies, implementing a set of mathematical and image processing methods customized for this specific purpose. The software wizard provides a user-friendly and semi-automated solution, where the medical end-user has only to intervene where medical judgment is required, such as in the fine tuning of the determination of the boundaries of the anatomical structures, being all mechanical error-prone tasks performed automatically by the software. The Cyclops Auris allows also the quadrant-wise measurement of the perforated relative area, which was shown to have clinical implications. Finally, Cyclops Auris' features that allow the direct feeding of a database with the measurement results or the export of data in statistical programs friendly formats allow the easy performing of retrospective and prospective studies. A complete description of this tool is beyond the scope of this chapter but its methodology involves five steps and is summarized in the Figures 5A to E.

ADJUSTING THE QUADRENTS 5: MAKING THE MEASUREMENTS

After validated in 2009, the Cyclops Auris was tested on our examination collection encompassing 950 patients with chronic otitis media, without any previous clinical or surgical treatment for whom examinations were acquired bilaterally, totalizing 19,000 video-otoscopic recordings. Around 700 patients were classified as presenting NCCOM and 166 (16.57%) of them were selected for having bilateral dry TM perforations as the sole alteration. The size and location of these perforations were calculated with the help of the software.

When the Spearman coefficient was applied on the sizes of the major perforation, called principal ear (PE) and the minor perforation, called contralateral ear (CE) of the 166 patients presenting a bilateral pathology, there was found a strong correlation ($r_S = 0,79$; P < 0,0001). When the perforation position of both ears of these patients were compared with the Wilcoxon test (P < 0.0001), there was also found a high concordance (P < 0,0001).

In a group of patients the similitude of the size and location of the perforations were so impressive that they could be considered almost as mirror images (Figures 6A to D and 7A to D).

The conclusions of this study again showed that the prevalence of NCCOM is high. Furthermore, in those cases where bilateral perforation were documented their size and quadrant distribution were strongly correlated. In short the findings of all the studies briefly presented above point to the same direction overlapping evidences that the bilateral chronic otitis media is much more than a coincidence.

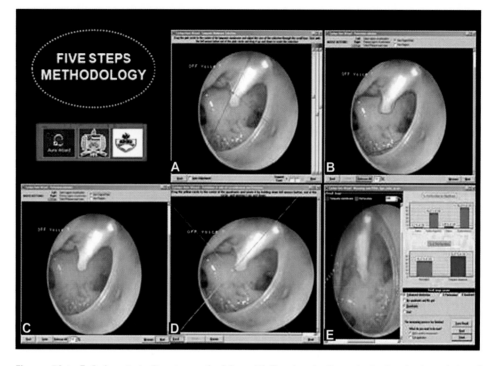

Figures 5A to E Cyclops Auris: Five step methodology: (A) Opening the file and selecting the boundaries of the TM; (B) Selecting the perforation area; (C) Fine tuning the perforation area; (D) Adjusting the quadrants and (E) Making the measurements

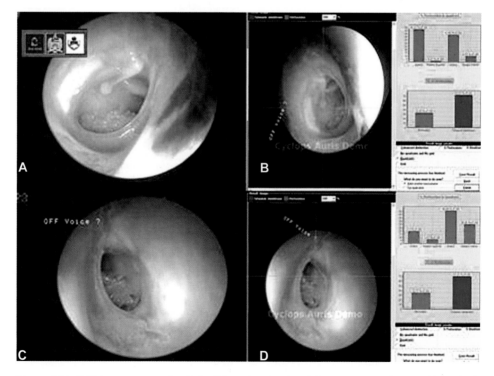

Figures 6A to D Video-otoscopy and analysis of bilateral perforations. It is easy to notice the resemblance, both in image and the parameters measured. (A) Video-otoscopy right ear; (B) Measures in the right ear; (C) Video-otoscopy left ear; (D) Measures in the left ear

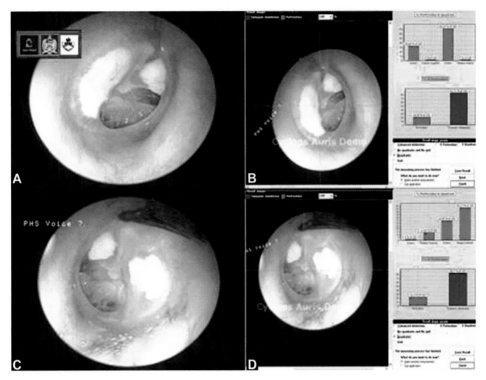

Figures 7A to D Video-otoscopy and analysis of bilateral perforations: (A) Video-otoscopy right ear; (B) Measures in the right ear; (C) Video-otoscopy left ear and (D) Measures in the left ear

Discussion and Practical Implications

A close analysis of the history of the procedures designed to treat COM and its complications clearly show that otological surgery gradually evolved during this last century with at least three different phases: (1) preservation of life (the 1853 simple mastoidectomy by Schwartz); (2) anatomical conservation (the 1910 Bondy operation) and (3) hearing improvement (the 1955 tympanoplasty by Wullstein and Zollner). Interestingly, these three phases bring us to current concepts which can be perfectly summarized under the contemporary objectives of chronic ear surgery: elimination of infection, preservation of the normal anatomical contours of the ear and, whenever possible, restoration of hearing function.

In fact, the last objective of COM surgery was set more than 50 years ago! During the same period there were major advances in the understanding of a variety of ear pathologies. These advances were spread over a variety of fields: from microbiology to the ultra-structure; from physiology to molecular biology and from the pathogenesis to technological breakthroughs. Essentially, the degree of scientific development from 1955 to 2010 highly exceeds the verified between 1853 (when the simple mastoidectomy was completely described) and 1955 (when the last objective—hearing restoration—was first proposed).

After all these years, the body of knowledge that has emerged coped with the accumulated experience mandates an important question: Is it possible to come up with a fourth objective in COM surgery? Our answer to that question is YES IT IS: to interfere and abort the natural history of the disease. The basic precondition for doing so is the correct understanding of the pathogenesis of the condition. In other words, to identify which direction the process will take from the precipitating etiology to the establishment of irreversible tissue pathology.

The body of studies defines a roughly standard natural history allowing us to forecast and possibly anticipate unfavorable end points since COM follows what we call a "predictable script".

Some interventions along the process are traditional and include:

1. Identifying and controlling risk factors
2. Clinical treatment during early phases
3. Close and careful follow-up
4. Management of diseases in the neighborhood

With this concept in mind we advance the discussion to a new level by considering a more vigorous and active intervention in the oligosymptomatic early steps.

The main dilemma is to appropriately decide between a passive or contemplative attitude or to undertake an early intervention to thwart progressive disease, despite the fact that an intervention is not devoid of intrinsic morbidity? Should one wait for a dry symptomless retraction pocket to become active cholesteatoma which then necessitates major surgery? Or, would a less invasive approach to an earlier stage have been better? Of course, the answers would be quite simple if we had confidence that this transition would be inevitable! Choosing the best option between these two extremes is our challenge! The circumstance that has brought us to this dilemma regarding the correct timing of intervention in ME disease is the lack of evidence-based information. Should we wait for a more traditional evidence-based model or should we venture into new alternative techniques?

When we take into consideration a patient that comes to our attention in the hope to be cured waiting for the evidences may become too late or no more appropriate. In the other hand, choosing a new technique in the hope of aborting the process may be ineffective and aggressive. The main difficulty to solve our impasse is the natural history of the disease itself since it moves freely among different stages, going through courses that are not necessarily unidirectional. Thus, as the active disease relapses for long periods, the silent sequel may emerge in acute outbreaks, at times, very close to complications.

Otitis media has traditionally been classified into two major groups: (1) suppurative (acute or chronic) and (2) nonsuppurative (serous or mucoid) otitis media. Chronic otitis media can be further distinguished according to the presence or absence of cholesteatoma.[20] Despite being generally accepted, this classification is not devoid of criticism since it neglects the so-called

silent chronic otitis media (irreversible inflammatory pathology in the ME associated with an intact TM)[14,16,36] and underestimates the potential aggressiveness of the subtype not associated with cholesteatoma (frequently referred as "simple" chronic otitis media).

In real-life practice, it is frequently impossible to determine the boundaries between subtypes of otitis media since the limits are thin if not overlapped.

We believe the importance of considering the CLE in conjunction with the most affected side in COM cannot be overemphasized. Regardless the presence of cholesteatoma, the astute analysis of both ears may shed some light into three key aspects of the disease process: where did it come from? (Etiology) what is the current condition (established pathology) and, more importantly, how fast and in which direction the disease is marching toward (natural history). The answer to these questions will illuminate and improve the true understanding of the pathogenesis of COM helping the treatment and the counseling of patients and relatives.

When we take into account the CLE, we can understand the dynamic pathologic process right before our eyes. There are many patients displaying similarity of both sides, at times one step ahead or behind the other.

For example, it is not rare to find a patient with a postero-superior cholesteatoma in one ear and a severe retraction of the pars tensa in the other; or with a classical pars flaccida cholesteatoma in one ear and a deep attic retraction pocket, but still cholesteatoma free in the other (Figures 8A and B).

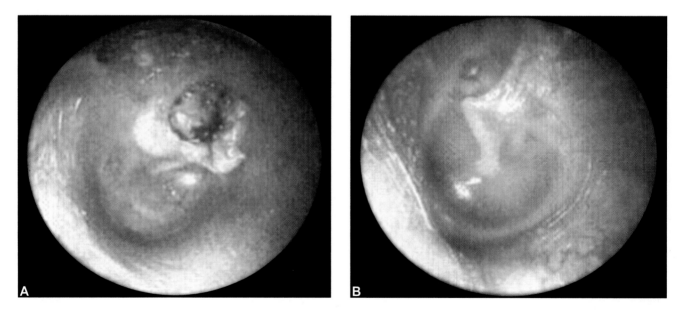

Figures 8A and B (A) Case 559 (Right Ear): Pars flaccida cholesteatoma; (B) Case 559 (Left Ear): CLE with a pars flaccida moderate retraction

5.2.6D
Congenital Cholesteatoma

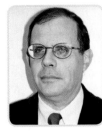

Carlos Ruah, Fernando V Mendonca

DEFINITION

According to Derlacki and Clemis,[1] a cholesteatoma may be considered congenital (CC) if it occurs behind an intact tympanic membrane (TM), in the absence of a history of otitis media or trauma. Levenson et al.[2] exclude from this definition intra-membranous cholesteatomas of the TM, giant cholesteatomas and those arising in atretic or stenotic external auditory canals (EACs). Since the incidence of congenital cholesteatomas overlaps the incidence of otitis media, it appears that the absence of a history of otorrhea, TM perforation or surgery to the ear is more relevant than the absence of a history of otitis media.

PATHOGENESIS

Several theories for the pathogenesis of CC have been proposed and which include the following.

Inclusion Theory

In this theory the CC may have its origin in epithelial embryonic cells misplaced during embryogenesis[3] or entrapped in fusion mesodermic lines[4] or in multipotencial germ cells being the simplest form of monodermic teratomas.[5]

Migration Theory

Aimi[6] suggested that the embryonic tympanic ring could act as a stop sign to the growth of the distal epithelial end of the EAC, by placing its annular plain ahead of its growth. He observed,

however, delays in the tympanic ring formation, which would allow epithelial remnants of the EAC to migrate into the middle ear, giving rise to the cholesteatoma.

Invagination Theory

Sadé[7] demonstrated histologically that inflamed mesenchyme or connective tissue under squamous epithelium could trigger the proliferation of the basal layer with the formation of cystic buds. These could become filled with keratin, grow into the middle ear and open to the surface of the TM.

Implantation Theory

Eavey et al.[8] have postulated that the persistence of amniotic fluid in the middle ear could produce an inflammatory reaction acting as a source of metaplasia, triggering the growth of invaginating keratinic buds from the TM. It was also speculated that the deposition and proliferation of the keratinocytes of the amniotic fluid could produce a CC.

Metaplasia Theory

Sadé et al.[9] suggested that CC could derive from metaplasia of the middle ear mucosa and proposed the term "primary cholesteatoma" instead of CC. This was based on two facts. The first is that any cell carries the information to form any other cell, and the second is the demonstration of the presence of small amounts of intracellular keratin in the cells lining the Eustachian tube and the middle ear. As such, all phenomena leading to metaplasia, such as middle ear inflammation, changes in CO_2/O_2 composition of middle ear gases or persistent amniotic fluid in the middle ear could be a source of cholesteatoma under an intact TM.

Epidermoid Formation Theory

Teed, in 1936,[10] described a small mass of epidermoid cells in the anterior superior quadrant of the middle ear and postulated that if this structure fails to resorb, it could give rise to a CC. This provocative speculation was not pursued until 1986 when Michaels[11] described an epidermoid formation occurring during the development of the middle ear, first in the posterior aspect of the tubotympanic recess (future Eustachian tube) in the fifth to seventh week embryo, and then in the anterior-superior quadrant of the middle ear at a later stage, disappearing around the 33rd week of gestation.[12] This epidermoid formation, however, was found in middle ears of temporal bones until the age of 2 years and 7 months.[13] It was again suggested that the persistence and further growth of this formation could result in a CC. Karmody et al.[14] described the first CC arising at the site where the epidermoid formation is usually found, in a temporal bone of a 3–6 year old child with congenital malformations. This finding reinforced this theory.

Acquired Inclusion Island Theory

Tos[15] noticed that the CC is usually attached to the malleus neck or handle, or to the long process of the incus. He suggested that during episodes of tubal occlusion, otitis media with effusion or acute otitis media, the TM could retract and adhere temporarily to any of these structures. Upon resolution of the ear disease, the TM would return to its original position, leaving behind a small island of epithelium that could proliferate and become a CC.

INCIDENCE AND CLINICAL FINDINGS

The incidence of CC is thought to be between 1% and 5%[16] or 0–12 children per 100,000 inhabitants.[15] The average age of

diagnosis is 4 years and 6 month, and varies between 9 months and 12 years of age, being more prevalent in the male than in the female (3:1).[17] The great majority occurs in the anterior-superior quadrant of the middle ear but it can be found anywhere in the middle ear and mastoid. In 3% of the cases it is bilateral, especially in children with congenital malformations of the head and neck.[18]

The natural history of CC explains its clinical findings. Initially they are assymptomatic and may be seen as white mass under the TM. As it grows, it may occlude the Eustachian tube and cause a middle ear effusion, or destroy the middle ear ossicles, leading to a conductive hearing loss. The facial nerve may be involved but erosion of the otic capsule is extremely rare. If they open to the EAC they are difficult to differentiate from an acquired cholesteatoma. The diagnosis is sometimes made at the time of myringotomy for the effusion when a whitish mass is seen under the TM. In the presence of effusion, the computerized tomography (CT) does not differentiate between the effusion and the CC, unless there is ossicular erosion. It certainly helps in the planning of surgery, showing the bony limits and thickness of the bony EAC, middle ear and mastoid. Magnetic resonance helps to differentiate the CC from other middle ear masses such as neuromas, adenomas, schwannomas or metastasis.[16]

STAGING

Although some staging systems have been proposed,[19,20] the classification of Nelson[21] appears the simplest which have been described hereunder.

Type 1

The CC is mesotympanic with no ossicular erosion. Around 15% of cases are of this type and no recurrence has occurred after surgical removal.

Type 2

The CC is mesotympanic or attical with ossicular erosion but no mastoid extension. Around 59% of CC are of this type and there were 34% of recurrences after surgical removal.

Type 3

The CC is mesotympanic and extends to the mastoid. Around 26% of CC are of this type and there were 55% of recurrences after surgical removal.

SURGICAL MANAGEMENT

1. The aim of surgery is to complete removal of the CC and optimal hearing outcome.
2. Although the average age of diagnosis is 4 years old, there is no minimal age for surgery. It may, however, be better performed if the child is one year of age or older for a more favorable anatomy of the EAC and middle ear.
3. Types 1 and 2 CC should be approached initially with a transcanal incision and flap. If the CC is seen extending into the mastoid, then a retroauricular incision is performed for mastoidectomy.
4. Due to the developing temporal bone, facial nerve may be exposed and if mastoidectomy is performed, exposure of dura may occur.

SURGICAL STEPS

1. After induction of general anesthesia, the child is positioned with slight hyperextension of the head for better assessment of the attic if necessary.
2. Infiltration of the EAC is performed with xylocaine and epinephrine in the four quadrants of the EAC (Figure 1).
3. A transcanal inferiorly based tympanomeatal flap is raised with a wide superior part to allow drilling of the scutum should the cholesteatoma extend to the attic (Figure 2).

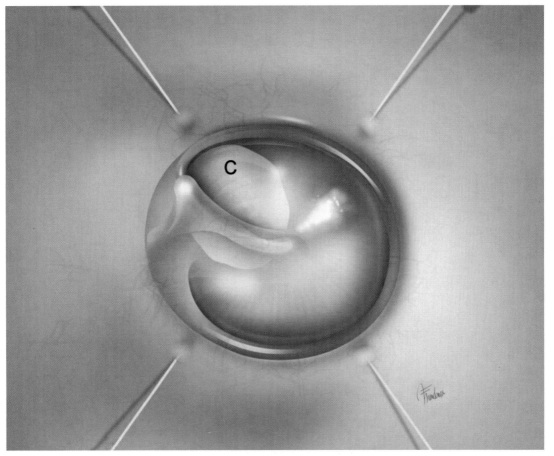

Figure 1 Infiltration of the EAC is performed with xylocaine and epinephrine in the four quadrants of the EAC. C: Cholesteatoma
© Copyright Fernando Vilhena de Mendonça

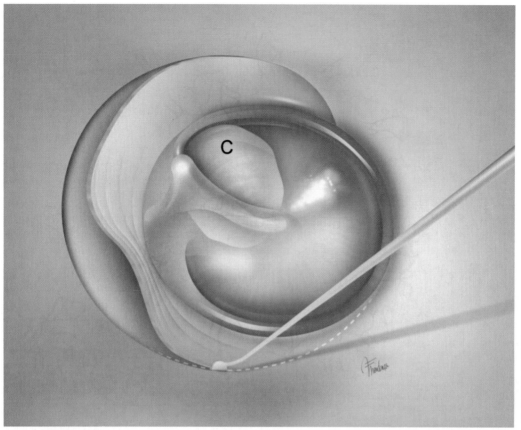

Figure 2 Raising a transcanal inferiorly based tympanomeatal flap with a wide superior part to allow drilling of the scutum. C: Cholesteatoma
© Copyright Fernando Vilhena de Mendonça

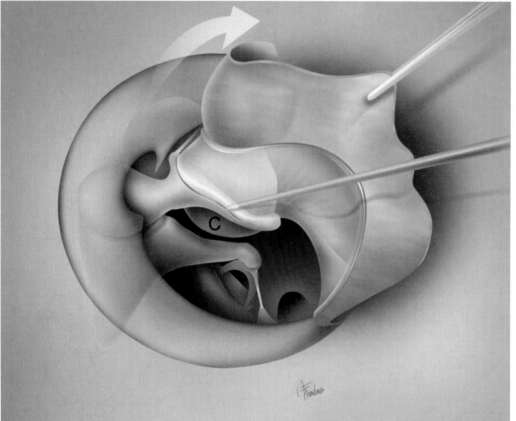

Figure 3A

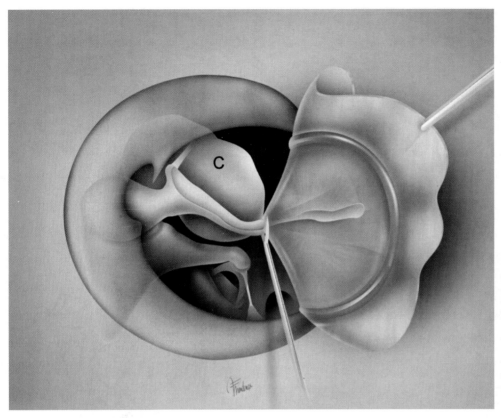

Figure 3B

Figures 3A and B The periosteum of the long process of the malleus is incised using a sharp sickle knife and stripped with the raised TM. It is important to separate the TM from the umbo using fine Bellucci scissors. C: Cholesteatoma
© Copyright Fernando Vilhena de Mendonça

4. If the EAC is too narrow, an endaural superior incision can be made to widen the EAC and allow the introduction of a larger speculum.

5. The flap should be raised from the posterior part, where the skin is thicker, to its anterior part where the skin is very thin and easily torned.

6. Do not try to raise the annulus until all the flap is completely raised to the bony tympanic sulcus.

7. Raise the tympanic annulus and tease off the TM from the lateral process of the malleus. Using a sharp sickle knife, incise the periosteum of the long process of the malleus and strip it with the raised TM. It is important to separate the TM from the umbo using fine Bellucci scissors (Figures 3A and B).

8. The tympanomeatal flap is pushed inferiorly, allowing full exposure of the middle ear (Figure 4).

9. The extension of the CC is then assessed. If it is only mesotympanic it should carefully be removed with great care not to rupture the matrix spilling the keratin contents into the middle ear. Caution should be taken in this step since the facial nerve may be dehiscent (Figure 4).

10. If the CC extends to the attic, drilling of the scutum is performed, exposing the attic and allowing the same carefully removal of the cholesteatoma (Figures 5A and B).

11. If it extends posteriorly to the ossicular chain and to the mastoid, and especially if there is erosion of the ossicles, a

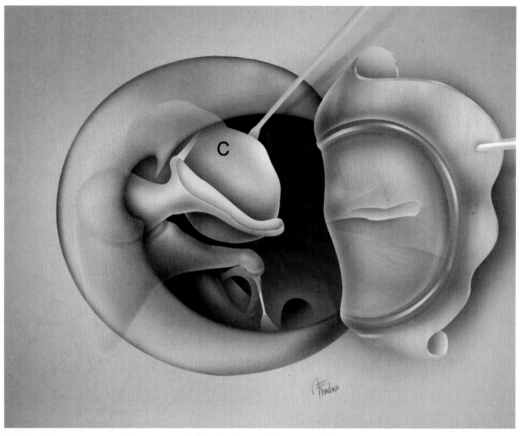

Figure 4 The tympanomeatal flap is pushed inferiorly allowing full exposure of the middle ear. C: Cholesteatoma
© Copyright Fernando Vilhena de Mendonça

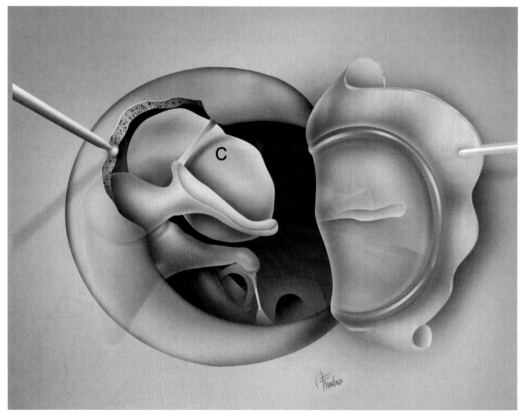

Figure 5A

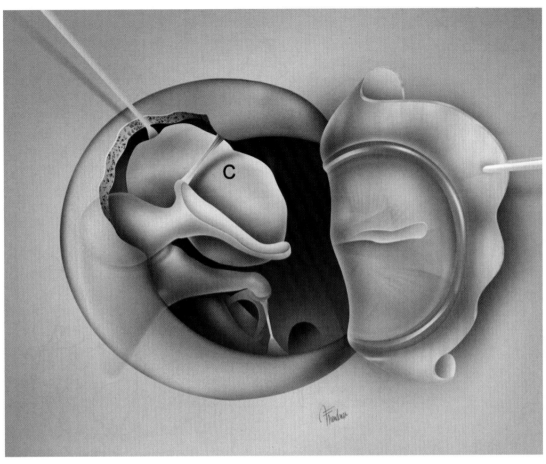

Figure 5B

Figures 5A and B Drilling of the scutum to expose the attic. C: Cholesteatoma
© Copyright Fernando Vilhena de Mendonça

retroauricular incision may be needed for mastoidectomy, complete removal of the cholesteatoma and ossicular reconstruction.

REFERENCES

1. Derlacki EL, Clemis JD. Congenital cholesteatoma of the middle ear and mastoid. Ann Otol Rhinol Laryngol. 1965;74(3): 706-27.

2. Levenson MJ, Michaels L, Parisier SC. Congenital cholesteatoma of the middle ear in children: origin and management. ORL Clin N Am. 1989;22(5):941-54.

3. Von Remak R. Ein Betrag zur Entwicklungsgeschichte dr Geschwiilster. Dtsch Klin. 1854;6:170.

4. Paparella MM, Rybak L. Congenital cholesteatoma. ORL Clin N Am. 1978;11(1):113-20.

5. Ruah C, Cohen D, Sadé J. Eustachian tube teratoma and its terminology correctness. J Laryngol Otol. 1999;113:271-4.

6. Aimi K. Role of tympanic ring in the pathogenesis of congenital cholesteatoma. Laryngoscope. 1983;93:1140-6.

7. Sadé J. Pathogenesis of attic cholesteatoma. In: McCabe BF, Sadé J, Abramson M (Eds). Cholesteatoma: First International Conference. Aesculapius Public Co.; 1977. pp. 212-32.

8. Eavey RD, Camacho AR, Northrop C. Chronic ear pathology in a model of neonatal amniotic fluid ear inoculation. Arch Otolaryngol Head Neck Surg. 1992;118:1198-203.

9. Sadé J, Babiacki A, Pinkus G. The metaplasic and congenital origin of cholesteatoma. Acta Otolaryngol (Stockh). 1983;96:119-29.

10. Teed RW. Cholesteatoma verum tympani. Arch of Otolaryngol. 1936;24:455-62.

11. Michaels L. An epidermoid formation in the developing middle ear: possible source of cholesteatoma. J Otolaryngol. 1986;15(3):169-74.

12. Michaels L. Evolution of the epidermoid formation and its role in the development of the middle ear and tympanic membrane during the first trimester. J Otolaryngol. 1988;17(1):22-8.

13. Levine JL, Wright CG, Pawlowski KS, et al. Postnatal persistence of epidermoid rests in the human middle ear. Laryngoscope. 1998;108:70-3.

14. Karmody CS, Byahatti SV, Blevins N, et al. The origin of congenital cholesteatoma. Am J Otolaryngol. 1998;19:292-7.

15. Tos M. A new pathogenesis of mesotympanic (congenital) cholesteatoma. Laryngoscope. 2000;110(11):1890-7.

16. Bennett M, Warren F, Jackson GC, et al. Congenital cholesteatoma: theories, facts, and 53 patients. ORL Clin N Am. 2006;39(6): 1081-94.

17. Friedberg J. Congental cholesteatoma. Laryngoscope. 1994;104(3 Suppl 62):1-24.

18. Peron DL, Schuknecht HF. Congenital cholesteatomas and other anomalies. Arch Otolaryngol. 1975;101:498-505.

19. Derlacki EL, Harrison WH, Clemis JD. Congenital cholesteatoma of the middle ear and mastoid. A 2nd report presenting 7 additional cases. Laryngoscope. 1968;78:1050-78.

20. Potsic WP, Sarmadi DS, Marsh RR, et al. A staging system for congenital cholesteatoma. Arch Otolaryngol Head Neck Surg. 2002;128:1009-12.

21. Nelson M, Roger G, Koltai PJ, et al. Congenital cholesteatoma. Arch Otolaryngol Head Neck Surg. 2002;128:810-4.

5.2.6E

Mastoidectomy Conserving the Posterior Canal Wall (Canal Wall Up)

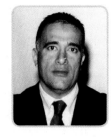

Marcelo Hueb

INTRODUCTION

The Eustachian tube/middle ear/mastoid complex is interconnected and communicates with the nasopharynx inferiorly and medially. Due to a complex embryologic origin and different tissue compositions it is subjected to many pathologic conditions, including otitis media on its various forms. Otitis media evolves in an inflammatory and/or infectious continuum highly related to etiopathogenic processes at epithelial, subepithelial, cavitary and fluid levels. It's evolution can be arrested in early stages but sequel and complications can occur in early or late stages.

Medical management and/or surgical procedures help to control otitis media and any controversy regarding techniques should not overcome the primary objective of a mastoidectomy, which is: removal or control of the disease as to have a dry, safe and well healed ear. Whether or not these goals can be achieved using an open or closed technique depends on the surgeon's skill and experience as well as the disease itself and patient particularities. Location and extension of the disease should be thoroughly assessed, especially regarding hidden areas such as the facial recess and sinus tympani [Figures 1(A and B) and 2]. Disease involvement or not in these places (Figures 3A and B) as well as pars tensa or epitympanic involvement extension (Video 1) and intracranial complications (Figure 4) are important in the preoperative assessment. The natural history of simple and cholesteatomatous chronic otitis media should be taken into consideration and the possibility of contralateral ear involvement should always be kept in mind (Figure 5 and Video 2).

Although some of these factors can suggest preoperatively which procedure to choose the surgeon should always be prepared to change it accordingly to what is preoperatively seen. A surgical view of the disease extension and anatomical conditions associated with a given patient characteristics give the final conditions for a conscious decision making. It is generally stated that open-cavity procedures help to achieve a better exposure and disease control while providing a poorer hearing

reconstruction. On the other hand closed-cavity procedures are generally believed to be associated with better anatomical and hearing results with a poorer disease control.

On these aspects, closed-cavity tympanomastoidectomy implies in middle ear and mastoid instrumentation conserving the separation between the ear canal and the mastoid (posterior canal wall up). By considering this technique as conserving this separation and not necessarily conserving the osseous canal wall opens a window for temporarily open tympanomastoidectomies. In this condition the posterior canal wall is drilled down (at bridge level or totally) and the preoperative advantages of an open technique are achieved. Reconstructing the drilled canal wall at the end of the procedure helps achieving the postoperative advantages of a closed-cavity procedure.

AIM

The surgical treatment of otitis media regarding its various procedures involving the middle ear and/or the mastoid and eventually the external auditory canal and pinna aims to achieve a "5 R" goal that comprises:
1. Removal, control or prevention (of the disease);
2. Recurrence (prevention of);
3. Restoring (of the hearing);
4. Reconstruction or modification (of the anatomy) and
5. Reintervention (when needed).

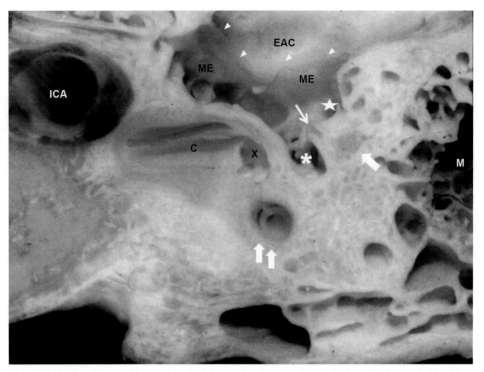

Figure 1A Unstained temporal bone section. EAC (external auditory canal), ME (middle ear), M (mastoid), C (cochlea), ICA (internal carotid artery), X (round window niche), tympanic membrane (arrow heads), facial nerve (thick arrow), posterior semicircular canal ampulla (two thick arrows), pyramidal eminence (thin arrow), facial recess (star) and sinus tympani (asterisk)

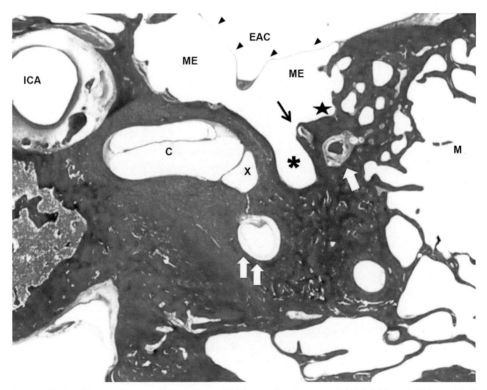

Figure 1B H and E stained temporal bone section. EAC (external auditory canal), ME (middle ear), M (mastoid), C (cochlea), ICA (internal carotid artery), X (round window niche), tympanic membrane (arrow heads), facial nerve (thick arrow), posterior semicircular canal ampulla (two thick arrows), pyramidal eminence (thin arrow), facial recess (star) and sinus tympani (asterisk)

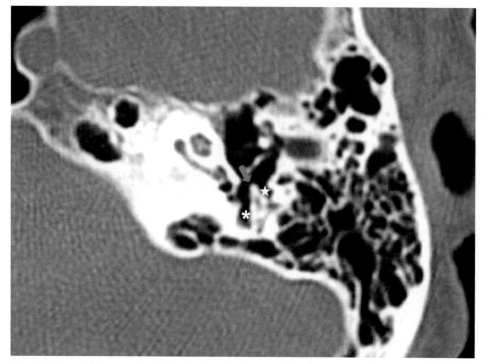

Figure 2 Computed tomography axial imaging showing the pyramidal eminence (arrow), facial recess (star) and sinus tympani (asterisk). The facial nerve is seen right behind the facial recess. The cochlea, round window membrane and niche and the middle ear are also seen. See Figures 1A and B for references

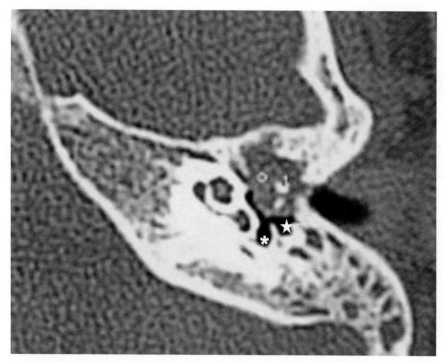

Figure 3A Cholesteatoma involvement in the middle ear/epitympanum is seen in this axial computed tomography imaging without involvement of the facial recess (star) or sinus tympani (asterisk)

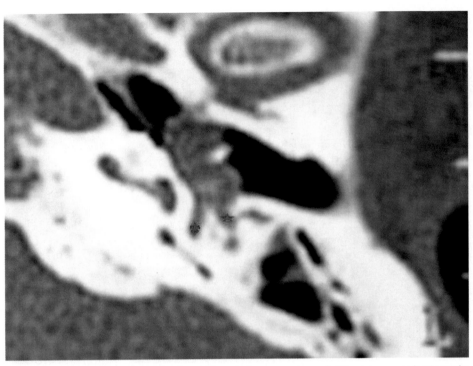

Figure 3B Cholesteatoma involvement in the middle ear/epitympanum is seen in this axial computed tomography imaging with involvement of the facial recess (star) and sinus tympani (asterisk)

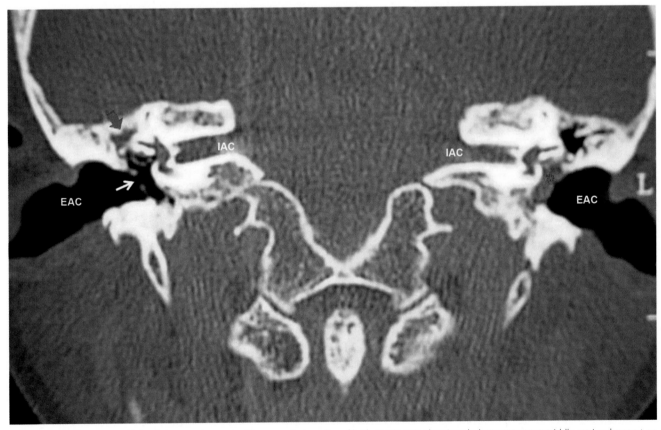

Figure 4 Same patient as in Video 2. A coronal computed tomography imaging of both ears is seen showing cholesteatomatous middle ear involvement on the left side and an "unexpected" epitympanic involvement on the right side (thick arrow). The atrophic central tympanic membrane area on the right ear is seen (thin arrow). EAC (external auditory canal), IAC (internal auditory canal)

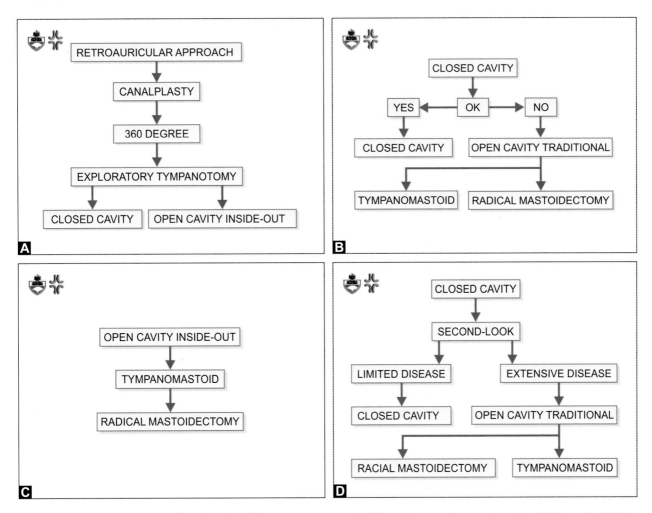

Figures 6A to D Surgical decision-making algorithm. (A) Retroauricular approach is followed by an ample canalplasty with a 360° view of the TM. The exploratory tympanotomy will dictate the further steps: closed or open technique; (B) If the option was a closed technique during the procedure it may be converted to a traditional open cavity (radical or not); (C) If the preoperative decision was for a CWD the inside-out technique is employed and the middle ear reconstruction will depend on the surgical findings; (D) After a CWU the findings during the second-look will dictate whether the posterior wall will be lowered or not

low the subdermal fat, leaving a layer of loose areolar tissue on the temporalis fascia. This plane is developed down to the mastoid tip. The attachments of the sternocleidomastoid muscle can be separated from the mastoid tip for increased exposure.[16] This dissection can be accomplished with the unipolar cautery leaving the periostium in place and delineating the posterior semicircle of the external auditory canal. A periosteal flap is then tailored to fit the surgical plan: if the CT scan has revealed a sclerotic mastoid, the flap may be triangular and anteriorly based. In those cases where the mastoid is expected to be drilled down to the tip, the flap is rectangular and inferiorly based. The reason for this modification is that at the end of the procedure the flap is returned to its original position filling in partially the surgical defect and decreasing the final size of the mastoid bowl (Figures 7A and B).

Exposure and Removal of the Temporalis Fascia

The postauricular incision extends up into the region of the temporalis fascia. A self-retaining retractor is inserted and by lifting it up, one can lift the scalp off the temporalis muscle.

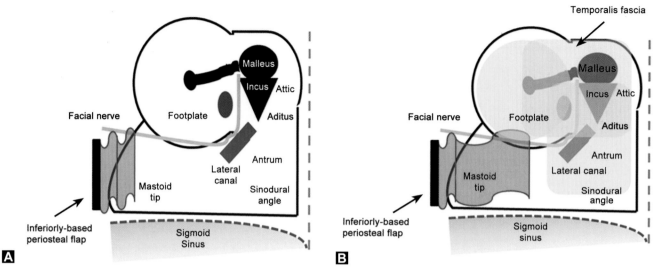

Figures 7A and B (A) The periostium of the mastoid cortex is elevated as an inferiorly-based flap and held in position by the self-retaining retractors; (B) At the end of the procedure, the flap returns to its original position filling in partially the surgical defect and decreasing the size of the mastoid bowl

The loose areolar tissue is then set apart from the true fascia through sharp and blunt dissection. Local anesthetic is injected under the fascia to elevate it from the muscle and with the scalpel the fascia is sectioned in a roughly ovoid shape and harvested. After being harvested, the fascia is spread on a polytetrafluoroethylene (PTFE) block, with the undersurface upward and any adherent muscle is removed. The PTFE block is placed under an electric lamp and after approximately 10 minutes, the fascia is dry.

Incisions in the Canal

After the elevation of the periosteal flap the bony landmarks of the mastoid cortex (spine of Henle, linea temporalis and cribiform area) are identified. Attention is directed to the posterior margin of the external auditory canal and the skin is gently elevated loose for a few millimeters. A number 11 blade knife is used in a straight angle to incise the skin from behind entering the lumen of the canal. A small Köerner flap is created and the self-retaining retractor repositioned. At this point the canal will become completely into view and the first incision is extended superiorly, inferioly and anteriorly around the 360° of the bony canal (Figure 8).

Elevation of the Meatal Flap

With the edges of the skin free, the surgeon uses a duckbill elevator or even a Rosen knife to separate the skin flap gently from the underlying bone. Separation must be slow and

careful to preserve the flap intact. A suction tip (finger off the hole) should be used against the elevator blade to keep the field free of blood. Care should be taken to avoid suctioning and damaging the flap. The skin is elevated evenly, avoiding tunneling, until it reaches the annulus (Figure 8). Sometimes this dissection is obstructed because of a narrow or sinuous, twisted external auditory canal. Regardless of the cause (e.g. stenosis, exostosis, or osteomas), the canal should first be surgically enlarged or straightened to improve or facilitate access to the middle ear. We always prefer to perform the canalplasty before entering the middle ear.

Canalplasty

After the flap has been elevated and the osseous canal exposed, the canal is drilled lateral to the annulus in a way that allows better exposure of the annulus and associated mesotympanum. When an anterior bump is present, the anterior osseous canal may be drilled, allowing better exposure of the anterior mesotympanum. Attention must be exercised to avoid entering the temporomandibular joint anteriorly or damaging the skin flap with the burr. For such, after the elevation of the flap, it is carefully folded and protected from the rotating burrs with a round shield fashioned previously with the external packing of the catgut suture. The shield is interposed between the flap and the burr protecting the first of being accidentally ripped off from the sulcus by the action of the high speed burr. An extra-protection is to switch to a diamond burr when the drilling gets close to the flap and the residual TM. During the posterior

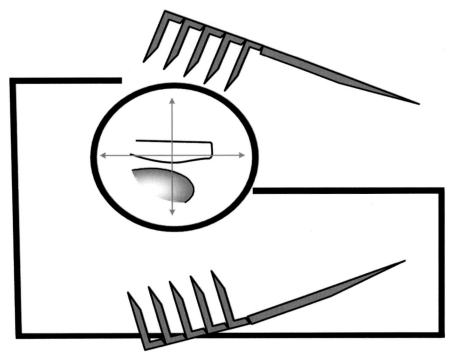

Figure 8 After repositioning of the self-retaining retractors the complete circumference of the external canal comes into view

canalplasty, the surgeon should watch for an anterior and more laterally located descendent portion of the mastoid segment of the facial nerve. During the course of posterior canalplasty, very often a few mastoid cells are opened thus, allowing a first glimpse of pathologic conditions in the mastoid. In fact we always overdrill the posterosuperior aspect of the canal opening the cells located lateral to the antrum. A prominent tympanosquamous and tympanomastoid suture lines are also taken off at this point to increase exposure of the pars flaccida.[10]

When the drilling is complete, the field should be rinsed with saline solution to wash out bone chips and so that the surgeon will have a panoramic 360° view of the tympanic membrane (Figures 9A to C).

Entering the Middle Ear

After the canalplasty is complete, the tympanomeatal flap is further elevated to the annulus. At this point, greater magnification can be used (10X or 16X) in the microscope. The annulus is positively identified and elevated with the elevator, working always against the bone. After the annulus is lifted away from the bony sulcus, a needle or the sickle knife can be used to open the mucosa, entering the middle ear always beneath the annulus and, if possible, inferiorly toward the round window. At this point, the duckbill can be passed through this initial hole,

pressed firmly against the bony annulus and moved downward to liberate completely the posteroinferior tympanic membrane. Upward, a needle or the sickle knife can be used to liberate the posterosuperior tympanic membrane gently, with care not to disturb the ossicles. The chorda tympani nerve should be identified and carefully moved out of the field of vision. As pointed out by Dornhoffer, this technique involves extensive drilling in close proximity and just lateral to the head of the malleus and the body of the incus, it is necessary to visualize the incudostapedial joint and the integrity of the lenticular process of the incus as an initial step. Except in cases of very limited retraction pockets, the incudostapedial joint is disarticulated to avoid trauma to the inner ear from the subsequent drilling.[10] The TM elevated up to the malleus. It is then grasped with the alligator forceps and peeled off the malleus neck exposing the lateral process which will serve as a pointer to the following bony removal of the scutum. At this point, the opening of the cholesteatoma sac will be brought into view (in a case of pars flaccida cholesteatoma) or exfoliated keratin will be identified in the posterosuperior quadrant (pars tensa cholesteatoma).

Atticotomy

The superior aspect of the bony canal is carefully removed with the drill. The atticotomy or amount of bone removed can be

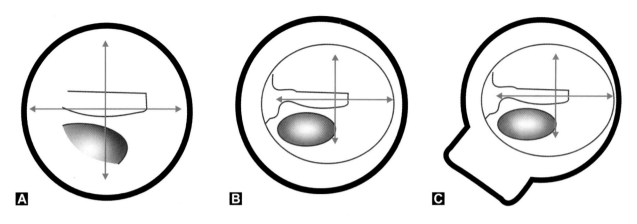

Figures 9A to C (A) TM view before the canalplasty; (B) After the canalplasty, a 360° view of the tympanic membrane with one position of the microscope; (C) During the canalplasty a preliminary notch is created in the posterosuperior aspect of the canal opening the cells located lateral to the antrum

small, medium, or large to facilitate exposure of the pathologic conditions at hand. This may be done to allow better exposure of the ossicles (i.e. the neck and head of the malleus and the incudomalleolar joint) or to follow mesotympanic disease extending toward the aditus ad antrum. Anatomic dimensions of the attic and its parts vary and pathologic conditions certainly can exist in the attic, contributing to obstruction at this site. Anatomic or pathologic obstruction of the attic or aditus ad antrum results in pathologic tissues that can occupy the mastoid, even with preservation of normal or near-normal findings in the middle ear. This is particularly true for pars flaccida cholesteatomas. When disease extends to the attic, the authors initially follow it, increasing the size of the atticotomy in an attempt to reach the end of the pathologic tissue. Working laterally to the ossicular chain, the bony removal continues until the incudomallear joint is perfectly visualized.

The next structure to be positively identified is the tegmen tympani or middle cranial fossa dural plate. It is important to know that the tegmen at the lateral external canal frequently is more inferior than the more medial tegmen at the level of the epitympanum, so care must be taken to avoid injury to the dura laterally. Preoperative CT helps to predict the height of the tegmen on the coronal view.[10] The final objective of the atticotomy is to bring into view the following landmarks: head of the malleus, the body of the incus and the tegmen (Figures 10A and B). These structures are frequently covered by the matrix of the cholesteatoma. When the disease is limited in this area and can be peeled off the ossicles, no further dissection is necessary, the surgical defect can be reconstructed using sculptured cortical bone chips, bone pate, or bone wax.

Retrograde Antrostomy

Frequently though, the cholesteatoma penetrates posteriorly from Prussak's space (following the embryologic course of the saccus medius), passing through the superior incudal space and then traversing the aditus ad antrum to enter deeply into the mastoid. In this situation, the fundus of the cyst cannot be reached through atticotomy. An inside-out antrostomy in sclerotic bones is the next step in the procedure. For such, the dissection should proceed backwards laterally to the ossicular chain and following and in close contact with the dural plate. The next landmarks to be identified are the short process of the incus medially and a few millimeters below it the solid bone of the dome of the lateral semicircular canal (Figure 11A). After opening a few more cells the final objective of the antrostomy has been achieved: the identification of the antrum itself (filled with cholesteatoma) the lateral semicircular canal and the dural plate. It should be emphasized that the inside-out technique offers a very safe approach to the antrum. It immediately exposes and thereby allows protection of important structures that may otherwise be subject to injury. First, the drilling is carried out lateral to the ossicular chain interposing the head of the malleus and the body off the incus between the burrs and the facial nerve (the possibility of an acoustic trauma is minimized since the incudostapedial joint has already been disarticulated as an earlier step). Second, the most flagrant landmark of the antrum is the dome of the lateral semicircular canal which protects the second genu of the facial nerve (located slightly medially and inferiorly) from an inadvertent and catastrophic drilling accident (Figure 11B).

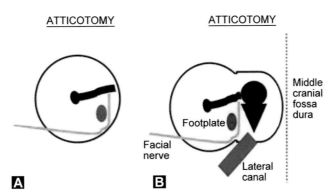

ATTICOTOMY   ATTICOTOMY

Figures 10A and B (A) The mesotympanic view before the atticotomy; (B) The final objective of the atticotomy has been achieved: identification of the head of the malleus, the body of the incus and the tegmen tympani

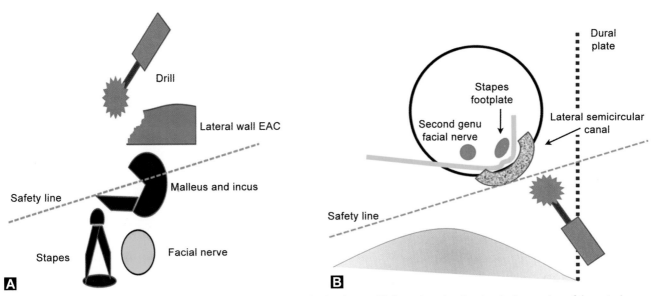

Figures 11A and B The inside-out mastoidectomy offers protection to the facial nerve. (A) Coronal section showing the interpositon of the ossicular mass between the burr and the tympanic segment of the facial nerve; (B) Axial section of the antrostomy with the lateral semicircular shielding the second genu of the facial nerve from the rotating burr

As the antrum is widely opened, the extent of the cholesteatoma can be appreciated. The goal is to remove only the bone necessary to expose the back edge of the sac and many times a complete mastoidectomy is not necessary. In a sclerotic mastoid, the surgeon may frequently find the cholesteatoma extending only to the antrum, so minimal drilling is needed. After drilling the bony bridge over the aditus the three upper compartments of the middle ear are completely identified: the attic (with the incudomallear joint), the transitional aditus and the antrum (with the lateral semicircular canal). The lateral and posterior wall of the epitympanum must be removed until the tegmen mastoid or tegmen tympani are continuous. The transition between the middle ear and mastoid must be smooth and uninterrupted.

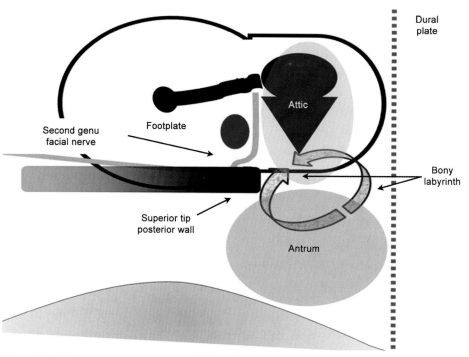

Figure 12 The three upper compartments of the middle ear are completely identified: the attic (with the incudomallear joint), the transitional aditus and the antrum (with the lateral semicircular canal). The tip of the posterior wall is still high blocking a better view of the tympanic facial nerve

At this point, the tip of the posterior wall is still high and with the malleus and incus in place prevents a better view of the tympanic segment of the facial nerve (Figure 12).

Mastoidectomy

Once this step is accomplished, it opens a large and safe two-way avenue. The first way goes (straight) all the way to the sinodural (Citelli's) angle; the second makes a right angle turn toward the bottom of the mastoid (Figures 13A and B). The cholesteatoma sac is followed back as posteriorly and inferiorly as necessary or until normal air cells are encountered.[10] Along the way, any cell filled with cholesterol granuloma should be explored and suctioned. Granulation tissue is also frequently found at this point either around the cholesteatoma or infiltrating the posterior wall. It should also be removed from the irregular bone which is then smoothed with the diamond burr. The amount of bone removal in the mastoid is dependent of how deep the disease penetrates into the bone. Conceptually,

we classify the degree of mastoid exenteration in three levels: (1) antrum; (2) mid-mastoid, and (3) tip (Figure 14).

When the pathology in the mastoid has been completely delineated, attention is directed back to the middle ear: first the incus is disarticulated from the malleus and removed. With the malleus nipper the head of the malleus is also removed gaining access to the medial wall of the attic (frequently lined by the cholesteatoma matrix). After drilling anteriorly and parallel to the dural plate the anterior attic (supratubal recess) is widely exposed and cleaned of any residual disease. It is important to dissect the dural plate all the way to the confluence of the anterior wall of the external auditory canal where a 90° angle is created and then rounded off (Figure 15). During this step, the tegmen tympani should be checked for areas of bony defects. Small or large dehiscence are common findings and may be either congenital or consequence of the bone erosion power of cholesteatoma and/or granulation tissue. Most of them are not clinically relevant and should be left alone. Larger areas especially when associated with dural herniation should be

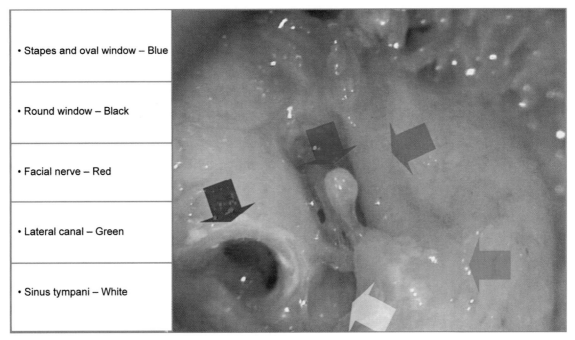

• Stapes and oval window – Blue
• Round window – Black
• Facial nerve – Red
• Lateral canal – Green
• Sinus tympani – White

Figure 17 Photo of the so-called posterior recesses of the mesotympanum

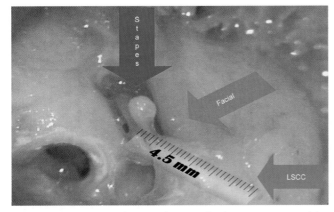

Figure 18 Along a linear distance of 4.5 mm the three components of the "critical triad": (1) lateral semicircular canal; (2) facial nerve, and (3) stapes and oval window
Source: Paparella MM. Personal communication

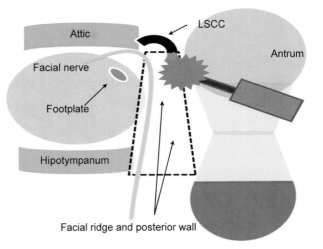

Figure 19 The superior pole of the wall will be completely lowered only after the perfect identification of the stapes (or the footplate), the facial nerve and its second genu

all epithelial remnants off the tip before repositioning the flap. To decrease the final size of the mastoid bowl it is also necessary to remove all the sharp edges around the surgical defect. Saucerization should be preferably performed at the beginning of the mastoidectomy because the enlarged cavity permits more light to penetrate to the depths of the cavity and creates more working room.[27]

Ossiculoplasty

After pathologic tissue in the middle ear has been eradicated, thorough attention is directed to assessment and reconstruction of the ossicular chain. Three prerequisites to obtaining

Open Mastoidectomy—Landmarks

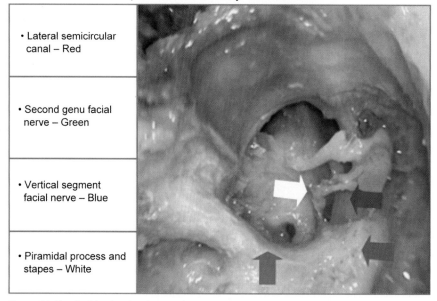

- Lateral semicircular canal – Red

- Second genu facial nerve – Green

- Vertical segment facial nerve – Blue

- Piramidal process and stapes – White

Figure 20 The final landmarks after a wide open mastoidectomy. Notice that the posterior wall has been reduced in all dimensions, the tympanic facial nerve, the genu and the vertical segment follow a smooth course and the hypotympanum and the anterior aspect of the wall have also been drilled

good functional restoration in cases of COM exist: (1) an intact tympanic membrane; (2) an air-containing, mucosa-lined middle ear space; and (3) a precise connection between the eardrum and fluids in the ear.[28] Materials often used for ossiculoplasty are grouped as autografts, homografts, or synthetic prostheses. Each material has advantages and disadvantages and no universal agreement exists concerning the most suitable prosthesis for ossiculoplasty.[19]

Bone and cartilage came into use in the 1960s and continues to be used alone or in combination with other materials. The authors believe that using the patient's own tissue (sculptured incus, malleus or cortical bone) is the best option. When these are not available, or when interpositioning of an ossicle is not reasonable we employ synthetic materials (hydroxyapatite or titanium). In cases in which the incus is absent, the stapes is normal and the wall has been taken down, decreasing the size of the middle ear cleft, the authors have used an autograft bony disk to bridge the gap between the stapes and eardrum. This disk is sculptured *in situ* using the drill and a small cutting burr in the mastoid cortex. The disk has a mean diameter of 3.5 mm and in its center an acetabulum is created to fit the head of the stapes. It is then carefully detached from the cortex using a small chisel, trimmed to its final form and positioned over the head of the stapes (Figure 21A). When only the footplate is remaining we also have used cortical bone. The only difference is that in this circumstance a T-shaped TORP is sculptured in the cortex of the mastoid. The window is lined with fascia or perichondrium,

the prostheses is trimmed to its final size, inserted in the niche and held in place with small pledges of Gelfoam® (Figure 21B).

Grafting the Tympanic Membrane

After final inspection and irrigation of the middle ear, the flap is folded fully anteriorly. Any debris or bone dust should be meticulously cleaned away. The dried temporalis fascia is removed from the block of PTFE and trimmed to fit medial to the remnant of the eardrum, the manubrium and the tympanomeatal flap. The graft is tailored to its final shape according to the surgical defect. When only the antrum has been exposed a bipedal graft is employed covering the middle ear and wrapping the attic, the lateral semicircular canal and the medial wall of the antrum (Figure 22A). When a level II or III defect has been created a kidney-shaped graft is fashioned covering the middle ear and lining the attic, antrum and the partially the mastoid [the tip has been removed or obliterated (Figure 22B)]. Gelfoam® soaked in saline solution is placed in the middle ear and the orifice of the ET to occlude the tube temporarily and to offer support for the graft anteriorly. Enough Gelfoam® should be used to create a true cushion in the middle ear to support the graft. Care should be used, though, to respect the limits of the fibrous and bony annulus because the moistened Gelfoam® tends to absorb liquid and expand. After the cushion is completed, a cotton ball is pressed against it, any solution or drops of blood are suctioned and the cotton is gently removed. The graft is grasped with an

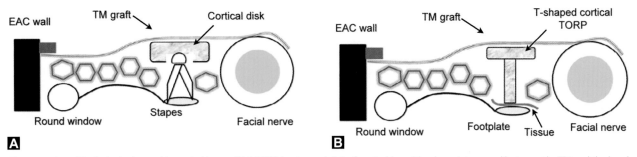

Figures 21A and B Ossiculoplasty with cortical bone. (A) A PORP (sculptured disk of cortical bone) has been interposed between the TM and the head of stapes; (B) A TORP replaces the chain (also sculptured with cortical bone). The footplate has been line with tissue (fascia, perichondrium or periosteum)

alligator forceps, rehydrated briefly with saline solution and placed as far anteriorly in the middle ear as possible and medial to the manubrium. The remaining base of the graft is spread over the Gelfoam® cushion and the mastoid walls contouring the dome of the lateral canal. The flap is returned to its original position with a duckbill and the surgeon's attention is directed to tucking the graft carefully into the margins of the remaining TM. Absolute control of the anterior border is critical to the final success of the entire surgery. A small, slit should be made in the anterosuperior quadrant of the TM so it may collapse over the graft (which will be resting over the Gelfoam®, the medial wall and the facial nerve) avoiding the formation of a cul-de-sac in the supratubal recess (which invariably will accumulate epithelial debris). Another cotton ball is inserted and moisture or blood is gently suctioned through the cotton. After its removal, the graft and flap are checked. After the flap has been meticulously returned to its original position, the cavity is packed firmly with Gelfoam® pledgets. The first piece of packing is a small, dry, rolled-up, tightly compressed piece of Gelfoam® placed in the sulcus anteriorly. The self-retaining retractors are released, a meatoplasty is carried out.

Meatoplasty

The meatoplasty is mandatory to widen the opening of external ear and to create a skin flap that will serve as a matrix for epithelization of the mastoid cavity. There is no question that meatoplasty strongly contributes to the functional recovery of the ear.[29] Its indispensable in open-cavity tympanomastoidectomies to monitor the conditions of the mastoid bowl in the postoperative period and to reach and clean all the newly created recesses. There are different ways to perform meatoplasty. We will describe a basic technique, most used in our experience which is a simple five steps procedure.

Steps

1. Incisions in the skin of the auditory canal
2. Dissection of subcutaneous tissue
3. Identification, release and partial ressection of the pinnal cartilage
4. Vertical incisions in the skin of the pinna (Köerner's flap)
5. Flap sutures

First step of meatoplasty is the initial incision of skin made in the beginning of the surgery. Thereafter, as mentioned before, two vertical incisions are done at 1 and 5 o'clock to prepare a Köerner's flap. Next step consists in dissecting soft tissues of Köerner's flap, leaving only skin. A smooth pressure with middle finger can support and guide this moment. It's important to remove a slice of conchal cartilage for the purpose of increased mobility of this skin flap.

After this, vertical incisions are prolonged. The higher they extend toward the free skin of the pinna, the greater the amplitude of meatus. A good parameter is the point when external meatus freely accepts the introduction of the index finger. Last stage is suturing the base of this flap in the adjacent subcutaneous tissue superiorly in order to pull it backward, which will promote healing tension forcing flap to meet bony wall of the cavity.[29]

Packing, Dressings and Postoperative Care

After the meatoplasty the self-retaining retractors are released and the ear is returned to its original position and sutured in place. A gauze impregnated in antibiotic ointment is used to line the cavity to prevent infection and to minimize adhesions of raw surface areas. Postoperative dressings generally consist of the standard mastoid dressing which is removed 24 hour after the procedure. Patients are instructed to change cotton

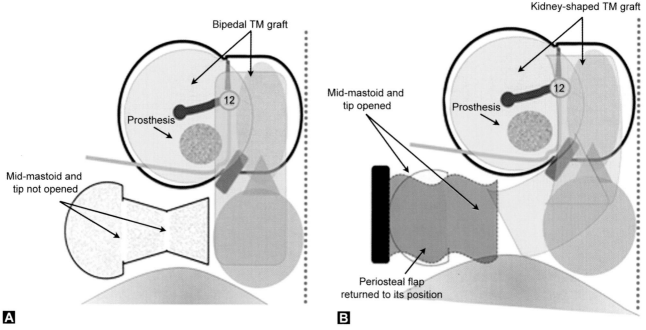

Figures 22A and B (A) A bipedal graft is employed covering the middle ear and wrapping the attic, the lateral semicircular canal and the medial wall of the antrum — Mastoid opening level I; (B) When a level II or III defect has been created a kidney-shaped graft is fashioned covering the middle ear and lining the attic, antrum and the partially the mastoid (the tip has been removed or obliterated by the periosteal flap)

balls in their ear and keep the postauricular incision clean. The internal gauze is left in place for 7 days. Both immediate and long-term care are vital for the surgical success.

We schedule at least three consecutive visits every ten days when the ear is inspected and manipulated accordingly until the cavity is completely healed.

Advantages of the Inside-Out Tympanomastoidectomy and Rules of the Thumb

Our accumulated experience in the last years with chronic ear surgery allows us to conclude that the inside-out tympanomastoidectomy has several advantages over the traditional OCTM:

- Low rate of recurrences and residual disease
- Similar hearing results
- Small postoperative cavities due to the hypopneumatization
- Postoperative otorrhea is rare if:
  - Cavity is well designed
  - No recesses
  - Eustachian tube is properly managed
  - Adequate meatoplasty
  - Rigid postoperative care

Finally the inside-out technique is:

- Safer
- Faster

- Follows cholesteatoma natural pathways
- More physiological
- Smaller cavities
- Customized meatus

REFERENCES

1. Alleva M, Paparella MM, Morris MS, et al. The flexible/intact bridge tympanomastoidectomy technique. Otolaryngol Clin North Am. 1989;22:41-9.
2. Costa SS, Souza LCA, Piza MRT. The flexible endaural tympanoplasty. Otolaryngol Clin North Am. 1999;32:413-41.
3. Sourdille M. New techniques in the surgical treatment of severe and progressive deafness from otosclerosis. Bull NY Acad Med. 1937;13:673-91.
4. Lempert J. Improvement of hearing in cases of otosclerosis. Arch Otolaryngol. 1938;28:42-97.
5. Shambaugh GE, Glasscock ME. Tympanoplasty. Surgery of the Ear, 3rd edition. Philadelphia: WB Saunders; 1980.
6. Friedmann I. Tympanosclerosis. Ann Otol Rhinol Laryngol. 1971;80:411-3.
7. Desai SB, Mehta PS. Imaging of the temporal bone. In: Souza SD, Claussen C (Eds). Modern Concepts of Neurotology. Mumbai, India: Prajacta; 1997. pp. 13-66.
8. Swartz JD, Hamsberger R, Mukherji SK. The temporal bone: contemporary diagnostic dilemmas. Radio1 Clin North Am. 1998;36:819-53.

9. Goycoolea MV, Paparella MM, Nissen RL. Atlas of Otologic Surgery. Philadelphia: WB Saunders; 1989.

10. Dornhoffer JL. Retrograde mastoidectomy. Otolaryngol Clin North Am. 2006;39:1115-27.

11. Smith JA, Christopher JD. Complications of chronic otitis media and cholesteatoma. Otolaryngol Clin North Am. 2006;39:1237-5.

12. Jackler RK. The surgical anatomy of cholesteatoma. Otolaryngol Clin North Am. 1989;22:883-96.

13. Cody DT, McDonald TJ. Mastoidectomy for acquired cholesteatoma: follow-up to 20 years. Laryngoscope. 1984;94:1027-30.

14. Costa SS, Silva MNL, Silva DP. Mastoidectomia Aberta e Fechada: Indicações e Técnicas. Pró-ORL 4(1):123-50.

15. Nelson RA. Temporal bone surgical dissection manual, 2nd edition. Los Angeles, CA: House Ear Ins; 1991.

16. Bennett M, Warren F, Haynes D. Indications and technique in mastoidectomy. Otolaryngol Clin N Am. 2006;39:1095-113.

17. Hough JVD. Malformation and anatomical variations seen in the middle ear during the operation for mobilization of the stapes. Laryngoscope. 1958;68:1337-79.

18. Moreano E, Paparella MM, Zelterman D, et al. Prevalence of facial canal dehiscence and of persistent stapedial artery in human middle ear: a report of 1000 temporal bones. Laryngoscope. 1994;104:309-20.

19. Chole RA, Kim HJ. Ossiculoplasty with presculpted banked cartilage. Operative Techniques. Otolaryngol Head Neck Surg. 1996;7:38-44.

20. Mutlu C, Costa SS, Paparella MM, et al. Clinical histopathological correlations of pitfalls in middle ear surgery. Eur Arch Otorhinolaryngol. 1998;255:189-94.

21. Neely JG. Tympanoplasty. In: Pillsbury HC, Goldsmith MM (Eds). Operative Challenges in Otolaryngology Head and Neck Surgery. Chicago: Year Book Medical Publisher; 1990. pp. 24-32.

22. Costa SS, Colli BO, Fonseca N, et al. Anatomia cirurgica da arteria carotida intrapetrosa. J Bras Neurocirurgia. 1996;730-43.

23. Overton SB, Ritter FN. A high placed jugular bulb in the middle ear: a clinical and temporal bone study. Laryngoscope. 1973;83:1986-93.

24. Moore PJ. The high jugular bulb in the ear: three case reports and a review of the literature. J Laryngol Otol. 1994;l08:772-5.

25. Graham MD. The jugular bulb: its anatomical and clinical considerations in contemporary otology. Laryngoscope. 1977;87:105-25.

26. Costa SS, Cruz OM. Exploratory tympanotomy. Operative techniques. Otolaryngol Head Neck Surg. 1996;7:20-5.

27. Meyerhoff WL, Kim CG, Paparella MM. Pathology of chronic otitis media. Ann Otol Rhinol Laryngol. 1978;87:749-61.

28. Costa SS, Paparella MM, Schachern PA, et a1. Temporal bone histopathology in chronically infected ears with intact and perforated tympanic membranes. Laryngoscope. 1992;102:1229-36.

29. Sousa LCA. Meatoplasty. Operative techniques in otolaryngology. Head Neck Surg. 1996;7:78-81.

5.2.6G(II)

Intact-Bridge Mastoidectomy

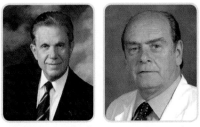

Michael M Paparella, Marcos Goycoolea

INTRODUCTION

There are advantages and disadvantages to both open-cavity and closed-cavity tympanomastoidectomy procedures. To optimize the advantages and minimize or eliminate disadvantages, we developed the intact-bridge technique (Paparella and Jung, 1983) which combines salient features of the other techniques. The closed-cavity procedure (or combined approach to tympanoplasty/posterior tympanotomy) is a modern version of the classically described simple mastoidectomy with posterior opening of the suprapyramidal (facial) recess. Our intact-bridge modification is another modern version of the classic modified or Bondy modified radical mastoidectomy, but it preserves sculptures and shapes the bridge.

An intact-wall or closed-cavity tympanomastoidectomy, as described in the late 1950s by Janssen (1968), requires a two-staged approach: first, removal of pathologic tissues and months later a second procedure for tympanoplastic reconstruction. Many authors have advocated a third stage to look for and remove any identified residual or current disease a year or more later. Major advantages of closed-cavity techniques are avoidance of postoperative problems with the cavity, preservation of the external auditory canal, preserved and enhanced hearing in tympanoplasty and development of a reservoir for air in the mastoid. Advantages of open-cavity techniques are provision for better visualization and for eradication of pathologic conditions during the tympanomastoid surgery. Disadvantages include loss of the ear canal and it is difficult for certain patients who have had open-cavity procedures to swim postoperatively.

These considerations led us to develop and use the intact-bridge tympanomastoidectomy (IBM), which provides some of the best advantages of both closed-cavity and open-cavity procedures. The IBM allows us to maintain and increase the width of the mesotympanic space, thus optimizing results from ossiculoplastic techniques by sculpturing and preserving the bridge. In large cavities that require it, mastoid obliteration is enhanced so that the obliterative tissue does not invade the middle ear space; it abuts cleanly against the bridge, which is shaped within. The IBM technique seems to provide the best features of the other methods, including adequate visualization

for eradication of pathologic tissue and desirable anatomic configurations for ossiculoplastic and tympanoplastic techniques. We find this procedure to be indicated for treatment of chronic otitis media and chronic mastoiditis with intractable pathologic tissue such as cholesteatoma, granulation tissue, or cholesterol granulomas in the mastoid and middle ear. Where the posterior wall of the canal remains, the IBM can be used as a first procedure. The steps for this procedure are as follows:

1. *Incisions:* In most cases, originating in chronic otitis media or mastoiditis, the mastoid is sclerotic or diploic. We use an endaural incision, but a postauricular incision can be used, or the two can be combined. The mastoid cortex is exposed in its entirety, a large tympanomeatal flap is elevated and the fascia is removed (Figures 1A to E).

2. *Meatoplasty:* A large piece of conchal cartilage is removed and can be preserved for ossiculoplasty later if desired. It is almost impossible to remove too much cartilage. Meatal skin rests on the bony wall below and the meatus always narrows postoperatively, so remove a generous amount of cartilage.

3. *Canalplasty:* First the posterior bony wall of the canal is drilled maximally, as has been described, so as to be able to see clearly the entire fibrous and bony annulus intraoperatively and also in follow-up.

4. *Mastoidotomy (optional):* The posterior bony meatus is enlarged. If pathologic conditions indicate, a small or larger atticotomy can be done. In most of these patients

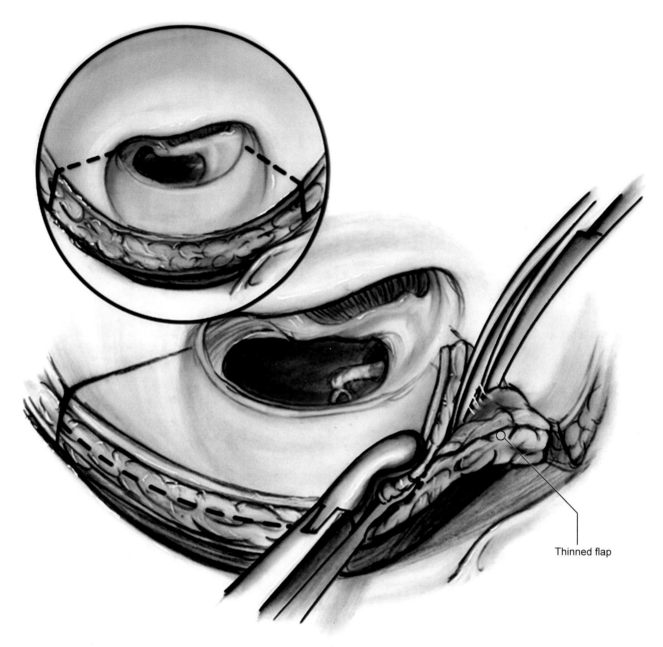

Thinned flap

Figure 1A

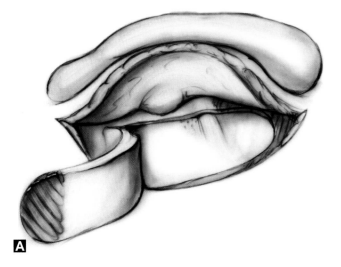

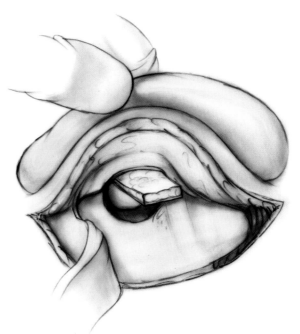

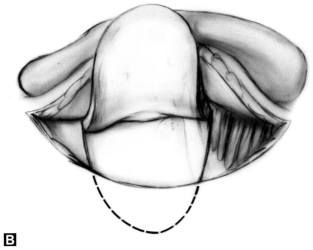

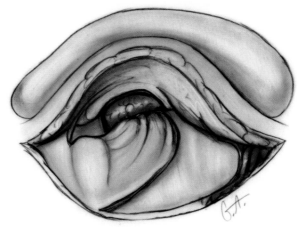

Figures 6A to E Procedure of grafting

all denuded surfaces in the mastoid cavity. If the tympanoplastic graft needs trimming and debriding, that can be done and the meatus can be enlarged if necessary (Figures of Thiersch graft are described in Section III; in Surgical approaches to the external ear canal, middle ear and mastoid).

CONCLUSION

The IBM procedure has been a satisfactory one-stage approach to tympanomastoid surgery, frequently achieving its primary objective of eradicating intractable pathologic tissue within the tympanomastoid cavity. Dry, safe healing results are routinely achieved and hearing results are proportional to the amount of ossicular reconstruction done.

BIBLIOGRAPHY

1. Goycoolea MV. Surgical Procedures in otitis media. Atlas of ear surgery. Philadelphia: WB Saunders Company; 1989.
2. Janssen CL. The combined approach for tympanoplasty. J Laryngol Otol. 1968;82:776.
3. Paparella MM, Jung TT. Intact bridge tympanomastoidectomy (IBM). Combining essential features of open vs. closed procedures. J Laryngol Otol. 1983;97(7):579-85.

5.2.6H
Mastoid Cavity Obliteration

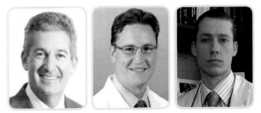

Marcus Atlas, Michael Gluth, Mauricio Cohen

AIM

The aim of canal wall down mastoidectomy is to produce a dry, self-cleaning ear. Obliteration of the mastoid cavity is a conventional technique, which is used to improve this result.

Many materials have been used for obliteration, including free grafts, cartilage, bone and synthetic materials. Many soft tissue flaps, which are used to obliterate the mastoid cavity, have been described as well.

INTRODUCTION

There has been a plethora of flaps described in the literature, probably indicating that there is not a perfect flap for this purpose. Kisch described an anteriorly based temporalis muscle flap in 1928, and multiple modifications from that technique developed, such as cavity "musculoplasty" by Rambo. The disadvantage of the anteriorly based flaps is that the critical attic area is covered by the bulk of the muscle and could also be a cause of narrowing of the meatus.

Palva popularized a posterior flap based on the pinnae with extension over the mastoid to include subcutaneous tissues. This flap is still used, but shrinkage is frequently noted.

Because of these shortcomings, the senior author developed a technique using two flaps for wall down mastoidectomy. The first is the middle temporal artery (MTA) flap; a superiorly based axial flap supplied by the MTA, and designed to obliterate the upper half of the mastoid cavity. The second is a musculoperiosteal flap (MPF), an inferiorly based random flap, which is supplied by the occipital and postauricular arteries, and is designed to obliterate the lower half of the mastoid cavity. Usually, a perfect result is achieved when bone pate is used first, to reduce the mastoid volume, and the flaps are applied over it.

These flaps provide vascularized tissue, which, in combination, obliterate the cavity and protect underlying bone, providing a stable surface for the re-epithelialization of the mastoid cavity.

HIGHLIGHTS

1. The middle temporal artery flap and the inferiorly based mucoperiosteal flap are simple to obtain with a reliable blood supply that is not compromised by previous mastoid surgery.

2. In our experience, a dry mastoid cavity is obtained in 86% of children and 95% of adults, and the average cavity volume achieved varies from 1.2 ml to 3.3 ml with an average of 1.6 ml, which is only twice that of a normal external auditory canal (0.7 ml).

3. Highly sclerotic, small mastoid cavities may not require significant obliteration, although they frequently benefit from the vascularized, thin MTA flap by aiding epithelialization.

4. On the other hand, highly pneumatized temporal bones usually require the use of fillers to reduce the mastoid cavity volume significantly. In our hands, this is best achieved with bone pate.

5. To properly understand how the flaps proposed here were developed, it is important to understand the vascular supply to the region.

ANATOMY OF REGIONAL VASCULAR SUPPLY

The Middle Temporal Artery

The middle temporal artery is a branch of the superficial temporal artery; arises from its medial surface in proximity to the zygoma. It pierces the temporalis fascia and the posterior fibers of the temporalis muscle, ascending in the temporal fossa, accompanied by two veins grooving the skull wall. Then, it anastomoses with the deep temporal branch of the maxillary artery.

The Posterior Auricular Artery

It arises from the posterior part of the external carotid artery, usually above the posterior belly of the digastric muscle. The artery passes superiorly and posteriorly to the notch between the external acoustic meatus and the mastoid process. Then it branches, supplying the medial surface of the auricle, the soft tissue posterior to it, and anastomoses with the occipital artery.

The Occipital Artery

Arises from the posterior aspect of the external carotid artery, at about the level of the facial artery, courses posteriorly along the lower border of the posterior belly of the digastric, then medially, grooving the base of the skull at the occipitomastoid suture, deep to the digastric notch and the mastoid process. The branches of the occipital artery include muscular branches to the sternocleidomastoid and adjacent muscles, a meningeal branch and an auricular branch, which ascends over the mastoid process to the posterior surface of the ear.

SURGICAL STEPS

1. Infiltration
2. Skin incision
3. Musculoperiosteal flap
4. Middle temporal artery flap
5. Removal of mastoid tip
6. Bone pate filling
7. Positioning of flaps
8. Closening

PITFALLS

Cholesteatoma Removal

Obliteration can only be applied if complete removal of cholesteatoma was achieved during modified radical mastoidectomy (MRM). Residual cholesteatoma has been found associated to inadequate exenteration of supralabyrinthine recess, inadequate lowering of the facial ridge, and a narrow meatoplasty. These findings illustrate how important it is to perform an open modified radical mastoidectomy correctly.

Cholesteatoma in children must be taken into consideration separately. Residual and recurrent disease is significantly higher than in adults. Meticulous surgical technique is even more relevant, and obliteration must be considered cautiously.

Overall, there is a minimal risk of residual and recurrent disease in well performed MRMs. Furthermore, in MRM, residual or recurrent cholesteatoma is usually limited to the tympanic cavity, where it can be seen by clinical inspection.

Inadequate Access

A small incision and anteriorly based incision, such as that performed in the postauricular sulcus compromises adequate exposure of the soft tissues surrounding the ear. But more importantly it also compromises exposure of the retrolabyrinthine and retrofacial cells, and therefore it is associated with higher failure rates.

Use of Bone Pate

Vascularized flaps cannot reduce the cavity volume adequately in highly pneumatized mastoids. In our practice, we have found that bone pate obtained from cortical bone at the beginning of mastoidectomy, is a safe and readily available material to assist reducing the cavity volume.

To ensure its asepsis, bone pate must be obtained before entering into the mastoid antrum and it is kept in antibiotic solution during the procedure until it is required.

Usually bone pate is used to fill the areas of the sinodural angle, retrolabyrinthine and retrofacial cells. It is rarely used in the attic or supralabyrinthine tract.

When used, bone pate is always applied first, over the mastoid bone, and the vascularized flaps are applied over it.

Protection of Flaps

Since the flaps are created at the beginning of the procedure, care must be taken to protect them properly throughout the whole surgery. We use fishhooks anteriorly and silk sutures posteriorly to secure the flaps out of the surgical field, attached to the edges of the incision.

PROCEDURE

Infiltration

Hemostasis is vital to perform safe ear surgery. It is facilitated by smooth and hypotensive general anesthesia, adequate local anesthetic infiltration before surgery and correct patient positioning.

We infiltrate using 20 ml of a 1:200,000 adrenaline and 2% lydocaine solution. Deep rather than superficial infiltration is performed at all areas of vascular supply. When properly applied, vasoconstriction helps significantly to the dissection that follows.

The postauricular incision must provide complete exposure to the structures of the tympanic cavity, mastoid and surrounding soft tissue (Figure 1).

The incision begins approximately 1 cm above the postauricular crease at the level of the anterior canal wall and curves posteriorly, extending as far as the mastoid tip. Placing the incision just behind the hairline results in the healed incision being almost invisible, and avoids postauricular contraction.

After incision, dissection is first carried out in a subcutaneous plane, lateral to the temporalis fascia, carefully preserving the inferior muscles and periosteum with some overlying fat.

Anterior extension of the incision provides adequate exposure of the anterior external auditory canal wall and attic.

This flap is inferiorly based, and extends superiorly behind the external auditory canal, and then inclines posteriorly to avoid the temporalis muscle and middle temporal artery. The flap is up to 5 cm width at the base and narrows superiorly including muscle and periosteum.

The incision for this flap begins at the level of the suprameatal crest and the inferior limit of the temporalis muscle. An anterior incision parallel to the posterior canal wall, and extending to the mastoid tip, is fashioned first (Figure 2).

From the superior edge of the anterior incision, a superior incision is created, curving gently in a posterior and superior direction around the temporalis muscle for approximately 3 cm (Figure 3). If necessary, this incision can be projected further, posteriorly to the temporalis muscle.

A posterior incision is then dropped inferiorly from the posterior edge of the superior incision to reach the muscles of the neck, so that the upper limit of the flap is approximately 3 cm in width and the lower limit of the flap is approximately 5 cm in width (Figure 4).

The flap is then raised in an anterior and inferior direction using sharp periosteal elevators and electrode cautery (Figure 5).

Mastoid emissary veins may require cautery or bone wax to control bleeding.

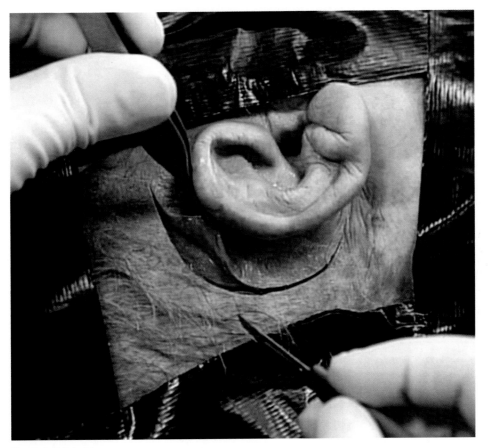

Figure 1 Skin incision

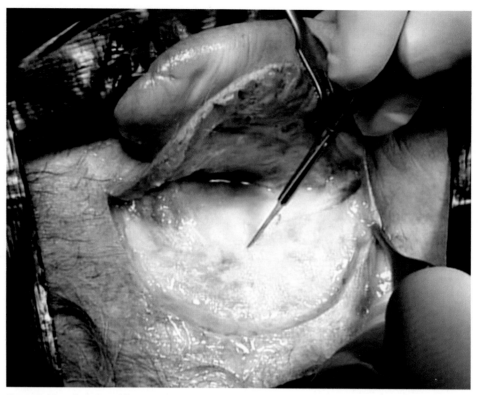

Figure 2 Musculoperiosteal flap—anterior incision

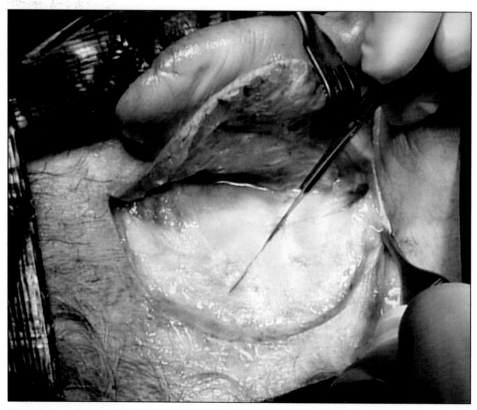

Figure 3 Musculoperiosteal flap—superior incision

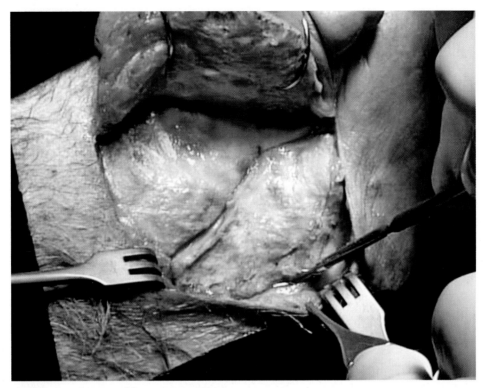

Figure 4 Musculoperiosteal flap—posterior incision

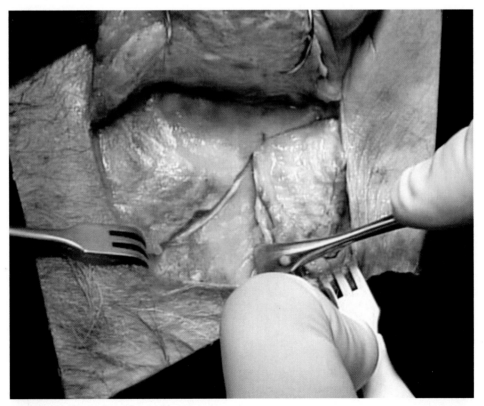

Figure 5 Musculoperiosteal flap—elevation

Dissection is carried out as long as the flap can be positioned to obliterate the mastoid cavity over the area of the retrofacial and retrolabyrinthine air cells and as far anteriorly as the facial ridge.

After temporalis fascia is harvested, an incision is made vertically through the posterior fibers of the temporalis muscle, taking care not to damage the periosteum. The temporalis muscle is then lifted forward over the underlying periosteum as far as the anterior canal wall (Figure 6).

The MTA presents as an almost invisible thin red line, passing in a posterior and superior direction, with a prominent vein on each side, giving a "railway track" appearance. Branches of the artery may be noted.

An axial flap is delimited with cold knife incision down to the squamous bone. It should be 5 cm in height above the suprameatal line at least, stretching out as far anteriorly as the anterior canal wall and the root of the zygoma. The flap should be at least 3 cm in width, but is often larger (Figures 7A and B).

The flap is then elevated in an anterior and inferior direction off the underlying bone using a sharp periosteal elevator (Figures 8A and B).

The creation of a well formed small MRM cavity requires removal of the mastoid tip before flap rotation (Figure 9). This facilitates soft tissue obliteration of the posterior mastoid cavity and maximizes their effectiveness. The digastric muscle is exposed, and drilling anterior and lateral to the facial nerve, leads to mobilization of the mastoid tip.

The mobile mastoid tip is removed by dissection (Figure 10) along the lateral border of the digastric muscle, rotating the tip away from the muscle. This plane is lateral to the clearly visible facial nerve.

An open cavity approach results in wide exposure of the middle fossa dura plate, the lateral and posterior semicircular canals, vertical portion of the facial nerve, attic, middle ear and tympanic bone region, retrofacial air-cells, sigmoid sinus and digastric muscle.

Here, all these structures are clearly visible in a highly pneumatized temporal bone.

After mastoidectomy, the musculoperiosteal flap is rotated to obliterate the lower half of the mastoid cavity, taking care that there will not be bare bone between the inferiorly based MPF and the superiorly based MTA flap (Figure 11).

The flap stretches as far anteriorly as the facial ridge adjacent to the MTA flap.

Then, the MTA flap is rotated into the cavity, obliterating the area of the mastoid antrum, and aditus, sinodural angle, and middle fossa dura, taking care not to cover the attic region (Figure 12).

Bone pate is commonly used to partially fill some areas of the cavity, further reducing its volume, and facilitating proper

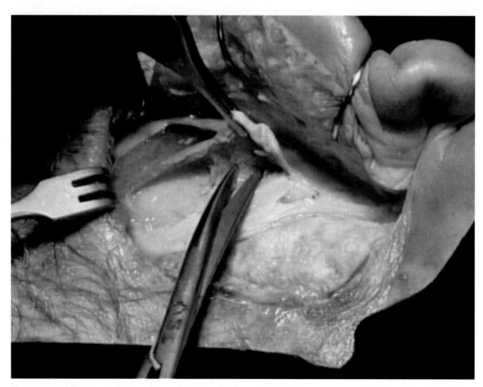

Figure 6 Middle temporal artery flap—elevation of temporalis muscle

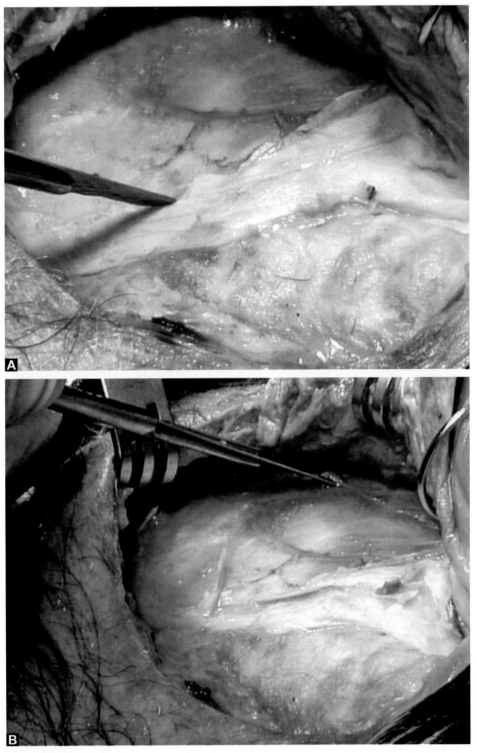

Figures 7A and B Middle temporal artery flap—flap incisions

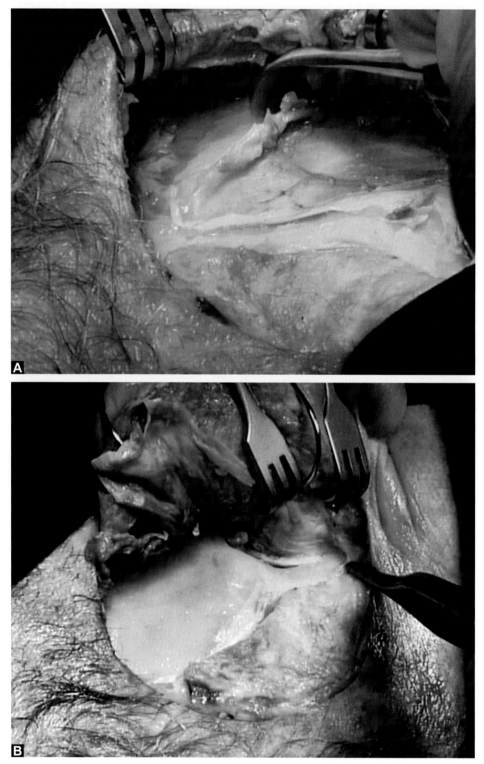

Figures 8A and B Middle temporal artery flap—elevation of the flap

5.3.1
General Concepts

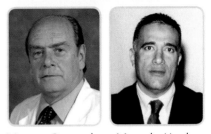

Marcos Goycoolea, Marcelo Hueb

Surgical procedures for stapes fixation aim to re-establish sound transmission through a stiffened ossicular chain, secondary to fixation of the stapes. These procedures involve partial or total removal of this ossicle and replacement with mobile portions of it or with a prosthesis.

By far, the most common cause of stapes fixation is otosclerosis. The term literally means "hardening of the ear" (in Greek, "ous" means ear; "skleros" means hard; "osis" means a condition), and is applied because there are evidences of one or more localized areas in which abnormal bone is deposited.

The term was described in 1881 by von Tröltsch who attributed these changes to interstitial middle ear catarrh. In 1894, Politzer described histological findings in 16 cases of stapedial fixation and suggested that this was "a primary disease of the bony labyrinthine capsule". In spite of the fact that the histologic lesion is bone deposit and not sclerosis, the term otosclerosis has prevailed because of tradition.

TERMINOLOGY

If the location is such that clinical manifestations are evident, the term "clinical otosclerosis" is used. The most classical manifestation is conductive hearing loss secondary to stapedial fixation due to otosclerotic changes in the area of the oval window (Figure 1).

If the bony changes are not translated into clinical manifestations, the term used is "histologic otosclerosis" (Figure 2). Obviously, this can only be determined by serial sectioning and microscopic examination of temporal bones. The term "cochlear otosclerosis" is used in cases of histologic otosclerosis in which there is invasion of the cochlear endosteum by the otosclerotic lesion.

ETIOLOGY

The etiology of otosclerosis is unclear; thus, multiple theories are available. Some of the theories that have been suggested are bone-cell dysfunction, viral (measles), hereditary, biochemical, endocrine, metabolic alteration of connective tissue, vascular, mechanic, type II collagen autoimmunity, and association of early lesions with remnants of embryonic cartilage* found in fissula ante and post fenestra, round window and semicircular canals.

The factors to be described (e.g. hereditary, age of onset, etc.) are analyzed based solely on clinical otosclerosis, therefore, strictly speaking they do not represent true prevalence of the disease.

Hereditary factors are reported in 37–55% of cases.

Gapany-Gapanavicius (1975) suggested that the otosclerosis gene has an autosomal dominant transmission with incomplete penetrance* and variable expressivity.**

The age of onset (of symptoms of conductive hearing loss) fluctuates between the reported extremes of 6 years and 54 years old.

More Frequent Ages of Onset

Age	Percentage
18–20	28%
21–30	40%
31–40	22%

Racial Factors

There is a definite racial predisposition in otosclerosis, being more common in Caucasians. The prevalence is estimated to be 10% histologically (the number is somewhat exaggerated

---

*It does not occur in all cases (can skip generations).

**It does not always express in the same manner.

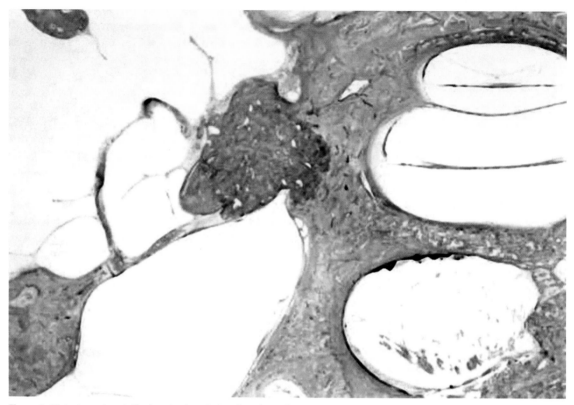

Figure 1 Clinical otosclerosis. The location is such that clinical manifestations are evident. Example: stapes fixation

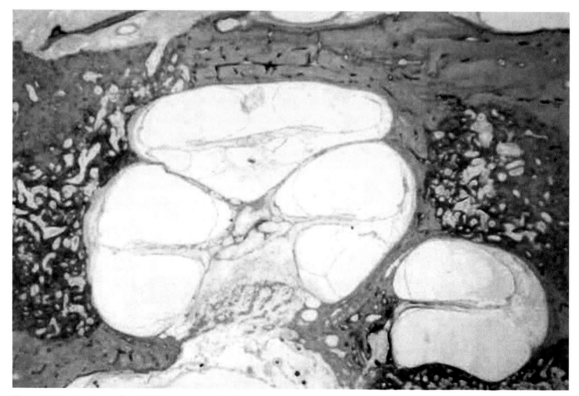

Figure 2 Histologic otosclerosis. The location is such that it does not manifest clinically. The diagnosis is histological

because there is a tendency to collect temporal bones with pathology) and 0.3–1% clinically. The prevalence is low in Blacks, Orientals and Polynesians. It is high in India, particularly in Todas, where the estimated prevalence is 17%. However, in this area 34% marriages are consanguineous and if marriages between distant relatives are included, consanguineous marriages rise to 45%. Prevalence in pure American Indians is practically nil (multiple studies from Canada to Chile). It is interesting to note that when there are racial mixtures, otosclerosis becomes evident. In studies done in Brazil, there were no cases of otosclerosis in Blacks or Indians in this study group. However, 22% of stapedectomies had been done in children of Black and Whites, and 6% in children of Indians and White.

Gender Factors

Women have a prevalence of 50–67%. Since otosclerosis is not a genetically sex-linked characteristic, one would expect a sex ratio prevalence of 1:1. This has prompted some authors to suggest endocrinologic factors (e.g. otosclerosis stimulated by pregnancy). In fact, 10–20% of cases appear during pregnancy and up to 63% have been reported to develop aggravation of their hearing loss during pregnancy. However, detractors point out that otosclerosis becomes evident during the child bearing period of life and that it is difficult to separate fact from coincidence.

In our temporal bone series (144 otosclerotic bones), there was no significant difference in prevalence between males and females; however, females had bilateral lesions in 89% of cases whereas males in 53%.

Sites of Involvement (Figures 3A to G)

Anterior to the oval window	81–95%
Round window	30–50%
Obliterated round window	2–6%
Apical and medial cochlear wall	22%
Anterior internal auditory canal	19%
Posterior to the oval window	14%
Stapedial	13%
Semicircular canals	11%

In decreasing order: cochlear aqueduct (3%), ossicles (3%), facial canal (1%), and other locations.

Otosclerosis is usually bilateral (70–85%).

Lesions are symmetric in 40% of cases.

HISTOPATHOLOGIC PROCESS

The circumscribed area of otosclerotic bone is clearly demarcated from normal bone. Early phases are characterized by resorption of bone around blood vessels with an increase of vascularity (Figure 4). Osteocytes become active and there is an increase in deposit of immature bone. This is an active lesion [otospongiosis (Figure 5)].

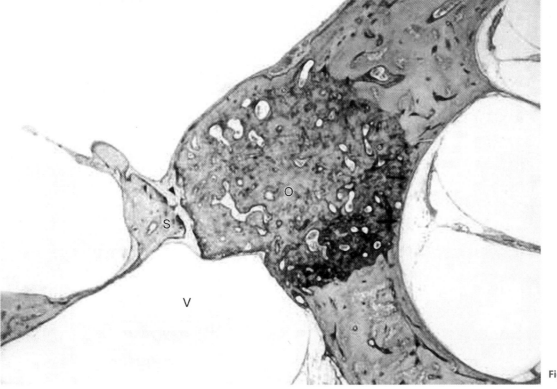

Figure 3A

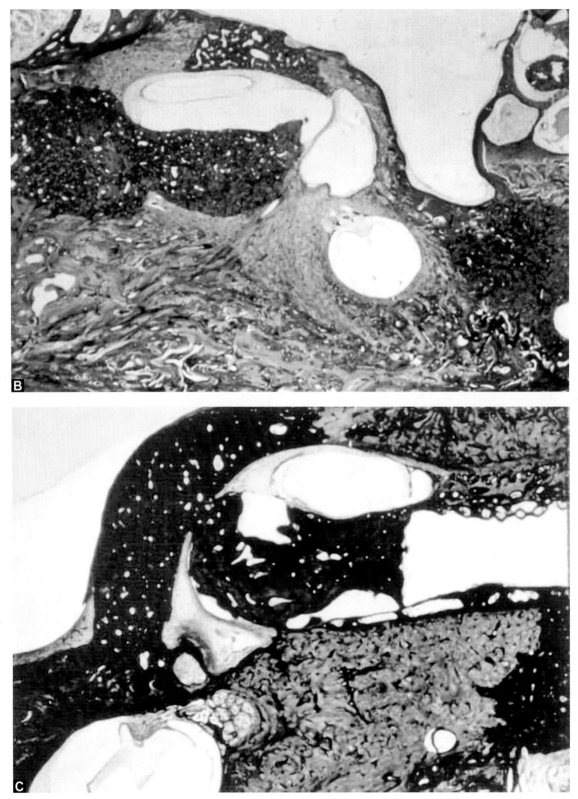

Figures 3B and C

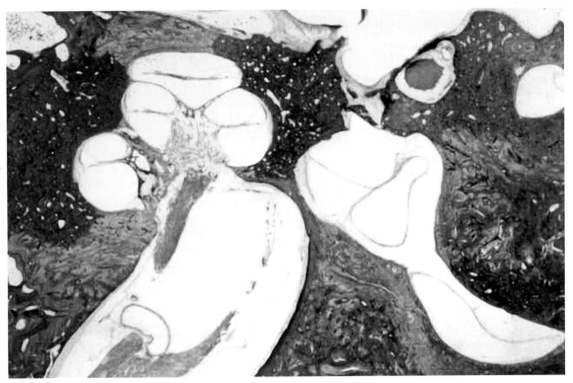

Figure 7 Different rates of activity in the same area

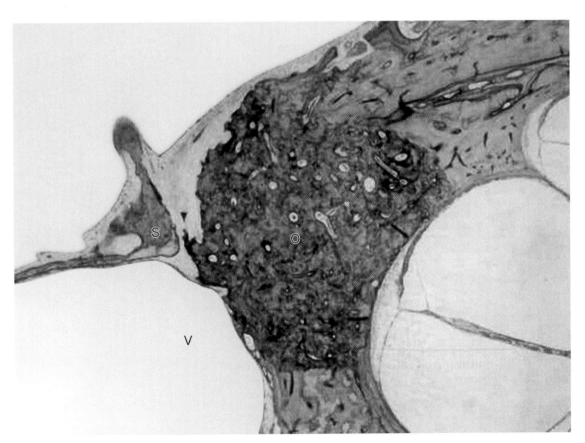

Figure 8A

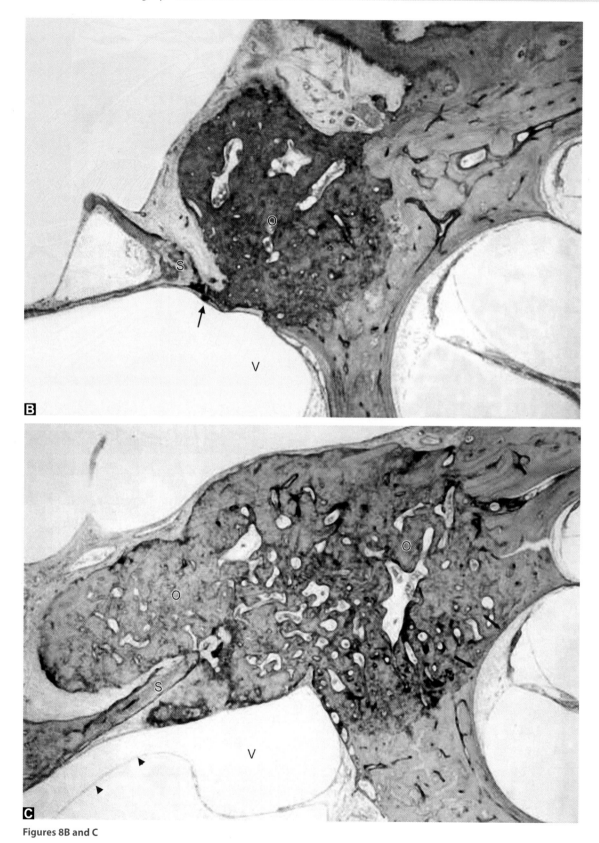

Figures 8B and C

Figures 8A to C Pattern of growth in a circular fashion involving the footplate of stapes

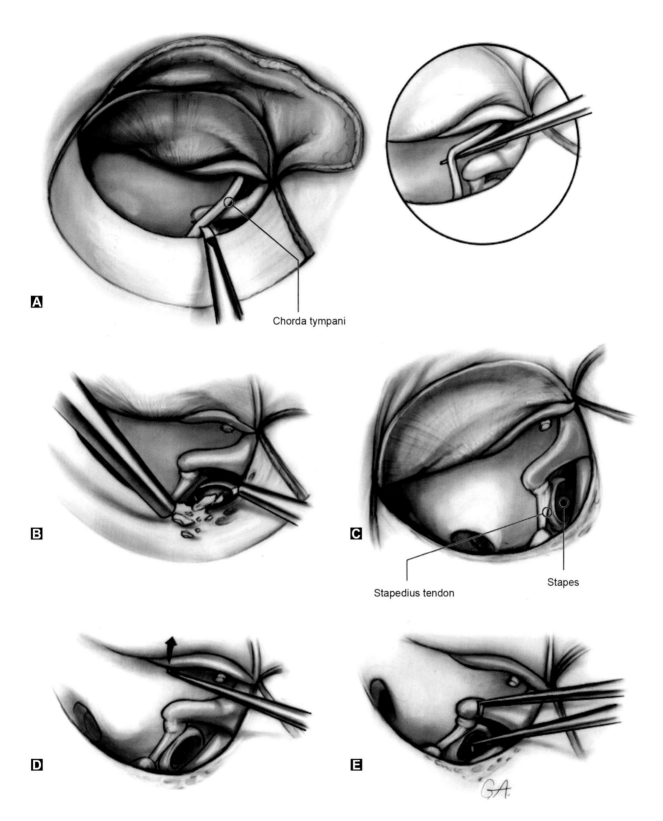

Figures 1A to E (A) A fine needle used to mobilize the chorda anteriorly toward the incus or sectioned sharply with a knife or Bellucci scissors; (B) Bone of the posterior canal drilled or curetted and bone chips removed; (C) All anatomic landmarks are inspected by visualization; (D and E) Ossicular chain is then palpated (using an angled hook or Hough hoe) in order to locate points of ossicular fixation

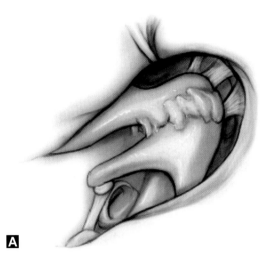

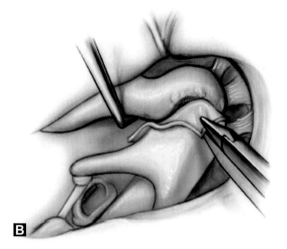

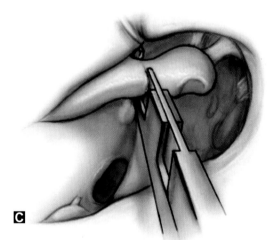

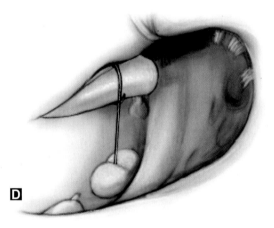

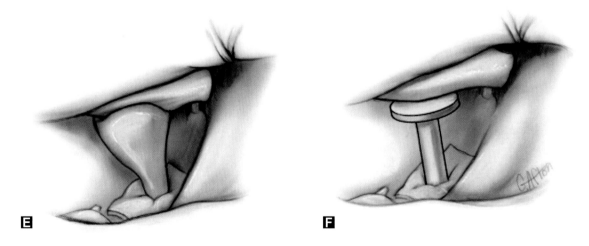

Figures 2A to F (A) Atticotomy and exposure of the head of the malleus; (B) Incus separated from the head of stapes with a joint knife in order to avoid acoustic trauma. Small pieces of Silastic® placed to avoid fixation; (C) Removal of head of the malleus with malleus nippers; (D to F) Placement of a malleus to oval window prosthesis, a bone strut, or a TORP

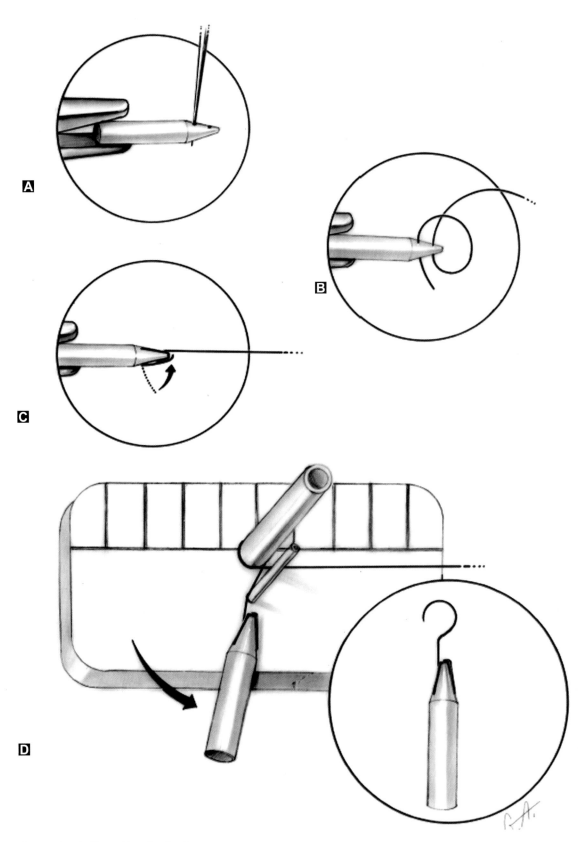

Figures 6A to D The making of a wire piston

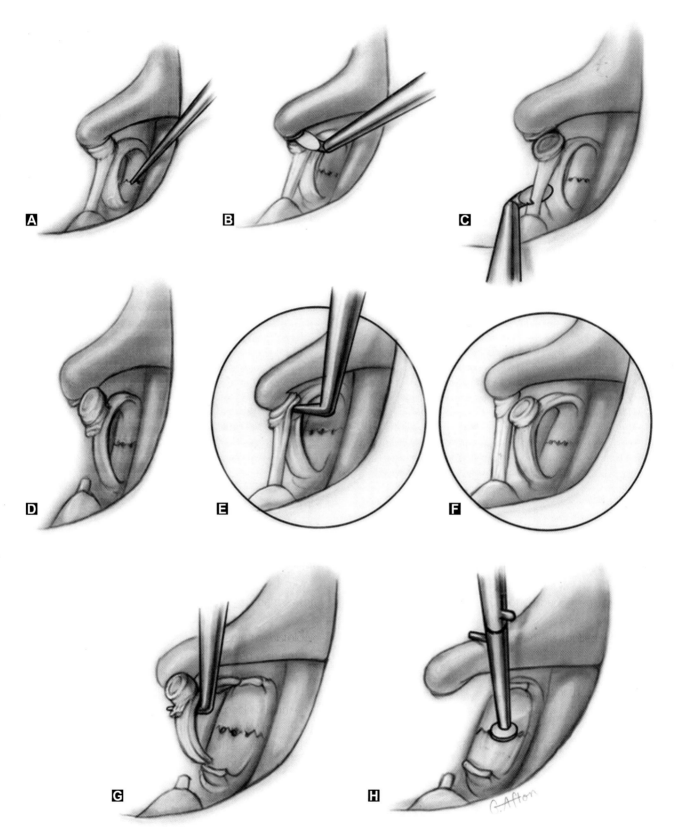

Figures 7A to H (A) The footplate fractured at the midline with a needle; (B) The incudostapedial joint; (C and D) The stapedial tendon is sectioned with the joint knife or a Bellucci scissors; (E and F) Stapedial tendon is peeled along with the mucoperiosteum and left attached to the long process of the incus; (G) Arch removed with the angled hook or a baby alligator forceps; (H) Measurements made

At this point, the patient is instructed not to move or talk. Similar recommendations apply to those in the operating room. The footplate is removed with a Hough hoe or a right angled hook (Figure 8A). It is important to place the instrument just barely beneath the fragments to be removed in order to avoid damaging the underlying vestibular structures. Bone fragments are either totally or partially removed (usually by removing the posterior two-thirds of the footplate), depending upon the procedure to be done (Figure 8A).

With an alligator forceps or a horizontal opening forceps (which allows better visualization) holding the bare edge of the wire, the prosthesis is placed (Figure 8B). If it cannot be placed easily in position, it is released and mobilized bimanually (for example, with the suction tip and a Hough hoe). If the wire is bent during positioning, it is better to use a new prosthesis than to fix it. The oval window should be left open for the shortest time possible; excessive time of exposure is directly related to effects on hearing. Once the wire connective tissue is well centered, additional connective tissue can be used to seal the window. If a prosthesis without connective tissue is used, the oval window graft is placed before the prosthesis (Figure 8C). Such a graft ideally should fit precisely; it cannot be too small or too large. If a piston is used, connective tissue is wrapped around it. Small pieces of Gelfoam® can then be placed over the connective tissue and around the prosthesis. Piston width in a stapedectomy is from 0.6 mm to 0.8 mm, whereas in a stapedotomy (described below), it is 0.4 mm.

The prosthesis is crimped with a McGee crimper or an alligator forceps. The crimper has the advantage of not closing completely; thus there is less chance of fracturing the long process of the incus (Figure 8D). It is also light and thin, and does not obstruct vision. Crimping is done in an anteroposterior direction and involves only the ring around the incus; otherwise, the prosthesis will be bent and will have to be changed. Teflon wire pistons bend very easily if not crimped properly. (Personally I use titanium pistons with a titanium ribbon prostheses. They are easy to handle, titanium has no spring when it is crimped, does not bend easily, and allows radiological studies with magnetic resonance). The round window reflex, the mobility of the ossicular chain, and the adequacy of the prosthesis position are checked at this point, after which the flap is repositioned. The patient is then asked if there is any improvement in hearing. Finally, the ear canal is packed (described below).

Problems and Variations During Surgery

Bleeding: Small vessels respond very well to topical application of cotton balls or Gelfoam® saturated with epinephrine. In the footplate, it is preferable to use Gelfoam® in order to avoid cotton strands. Lidocaine (Xylocaine) with epinephrine should not be used in the open vestibule since it can cause marked vestibular disturbances. The presence of an abnormal jugular bulb has been described in another chapter; if its location allows a safe exploration and stapes procedure, it should not be a contraindication. A persistent stapedial artery (running over the footplate) is a very unusual finding. This artery is fairly large and should not be confused with small, but prominent mucoperiosteal vessels in the footplate. If a small opening on the footplate can be made and a small piston placed, the procedure can be done; otherwise, the operation should not take place.

Obliteration of the round window and fixation of the malleus has been described.

Accidental dislocation of the incus: The incus should be palpated. If the dislocation is partial and the incus moves with the malleus, the prosthesis is placed as usual. If it is totally luxated, a malleus-to-oval window prosthesis (or an equivalent prosthesis) is placed.

Fracture of the long process of the incus while crimping the prosthesis is rare; if it happens, the prosthesis can be crimped on the remaining strut (Figure 9A). If this is impossible, a malleus-to-oval window prosthesis (or its equivalent) can be used instead (Figure 9B).

Pain: An occasional patient might complain of pain when the middle ear mucosa is touched. Topical application of 2% lidocaine in cotton or Gelfoam® pledgets suffices. If the oval window is exposed (partially or completely), lidocaine should be avoided since postoperative vertiginous symptoms might be severe.

Prominent promontory: This can be drilled carefully in order to provide adequate visualization (Figure 9C). Depending upon the visualization obtained, a small piston or wire connective tissue prosthesis is placed. An abnormal (open or redundant) seventh nerve in itself is not a contraindication. It may be possible to mobilize it gently with a blunt hook, allowing an opening to be made in the footplate for placement of a prosthesis. Sometimes, depending upon the anatomic conditions, wire connective tissue prosthesis can be bent to fit. On occasion, an offset Robinson prosthesis fits precisely. Flexibility and use of prosthesis to fit the need are paramount; the course of action should reflect the anatomic and functional needs of the patient, and the rational and safe approach of the surgeon.

Narrow oval window: A narrow window can be secondary to a prominent overlying promontory; it can also represent a congenital defect, which not uncommonly leads to a perilymph "gusher". It is also very important to assess the facial nerve and its relationship to the footplate (Figure 9D). If the window itself is quite narrow and a congenital defect is suspected, a small

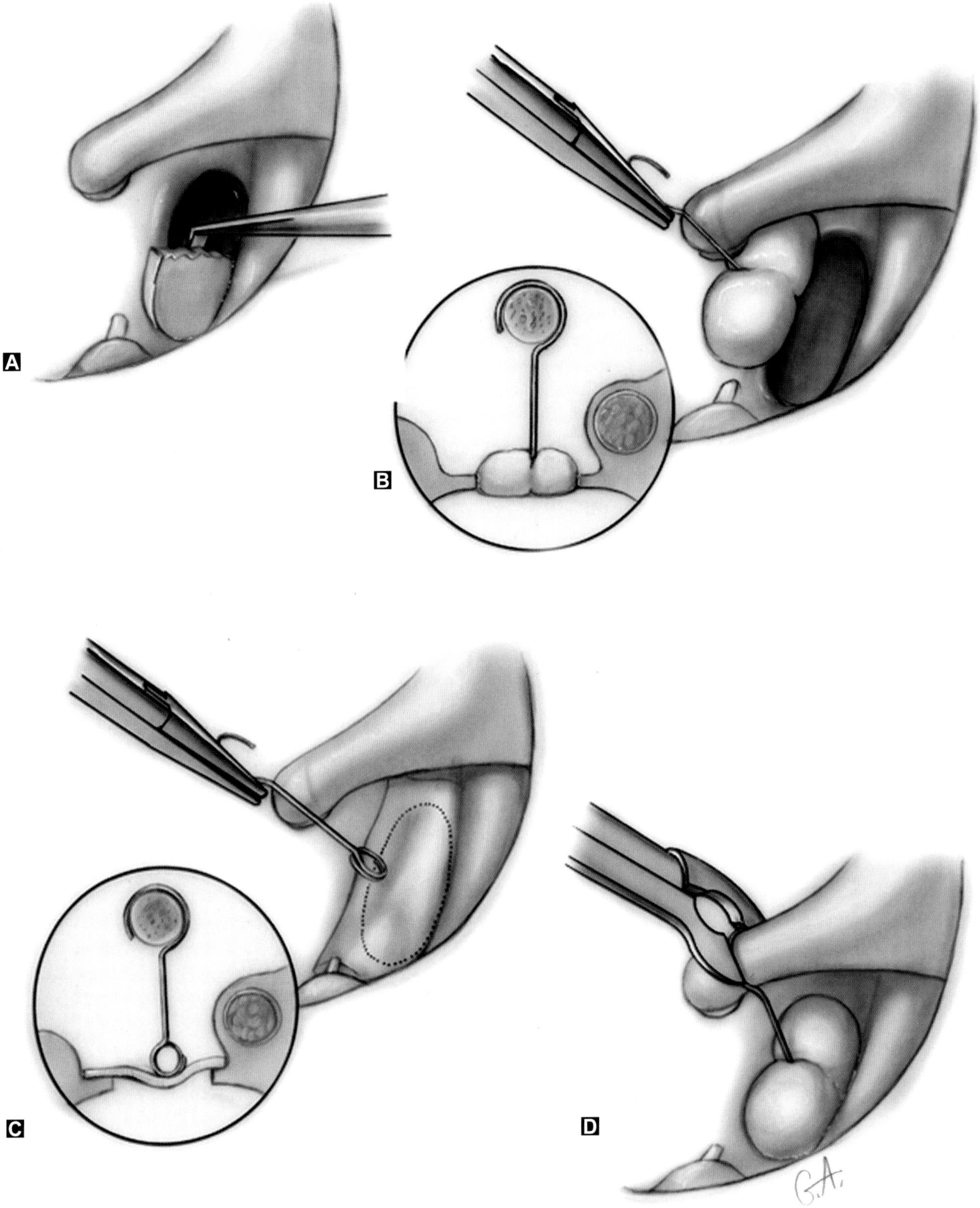

Figures 8A to D (A) Footplate removed with a Hough Hoe or a right-angled hook; (B) Prosthesis placed; (C) Connective tissue used to seal the window; (D) Prosthesis crimped with a McGee crimper or an alligator forceps

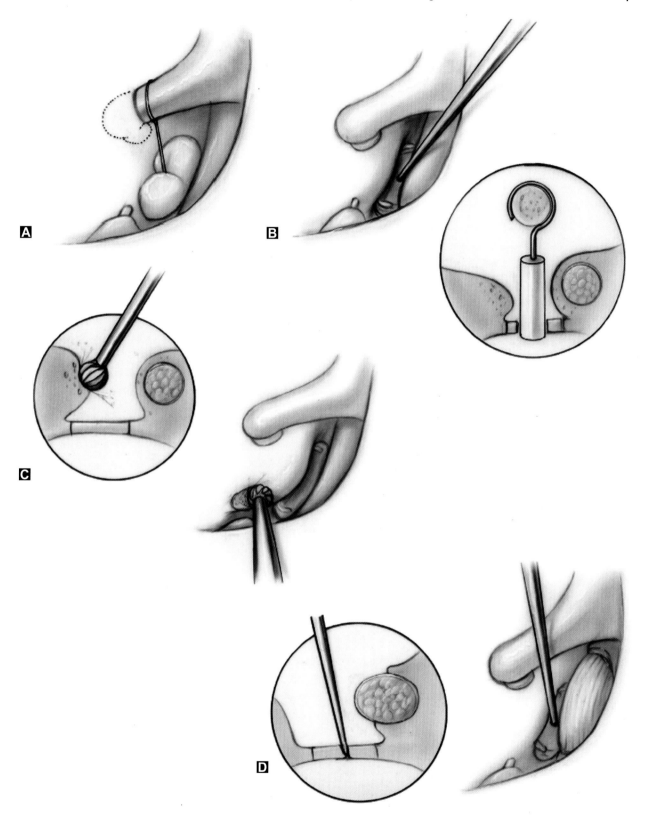

Figures 9A to D (A) During fracture of the long process of incus, prosthesis crimped on the remaining strut; (B) Malleus-to-oval window prosthesis used; (C) Prominent promontory drilled in order to provide adequate visualization; (D) Assessment of facial nerve and its relationship to the footplate opening can be made with a small, sharp needle; if a gusher is found, it is covered with connective tissue and Gelfoam®. The head of the patient is raised. If there is no gusher, the small opening can be enlarged to place a 0.4 mm piston or a thin prosthesis.

Cerebrospinal fluid leak: A "gusher" is uncommon, and is generally (but not exclusively) seen in cases of a congenitally fixed stapes (and a patent cochlear aqueduct). The patient's head is elevated and a large connective tissue wire prosthesis used for a seal, with additional connective tissue.

Dry vestibule: If the perilymph is accidentally suctioned out of the oval window [the suction tip should never be put into the oval window (Figures 10A and B)], the window will refill. If it does not, a few drops of saline are used to fill it. Blood might stimulate an inflammatory reaction in the vestibule.

Floating footplate: This refers to a footplate that becomes mobile before an opening is made in it and after removal of the arch (the superstructure consisting of the head and crura). This is a difficult challenge. One way to avoid it is to fracture the footplate before removing the arch. A floating footplate tends to occur in a stapes that has been previously mobilized or in one with poor fixation.

Sometimes the footplate can be carefully removed with an angled hook. If this is impossible, an opening can be made with a diamond burr or small burr in the anteroinferior margin, and the footplate removed with a hook (Figures 10C and D). If this too is impossible and the footplate is not depressed, fascia can be placed over it and a shorter piston placed. If refixation occurs (which is likely), the footplate can be revised with better chances of success (Figure 10E).

Depressed fragments: Depressed fragments can be removed carefully with a hook, but "fishing" in the vestibule should be avoided; it is better to leave the fragments in the vestibule and use ample amounts of steroids, topically and parenterally. Some authors recommend placing a few drops of blood in the vestibule and allowing them to clot; when the clot is removed the fragments may come out with it (Figure 10F).

Obliterative otosclerosis: If an obliterative focus is found, for example if the oval window has no discernible footplate owing to otosclerotic change (Figure 11A), the procedure is different. If the patient is a child with an active focus, it is better to delay this procedure. (The question of operating on children with otosclerosis is not an easy one; in general, it seems better to delay such procedures but some surgeons do perform them reportedly with good results.)

A thick footplate must be thinned with a 0.6–1 mm cutting or diamond burr with slow rotation (Figure 11B). This is done anteroposteriorly, saucerizing evenly and applying just enough pressure over the footplate to be effective. Bone dust is meticulously removed. If the footplate is thinned evenly (to a thin bluish plate) then a small (0.5 mm) opening is made and a piston surrounded by connective tissue is placed (Figures 11C to E). Less commonly, the footplate is fractured and removed and a graft is placed. Laser and drill use in these cases will be described.

Stapedotomy

This procedure has many advocates because it should involve less risk of inner ear damage, less chance of adhesions between the graft and vestibular contents, and less mobility of the oval window as a whole. The procedure also can be done with a laser (see special description). The operation is similar to a classic stapedectomy, up to the point of opening the footplate. Then the footplate is perforated with a sharp needle, or special microdrill or laser in three different spots. Enlargement of these openings is done very carefully with angled hooks, trying to leave a single central opening that is slightly larger than 0.4 mm. The size can be measured with a 0.4 mm measuring rod. This step can be done without removing the stapes arch, avoiding mobilization of the stapes. Once this is done, the incudostapedial joint is separated and the crura are sectioned with crurotomy scissors; the prosthesis is then placed over the incus and into the footplate opening, and surrounded with connective tissue.

Stapes Interposition

In the presence of a wide niche, an anterior fixation and healthy posterior crus, an interposition procedure is a rational alternative. It represents a safe and logical approach, but is difficult to perform properly requiring ability and experience. The procedure involves removing a portion of the footplate (fixed) and mobilizing the posterior crus (as "prosthesis") over an underlying graft, thus re-establishing the continuity and mobility of the ossicular chain.

Initially the anterior crus is sectioned with angled crurotomy scissors (Figure 12A). M Portmann (an advocate of this procedure) recommended sectioning in the main axis of the stapes, introducing the scissors between the malleus and the incus, since the simpler approach through the promontory carries the risk of fracturing the stapes at another site. This is followed by sectioning of the stapedial tendon. The posterior crus is then carefully fractured with a microhook at its junction with the footplate. When the posterior crus is free (from mucosal adhesions as well), it is mobilized anteriorly while the incus is lifted with a Hough hoe [thus avoiding fractures in the posterior

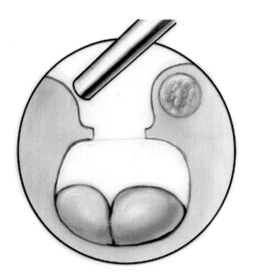

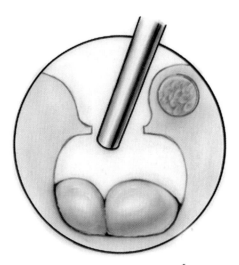

A

B

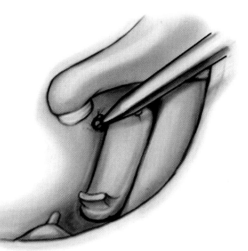

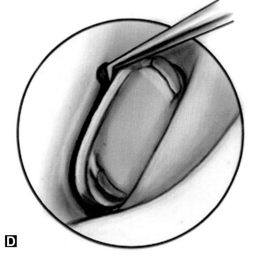

C

D

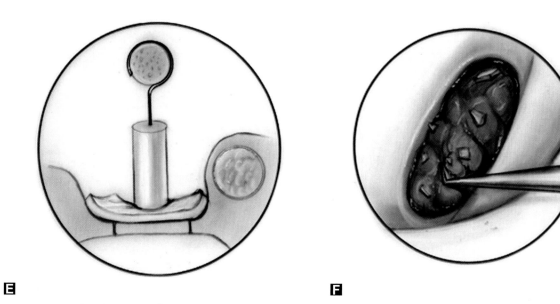

E

F

Figures 10A to F (A and B) Position of the suction tip in relation with the oval window. A. correct, B. incorrect; (C and D) An opening is made in the footplate with a diamond burr and the footplate is removed with a hook; (E) Fascia is placed over the footplate and a shorter piston is placed; (F) Blood clot in the vestibule is removed along with the fragments

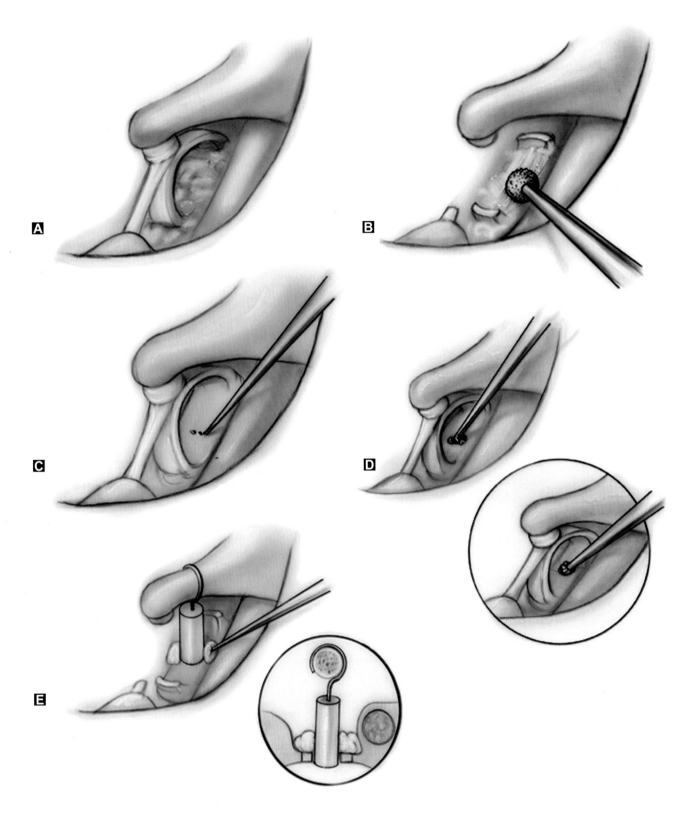

Figures 11A to E Obliterative otosclerosis. (A) Oval window with no discernible footplate owing to the otosclerotic change; (B) Thick footplate thinned with cutting or diamond burr; (C to E) Opening made in the footplate and a piston surrounded by connective tissue is placed

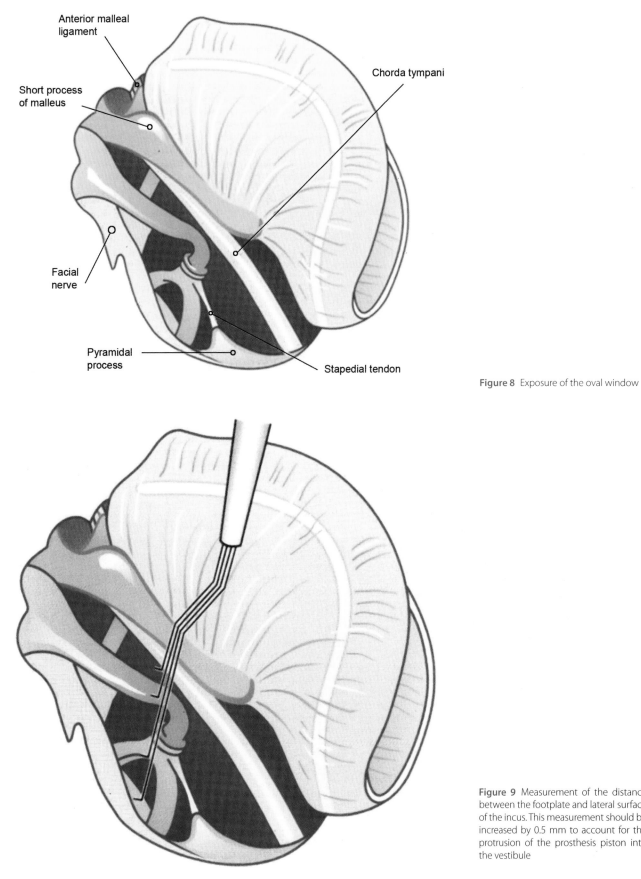

Anterior malleal
ligament

Chorda tympani

Short process
of malleus

Facial
nerve

Pyramidal
process

Stapedial tendon

Figure 8 Exposure of the oval window

Figure 9 Measurement of the distance
between the footplate and lateral surface
of the incus. This measurement should be
increased by 0.5 mm to account for the
protrusion of the prosthesis piston into
the vestibule

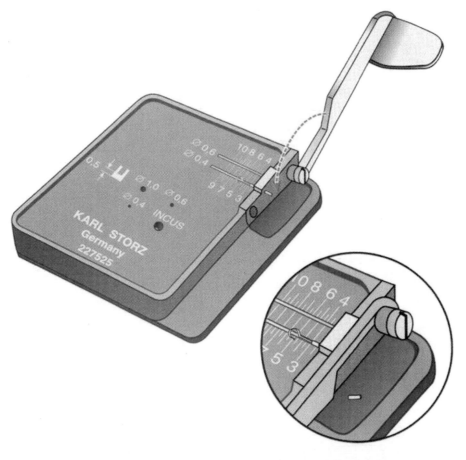

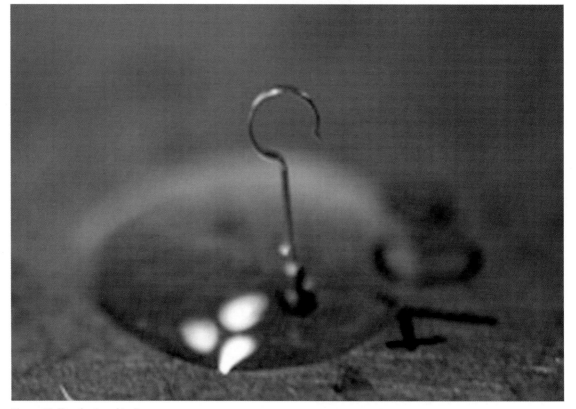

Figure 10 We use only one prosthesis which is trimmed on a special titanium cutting block and placed in the preformed 0.4 mm hole for later use

Figure 11 "Prosthesis parking"

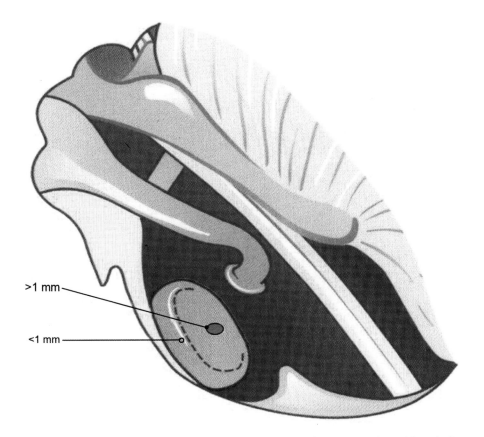

>1 mm

<1 mm

Figure 12 Perforation of the footplate: Made in the safe area (the central area between the middle and inferior third of the stapes footplate where the saccule and utricule lie more than 1 mm below footplate level); the prosthesis will remain perpendicular to the footplate

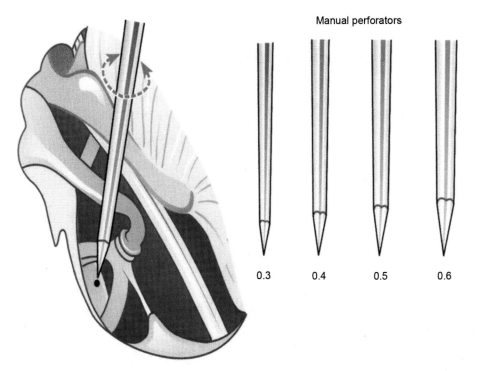

Manual perforators

0.3   0.4   0.5   0.6

Figure 13 The perforators are rotated back and forth between thumb and index finger. The tip of each perforator is only partially introduced into the vestibule

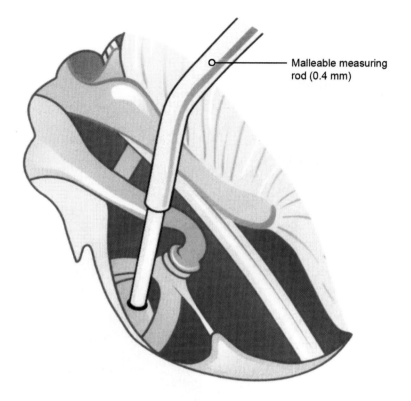

Figure 14 Measurement of the opening of the footplate

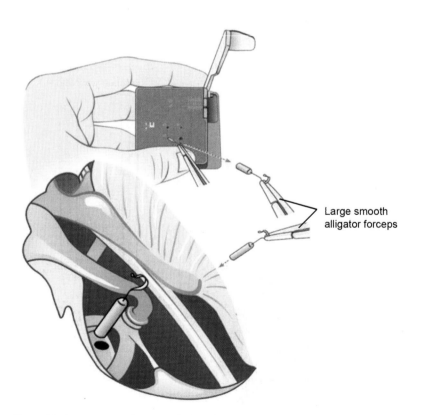

Figure 15 The stapes prosthesis is picked up from the cutting block, using large smooth alligator forceps. Note the way to pick the prosthesis up

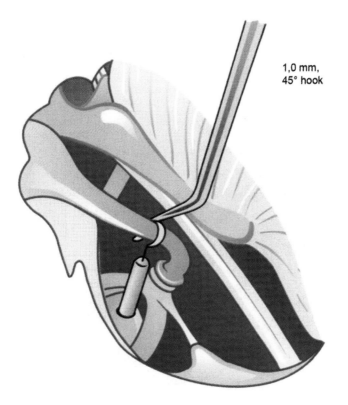

1,0 mm, 45° hook

Figure 16 Introduction of the prosthesis into the stapedotomy opening. Note the flatness of the prosthesis loop, which facilitates to crimp it

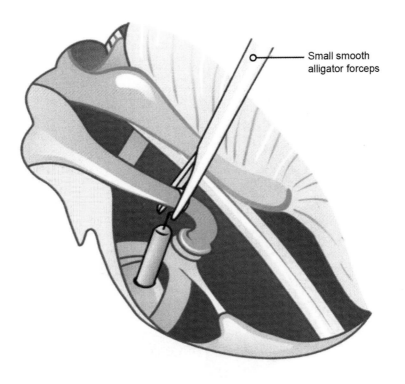

Small smooth alligator forceps

Figure 17 The loop of the prosthesis is crimped over the incus with the small smooth alligator forceps. Note that in Fisch technique, the prosthesis is placed and fixed previous to remove the suprastructure of the stapes

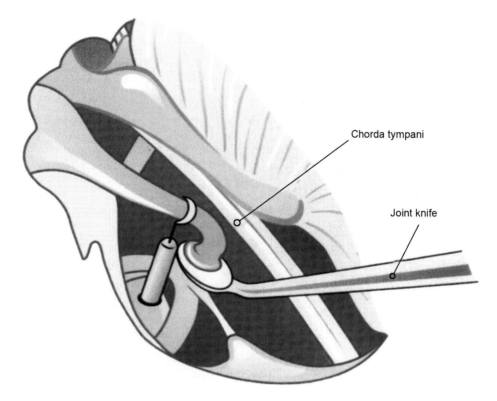

Figure 18 The incudostapedial joint is separated with a joint knife, leaving the stapedial tendon intact for better stability of the maneuver

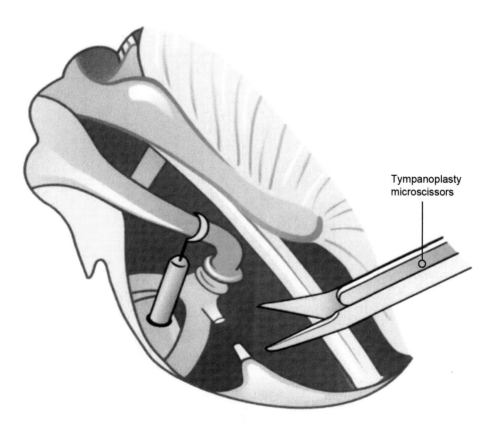

Figure 19 The stapedial tendon is sectioned with tympanoplasty microscissors

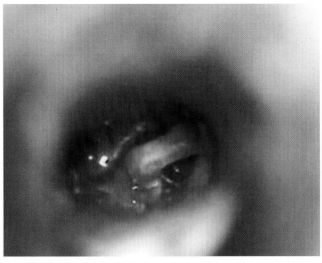

Figure 6 The chorda tympani has been displaced forward

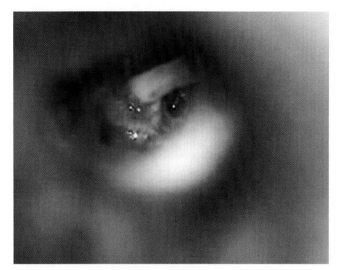

Figure 8 Drilling of the posterior osseous wall

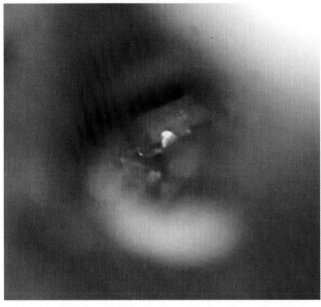

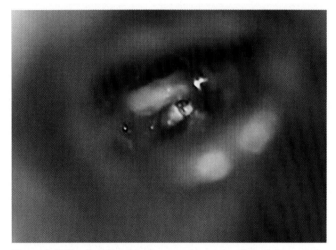

Figure 9 Drilling is initiated in the posterior canal wall that obstructs the view of the incudostapedial joint. The chorda tympani is protected with Spongostan™ and displaced outward and forward. Diamond burrs are used

Figure 7 In this right ear, the flap has been developed and placed forward. Incus, incudostapedial joint, stapedius tendon and chorda tympani can be seen

scissors than to stretch it. The sequelae of sectioning this nerve involve metallic taste in the border of anterior two-thirds of the tongue. These are transitory and generally resolve spontaneously in a few weeks.

7. At this moment it is important to measure the distance from the footplate to the inferior surface of the incus (approximately 4.5 mm). This is useful in order to select the size of the piston prostheses to be used (Figure 10). For the length of the prostheses, 0.25 mm should be added in order to compensate for the ring that is to be crimped around the long process of the incus plus 0.5 mm to be introduced in the vestibule (total 5.25 mm). The diameter of the Teflon wire prostheses that we use is 0.5 mm (Figure 11).

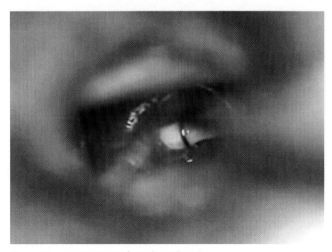

Figure 10 Measurements of prostheses length

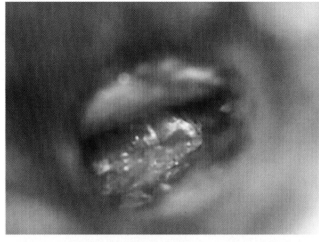

Figure 11 Placement of a teflon stainless steel piston of 0.5 by 5.25 mm

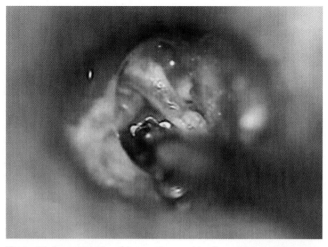

Figure 14 Accomodation of the prostheses with a Rosen pick and adjustment with McGee forceps

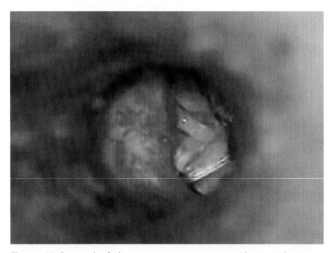

Figure 12 Removal of the stapes superstructure with a crochet type instrument. Opening of a triangular orifice of 0.6–0.8 mm for the placement of a prosthesis. This is useful in obliterative footplates. A diamond burr can also be used

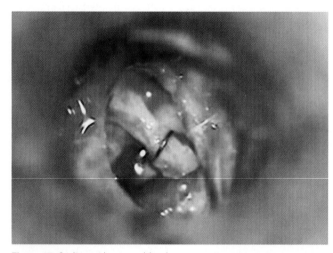

Figure 15 Sealing with venous blood

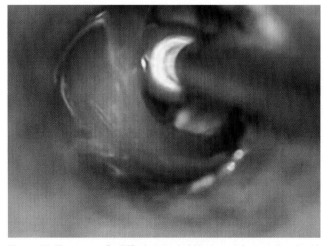

Figure 13 Placement of a Gilford piston held by its stainless steel neck with Wullstein forceps

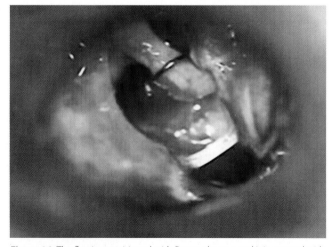

Figure 16 The flap is repositioned with Rosen elevator and it is covered with Spongostan™ and gauze

5.3.3
Stapedectomy Revision

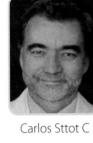

Carlos Sttot C

As it has already been described in previous sections of this book, otosclerosis surgery requires a surgeon with expertise. This is especially true for revision surgeries, where new problems with difficult solutions arise, and where good surgical decisions are needed. This surgery should only be done by expert surgeons either in charge of the surgery itself or close by in order to give advice, if needed.

First of all, we should have a thorough adequate history of our patient including disease background before the surgery and, if possible, the previous surgical protocol with details found by previous surgeons, as well as pre- and postoperative audiograms, and imaging studies.

PAST HISTORY

This information will lead us to much more precise information of the disease previous to the surgery, and will help us define whether the disease is bilateral or unilateral. This will also give us information about the patient's hearing before and after the surgery, and will help us know if there was any improvement and how long it lasted, or whether the hearing result was inadequate from the beginning.

SURGICAL PROTOCOL

Although it is not always possible to obtain one, when we do, it guides us toward the difficulties encountered, how they were faced, the techniques that were employed and the type of prosthesis used.

HEARING STUDY

It is essential, even more when it is done previous to the surgery. It is very different to deal with a persistent conductive hearing loss, than with a post surgical mixed or neural sensory hearing loss.

IMAGING

It is this author's firm belief that a computerized tomographic study with fine cuts provides valuable information of the ear's state previous to a revision surgery. It is possible to suspect a granulomatose lesion, a misplaced or too long prosthesis, an empty vestibule syndrome, a chain lesion or a malleus fixation.[1,2]

Once we have our problem clearly identified and a finished study of it, we can take the decision of revising the previous surgery. This can be a tough decision because we won't always have all the information we would want. It is also very important to know when not to perform surgery, because if options are not good, we still have the possibility to adapt a hearing prosthesis to our patient. At the end of this chapter, we will deepen into our philosophy of when not to operate.

This is the moment to clarify that, in general terms, revision surgeries do not have the same results as primary surgeries. In different statistics, positive results oscillate between 16% and 80% with an average of 53%.[3] It is very clear nowadays that the use of Laser in revision surgery is advisable as it is shown by the results from different publications and clinical experiences.[4,5]

When should we revise an otosclerosis surgery? It is a tough question, as it has to be analyzed on a case by case basis. In general, it can be said that the best case is a persistent or recurrent conductive hearing loss. Other candidate for revision is a patient who, after 7–10 days of surgery, starts with vertigo, instability and fluctuating hearing loss. Nevertheless, this patient does not have the best options because he could have a fistula and/or granuloma.

The causes of revision of an otosclerosis surgery can be divided, in a personal manner, between proximal prosthesis problems, distal prosthesis problems and oval window problems. In this classification, "proximal" is the junction of the prostheses with the incus, and "distal" is the junction of the prostheses with the oval window.

Leaving aside the bad results of an otosclerosis surgery caused by a bad evaluation and/or a misdiagnosis, the following diagnosis are also revision candidates, but are not included in this chapter:

- Osteogenesis imperfecta
- Superior semicircular canal dehiscence
- Fixation of the ossicular chain (Ex. fixation of the anterior malleus ligament)
- Ossicular discontinuity
- Round window niche obliterated by otosclerosis
- Otitis media with effusion.

Nowadays, otosclerosis surgery is highly regulated, its steps and technique are well known. Revision surgery, however, is neither regulated nor are there norms, leaving its process to the criteria of each surgical group. Controversies arise from the very beginning, starting from the definition of which type of anesthesia should be used. While some prefer the use of local anesthesia, others (including this author) prefer general anesthesia.

REVISION OF PROXIMAL PROSTHESIS PROBLEMS

Among the most frequent problems in revision surgery we find prosthesis that are not well adjusted to the incus because they are not well anchored; prosthesis out of position in the incus and leaned over the promontory or in other place of the tympanic cavity. A big number of revisions will occur because of partial necrosis of large portion of the incus or simply because of its total necrosis.

REVISION OF DISTAL PROSTHESIS PROBLEMS

In this group, we find lesions made by prosthesis—either long or short, some of these being associated with perilymph fistulas. The prosthesis could have also moved and be located outside the small fenestra (in the case of the stapedotomy) (Figure 1), or could have been in contact with a bony edge of the oval window (in the case of the stapedectomy) (Figure 2). Another possible revision causes are the adhesions around the prosthesis (Figure 3).

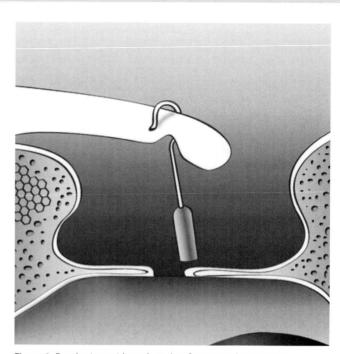

Figure 1 Prosthesis outside oval window fenestra with incus erosion

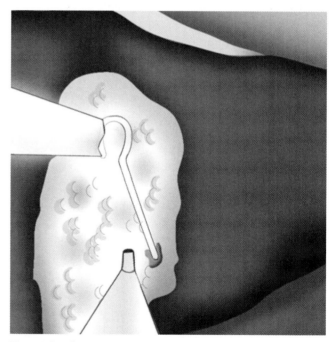

Figure 2 Prosthesis migration in stapedectomy with complete incus erosion

REVISION OF OVAL WINDOW PROBLEMS

In this group, we find more serious and complex problems. Here we find granulomas, fistulas, new bone formation in the fenestra or under it, and membranous labyrinth lesions.

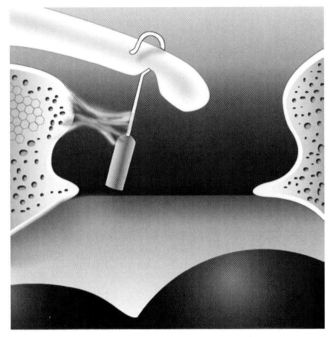

Figure 3 Adhesion of the prosthesis to the Fallopian canal

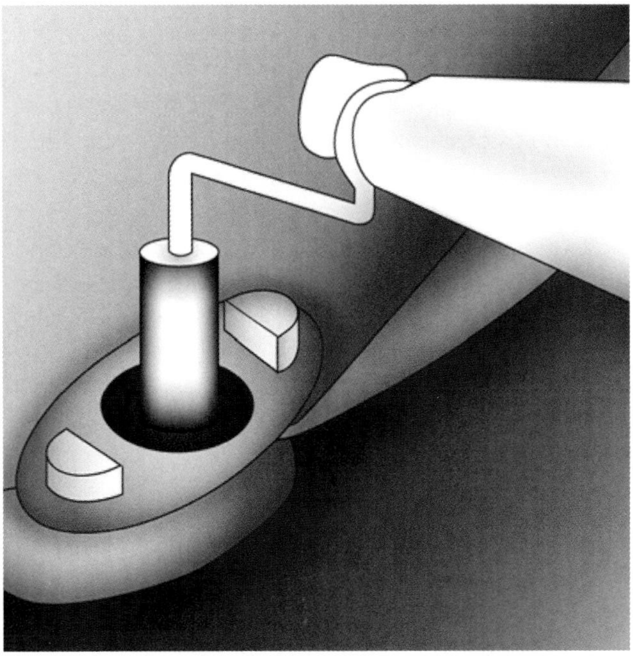

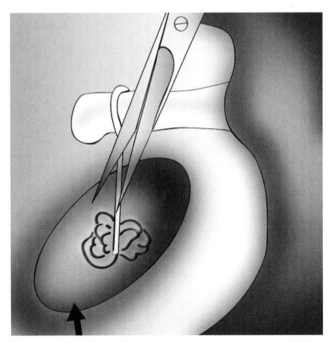

Figure 4 A surgical solution to the incus erosion

Each of these causes can be found alone or accompanied. For that reason, the surgeon must be prepared to find more than one problem. The ideal is that the same surgeon is in charge of both procedures. The use of Laser in this procedure is also advisable.

Proximal problems have an excellent result overall, except with the total necrosis of the long arm of the incus. In this situation, the solution consists on replacing the prosthesis in the incus if it has loosened; adjust it well or locate it in a higher position than the incus, in case of partial incus necrosis (Figure 4). In the latter case, there are surgeons who use reinforcing materials on the incus, such as bone cement or perichondrium.

It is this author's belief that both partial and total incus necrosis are not caused by an over crimping of the prosthesis only. On the contrary, a loose prosthesis, one that has an incomplete contact, or a re-fixation of the prosthesis at its distal end, with the movement of the incus proximally in a persistent manner is the cause of erosion of the incus.

In the case of a total incus necrosis, the solution is a malleo-vestibulopexy. There are different prostheses in the market for this purpose, being Kurz Corporation, the brand chosen by this author.

The problems that arise from the distal portion of the prosthesis must be evaluated cautiously. In occasions, it is preferable to leave in its place an eccentric prosthetics of the oval window and then cut it to replace it for a new one, than change it and face the risk of damaging the hearing ability (Figure 5). Now, if the length of the prosthetics is inadequate and the maneuver

Figure 5 Cutting the prosthesis with micro scissors

is not risky, it can be removed and changed for another one with an adequate size. It should be noted that if prosthesis is too long, it cannot only cause vertigo because of the contact with membranous structures, but also a fistula in the same place as the platinostomy that is not covered by the prosthesis embolus.

A possible solution for adhesions is to section them with micro scissors or vaporize them with a Laser.

In case of perilymph fistula and granuloma symptoms, the surgeon must be put in alert and reoperate them promptly. A persistent vertigo, of more that 7–10 days and a fluctuating or descendent sensorineural hearing loss are cause for alarm. The use of Gelfoam® and the technique of totally removing the footplate carry more risk to have these problems than the stapedotomy. In the case of fistula, the mucosa that surrounds must be reamed and covered with perichondrium and blood clot, which gives an excellent result and avoids a larger deterioration of the hearing, but not necessarily its recovery. For the granulomas, to avoid larger damage to hearing, the only solution is its total removal.

It is possible that the number of revision stapedotomies will increase over the years because of the rising numbers of professional formative centers and, for that reason the amount of surgeries will diminish yearly in each center. This gives less chance for our fellows to gain practice in this technique. It also has a great impact in the overall survival rate of our population. Nowadays, the revision rate is in between 4% and 20% depending on how big the sample is.

When not to Consider Revising

By experience, it is advisable to abstain from ear revisions that have been operated in more than two occasions since the success diminishes with each surgery.[6,7] It is also not advisable to operate patients that already have a deep sensorineural lesion, which has been installed for a while. Also, patients with a suspected infectious type of inflammation of the middle ear and/or perforated eardrum should never be operated.

Last, one should never forget the possibility to advise the use of hearing aids in our patients.

REFERENCES

1. Naggara O, Williams T, Ayache D, et al. Imagerie des echecs et complications post-operatoires de la chirurgie de l`otospongiose. J Radiol. 2005;86:1749-61.

2. Kosling S, Woldag K, Meister EF, et al. Tile value of computed tomography in patients with persistent vertigo after stapes surgery. Invest Radiol. 1995;30:712-5.

3. Battista R, Wiet R, Joy J. Revision stapedectomy. Otolaryngol Clin N Am. 2006;39:677-97.

4. McGee TM, Diaz-Ordaz EA, Kartush JM. The role of KTP laser in revision stapedectomy. Otolaryngol Head Neck Surg. 1993;109:839-43.

5. Silverstein H, Bendet E, Rosenberg S, et al. Revision stapes surgery with and without laser: a comparison. Laryngoscope. 1994;104:1431-8.

6. Lippy WH, Battista RA, Berenholz L, et al. Twenty-year review of revision stapedectomy. Otol Neurotol. 2003;24:560-6.

7. Farrior J, Sutherland A. Revision stapes surgery. Laryngoscope. 1991;101:1155-61.

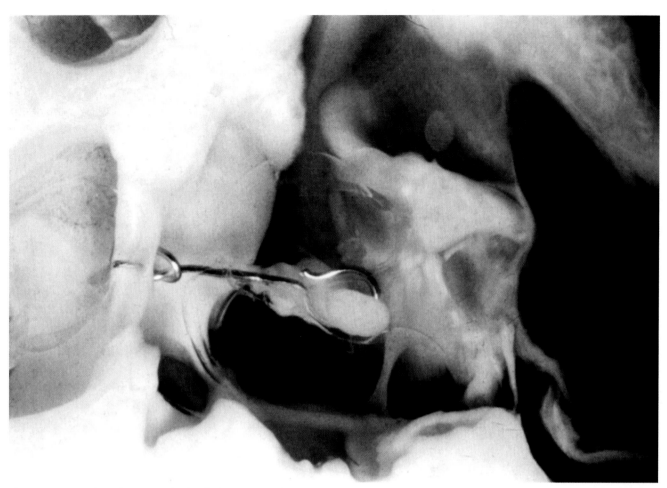

Figure 6 Wire prostheses loosely attached to the long process of the incus. Notice the small peg that is present at the oval window immediately below the wire knot

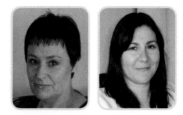

Raquel Levy, Viviana Orellana

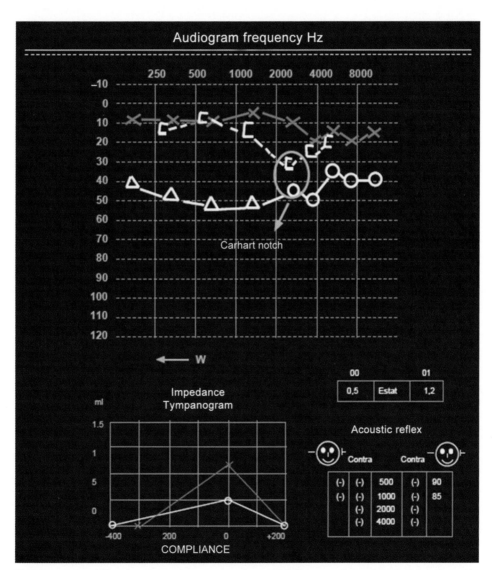

Figure 1 38-year-old female with otosclerosis in the right ear. Audiologic tests show a right conductive loss with a Carhart notch (audiologic artifact simulating sensorineural hearing loss at 2 kHz) and type A tympanograms with negative acoustic reflexes. Weber lateralizes to the right (affected) ear

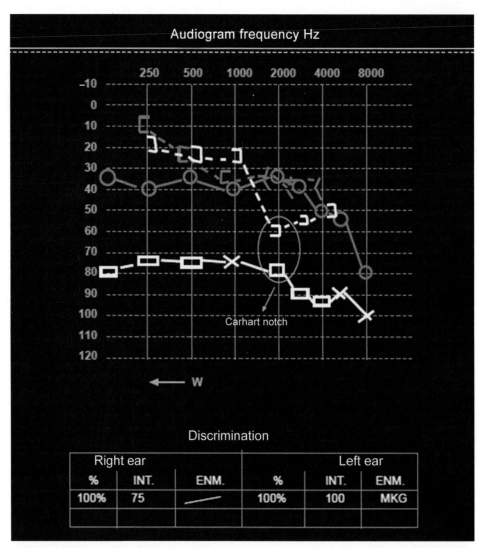

Figure 2 63-year-old male with bilateral otosclerosis and stapedectomy on right. Audiological tests show a moderate hearing loss on the right where the "gap" disappears at 2 kHz. There is a large gap on the left ear. Weber lateralizes to the ear with a larger air bone gap

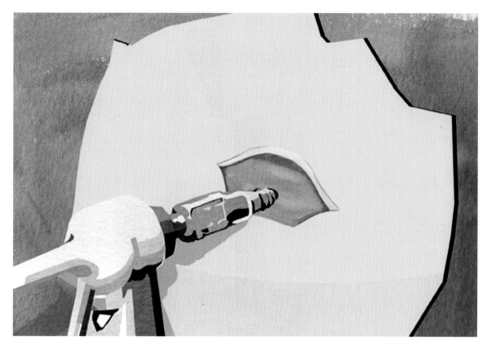

Figure 21   Visualizing and checking the depth of the implant site using the blunt dissector

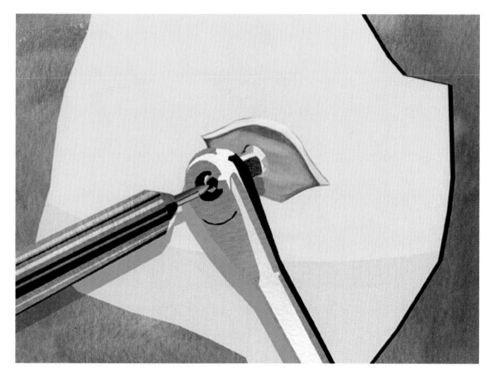

Figure 22   Placing the self-tapping fixture with premounted fixture mount to the handpiece

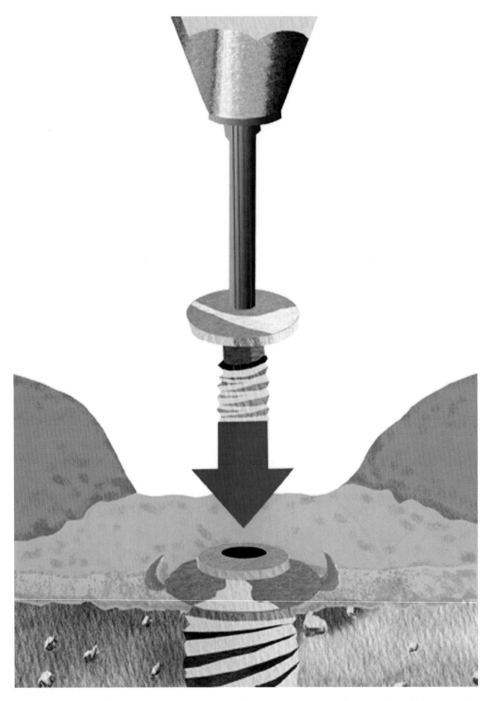

Figure 23   Lifting off the handpiece and removing the fixture mount using the screwdriver Unigrip and the surgical wrench

and the at least four month waiting period of osseointegration.

- Skin overgrowth:
  - Always remove all subcutaneous tissue
  - Use of Clobetasol (steroid cream used for psoriasis) has proved to be effective in treating skin overgrowth
  - Educate your patient to detect early skin overgrowth and seek for treatment as soon as possible.

PITFALLS AND PEARLS OF WISDOM

- Always observe the quality of the cortical bone during drilling process in order to avoid penetrating the wall of sigmoid sinus or dura
- Always remember that cooling while drilling is critical. An osteocyte will die after 1 minute at 42°C making osseointegration more difficult

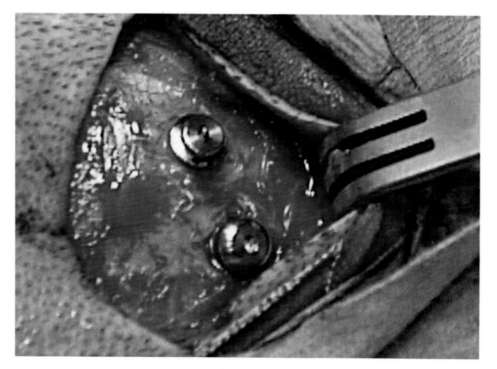

Figure 24   Putting the cover screw to the implant by using the unigrip screwdriver

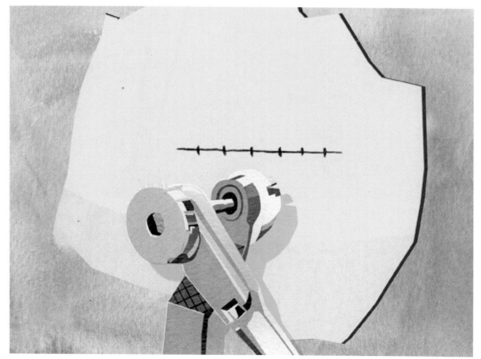

Figure 25A

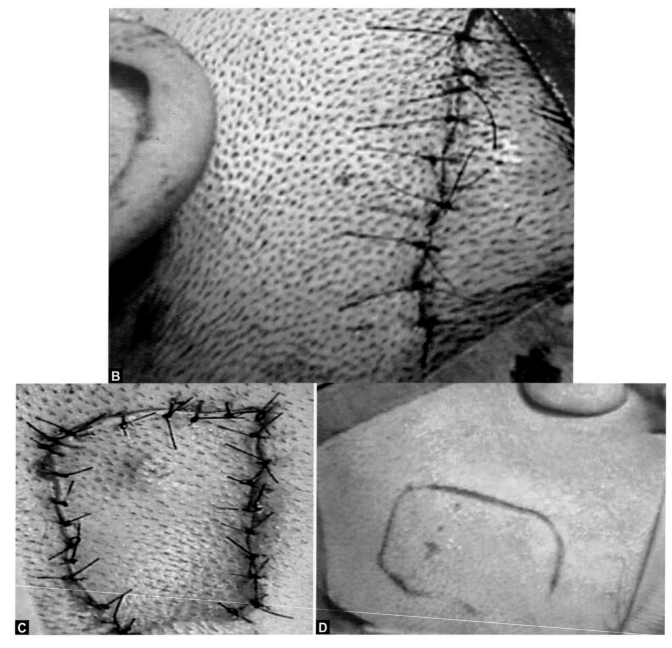

Figures 25B to D

Figures 25A to D Once the abutment is in place and tightened with the Unigrip screwdriver using the counter torque wrench, place the healing cap and dressing as in the one-stage surgery

- Never over countersink as this will result in an abutment/implant interface below bone level, which can produce bone overgrowth and infection
- Try not to use electrocoagulation in irradiated patients
- Never touch the implant with nontitanium instrument or gloves. It can contaminate the implant oxide layer needed for osseointegration
- If the implant is placed incorrectly you may reverse the drill and unscrew the implant in order to place it again in the correct position
- In children with craniofacial anomalies the placement of the implant may be on the parietal cortex
- MRI is not contraindicated with the titanium implant. Attached components must be removed before the MRI.

BIBLIOGRAPHY

1. Badran K, Ayra AK. Long-term follow-up of bone-anchored hearing aids a 14 year experience. The Journal of Laryngology and Otology. 2008:20;1-7.
2. Christensen L, Dornhoffer JL. Bone-anchored hearing aids for unilateral loss in teenagers. Otology and Neurotology. 2008:29;1120-2.
3. Della Santina CC, Lustig LR. Surgically Implantable hearing aids. Cummings: Otolaryngology: Head and Neck Surgery, 4th edition. St. Louis: Mosby, Inc; 2005.
4. De Wolf MJF, Hol MKS. Clinical outcome of the simplified surgical technique for Baha implantation. Otology and Neurotology. 2008;29:1100-8.
5. Falcone MT, Kaylie DM. Bone-anchored hearing aid abutment skin overgrowth reduction with clobetasol. Otolaryngology-Head and Neck Surgery. 2008:139;829-32.
6. Holgers KM, Tjellstrom A. Soft tissue reactions around percutaneous implants: A clinical study of soft tissue conditions around skin penetrating titanium implants for bone-anchored hearing aids. American Journal of Otology. 1988:1;56-9.
7. Hounse JW, Kutz JW. Bone-anchored hearing aids incidence and management of postoperative complications. Otology and Neurotology. 2007:28;213-7.
8. Newman CW, Sharon A. Longitudinal benefits from satisfaction with the Baha system for patients with acquired unilateral sensorineural hearing loss. Otology and Neurotology. 2008:29;1123-31.
9. Stahfors J, Tjellstrom A. Skin reactions after Baha surgery: A comparition between the U-graft technique and the Baha dermatome. Otology and Neurotology. 2008:29;1109-14.
10. Tjellstrom A, Granstrom G. How we do it. Frequency of skin necrosis after Baha surgery. Clinical Otolaryngology. 2006:31;216-7.
11. Verhaegen VJO, Mylanus EAM. Audiological application criteria for implantable hearing aid devices: A clinical experience at the Nijmegen ORL Clinic. Laryngoscope. 2008;118:1645-9.

5.4.3

Surgery for Implanted Electronic Implants (Vibrant Sound)

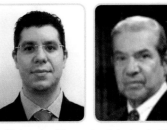

Alejandro Rivas, José Antonio Rivas

INTRODUCTION

Amazing technological advances have been witnessed over the past decade in the field of hearing aids, including implantable and semi-implantable devices for the rehabilitation of severe to profound sensorineural hearing loss, as is the case of cochlear implants. Prostheses whose active stimulation components are localized in the middle ear are being used for sensorineural and moderate mixed hearing losses.

Certain biomechanical aspects must be taken into consideration when implanting hearing aids in the middle ear. First of all, the device must not affect the normal functioning of the middle ear. In the ideal scenario, the device must not alter air conduction thresholds. In the event the prosthetic device is unsuccessful, the added mass that is connected to the ossicular chain should not affect its vibratory function. Another important aspect is the fixation of the stimulator when it is placed on the ossicular chain. Even when there is slight laxity in the interphase between the stimulator and the bone, transmitted power may be diminished, leading to reduced effectiveness. This has an effect on the stability and longevity of the device. The mechanical forces acting on the interphase may affect the life expectancy of the device. Finally, the vibration direction of the transducer must be aligned with the normal transmission axis of the ossicular chain or of the vibratory structure to which it is attached.

Middle ear implants were developed for the treatment and rehabilitation of conductive or mixed and mild-to-severe sensorineural hearing losses. The development of these middle-ear implants was based on several considerations. These devices improve sound quality as a result of the direct stimulation of the ossicles or another vibratory structure (round or oval window), enabling the amplification of a vibratory stimulation, while the external auditory canal remains open. This practically eliminates feedback, a frequent adverse effect in users of conventional hearing aids. Another important effect is improved cosmesis

as a result of the miniaturized electronics. This has made it possible to hide the external component which, in these types of prostheses, is usually a processor of the size of a coin that is placed behind the ear. At present there is a middle-ear implant that does not require this type of external component and enables the patient to benefit from amplification even while showering or swimming.

In general terms, these devices utilize the physical properties of certain materials that, stimulated by an electrical current, change their length or vibrate in response to the induced electric or magnetic field coming from the receiver-stimulator or demodulator, depending on the system. There are two main types: (1) piezoelectric and (2) electromagnetic [Figures 1(A to C) to 3].[1,2,3]

In this chapter we discuss the surgical technique for two middle ear implants: (1) the vibrant soundbridge (VSB) system of the European company Med-El[4] and the fully implantable (2) Carina® hearing-aid system by the American company Otologics, LLC.

AUDIOLOGIC INDICATIONS

Middle ear implants are designed for the rehabilitation of conductive hearing losses with bone conduction thresholds not lower than 56 dB in average and for sensorineural hearing losses[5] with air conduction thresholds not lower than 76 dB in average, at least 50% in open word tests with the most

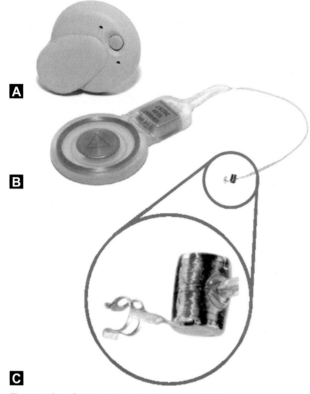

Figures 1A to C Vibrant Soundbridge system: (A) External sound processor; (B) Internal receiver-stimulator (VORP); (C) Detail of the floating mass transducer (FMT)

comfortable listening level, or at 65 dB SPL in aided free field. It is also recommended that the hearing loss must be stable and that the patient has experience with conventional hearing aids.

Other indications include absence of cochlear, retrocochlear or central hearing abnormalities, having realistic expectations and not having any skin conditions that may preclude fixation of the external processor if required (Figures 4 and 5).

GENERAL CONSIDERATIONS FOR MIDDLE EAR IMPLANT SURGERY

In our practice, all procedures for implanting middle ear electronic hearing aids are performed under general anesthesia, both in children and adults. Average surgical time is 2.5–3 hours, depending on the anatomical and pathological conditions of the middle ear at the time of implantation—chronic ears with more than one intervention, or congenital malformations (e.g. atresia). These are usually out-patient procedures (Figures 6 and 7).

Vibrant Soundbridge System (VSB-Med-El)

This system belongs to the group of electromagnetic devices. These devices work by passing an electrical current to a coil that creates a magnetic flow. This magnetic flow is conducted to a magnet that, in turn, vibrates depending on the amount of magnetism generated. This vibratory activity in the terminal magnet is the one used to stimulate the corresponding structure in the middle ear.

The VSB middle ear implant is a semi-implantable device consisting of an external sound processor and amplifier, an internal receiver containing a demodulator and the vibrating ossicular replacement prosthesis (VORP) that is surgically implanted. The sound is digitally encoded by the processor and then picked up by the internal receiver coil that relays the signal through the demodulator to the stimulating element or floating mass transducer (FMT). The FMT is placed on the long process of the incus (incus vibroplasty) or on the round window membrane (round window vibroplasty). The placement of the FMT on the oval window has also been described recently. The digital processor enables programming for optimal gain.

The surgical technique used for implanting the VSB system[6,7] is similar in many ways to the procedures performed for approaching the middle ear through the facial recess after making the same type of mastoidectomy used for cochlear implants. The approach is made through a "C"-shaped incision along the retroauricular fold down to the periostium. Skin and subcutaneous tissues are repaired and, using a periosteum elevator, a subperiosteal pocket is created up to the temporal and lambdoid sutures for placement of the VORP. Next, the mastoidectomy cavity is marked and a surgical chisel is used to lift a fragment of cortical bone that will be used at the end of the procedure to occlude the cavity. Then a limited mastoidectomy and posterior tympanotomy are performed, creating enough room to work on the long process of the incus or in the area of the round window, depending on where the FMT will be positioned. If a round window vibroplasty is performed, this structure is rendered totally visible using a diamond burr, but preserving the membrane. The VORP is then placed inside the subperiosteal pocket and the wire is secured under a bone ledge prepared on the posterior-superior edge of the mastoidectomy cavity. Before that, a 3 mm punch is used to prepare several temporal fascial fragments, one of which will be placed on the round window membrane. It is on top of this fragment that the FMT is positioned in order to ensure that the vibration is directed

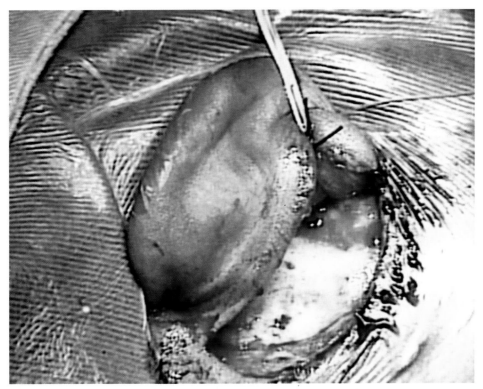

Figure 2 Limited incision along the retroauricular fold. A power scalpel is used to incise the subcutaneous tissues, the muscle and the periosteum, under careful hemostatic control

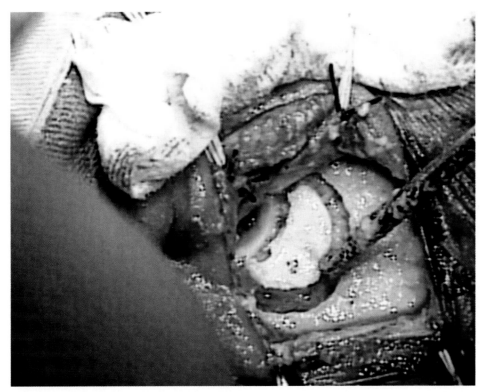

Figure 3 After soft tissue repair and once good hemostasis is accomplished, the area for the mastoidectomy cavity is delineated, preserving the cortical bone plate

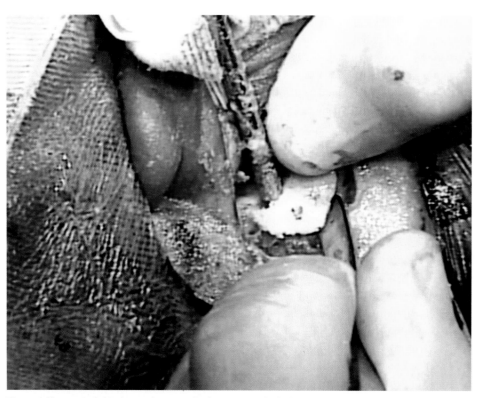

Figure 4 The surgical chisel is used to tease the fragment marked, taking care not to injure the sigmoid sinus or the dura mater of the medial cranial fossa while pushing under the edges of the fragment. After the fragment is detached, it is set aside for use at the end of the procedure to close the mastoidectomy cavity

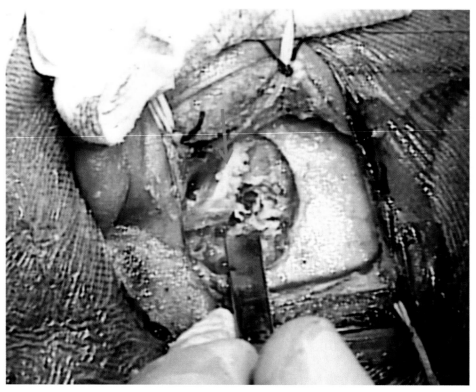

Figure 5 The cortical bone fragment is obtained (arrow) and the mastoid cells are exposed

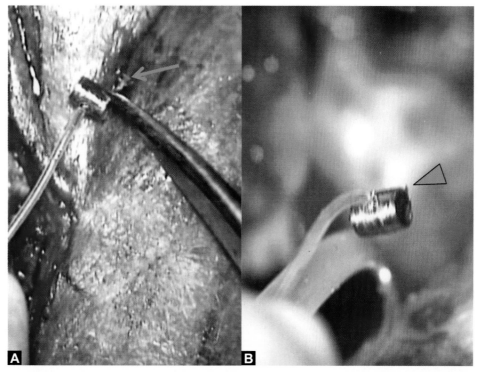

Figures 15A and B (A) The fixating clip is removed using the tip of the scissors (arrow). (B) The lower end of the FMT must be placed opposite to the round window membrane and the small remnant of the site, where the cut is made serves as a guide for this purpose (tip of the arrow)

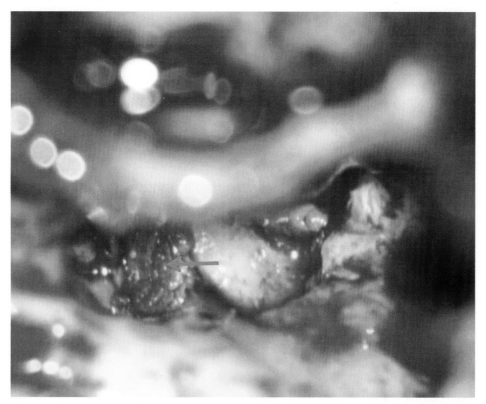

Figure 16 The round window membrane is protected interposing the 3 mm diameter fascia fragment (arrow) previously obtained with the punch

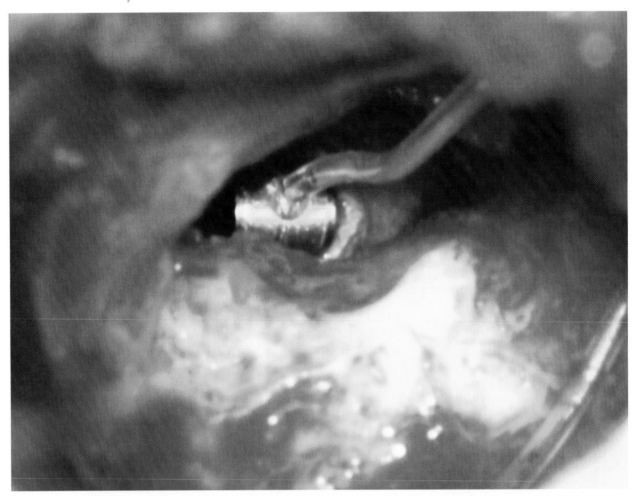

Figure 17 The FMT is positioned in such a way that the end that contained the fixation clip is making good contact with the fascia fragment previously placed on the round window membrane

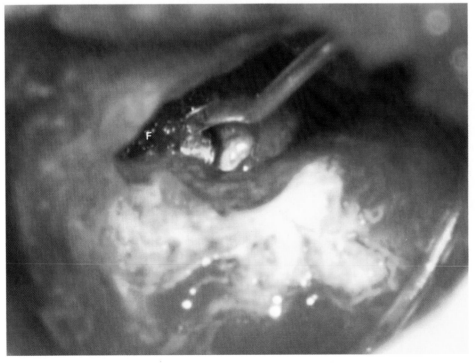

Figure 18 Additional fascia and/or cartilage fragments can be used to stabilize the FMT in its optimal position. The FMT is then covered with gelfoam®. Notice a fascia fragment (F) inferior to the FMT

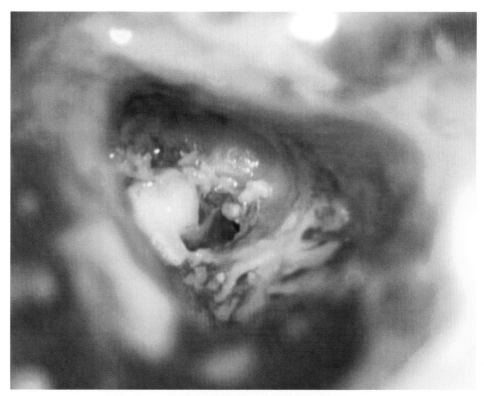

Figure 19 The VSB system has also been used in cases of external auditory canal atresia. The figure shows access to the middle ear, created through an atresia plate under constant facial nerve monitoring

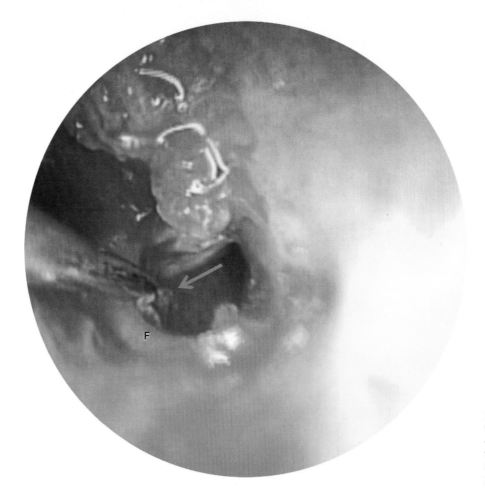

Figure 20 Endoscopic view to visualize the head of the stapes (arrow) and the course of the facial nerve (F). The dysplastic fused malleous and incus, with absent incudal-stapedial joint have been removed previously

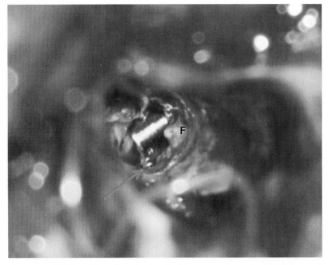

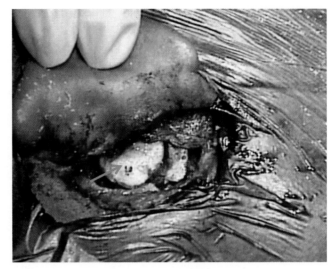

Figure 21 FMT positioned on the head of the stapes (arrow) with the help of the fixation clip. The stimulator is stabilized using fascia fragments (F)

Figure 22 Tissue repositioning over the mastoid cavity previously filled with gelfoam®. Notice the cortical bone occluding the mastoidectomy cavity (arrow)

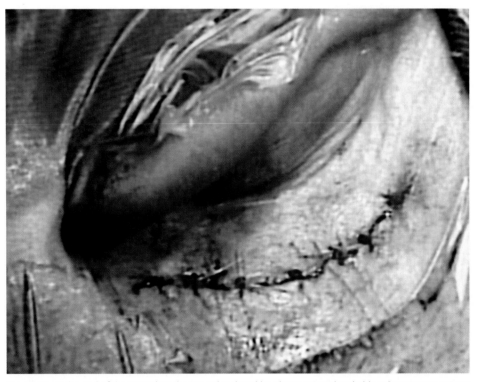

Figure 23 At the end of the procedure the wound is closed by planes using absorbable subcutaneous sutures and external stitches that are removed in the next few days. The incision is covered with antibiotic ointment and a protective dressing

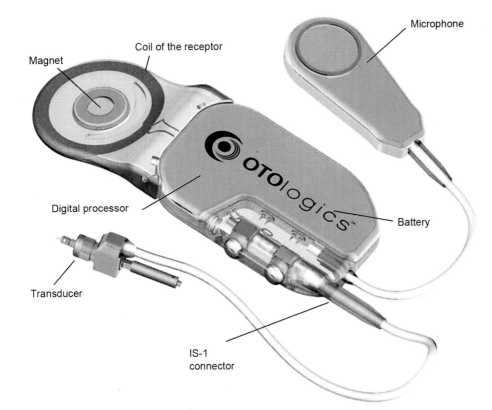

Microphone

Coil of the receptor

Magnet

Digital processor

Battery

Transducer

IS-1
connector

Figure 24 Surgically implantable
component of the Carina® prosthesis

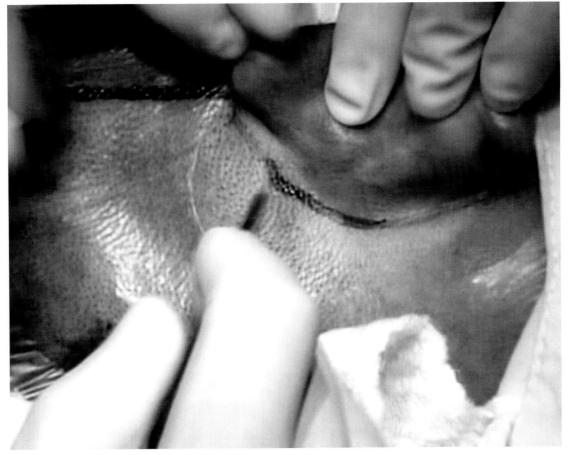

Figure 25 Incision line along the retroauricular fold, extending 3 cm superiorly

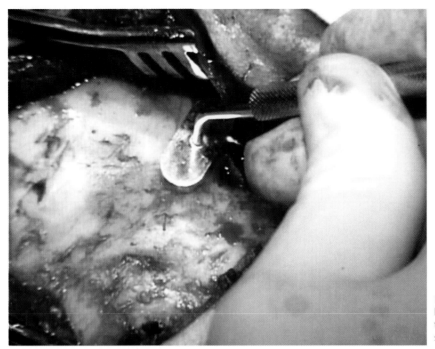

Figure 26 Once skin, muscle and periosteal flaps have been repaired, the site to approach the middle ear through a limited atticotomy is delineated using the special design template

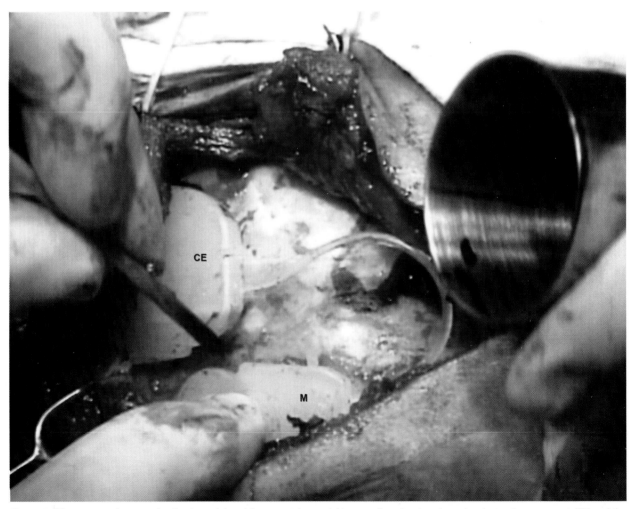

Figure 27 The next step is to use the silastic model to delineate on the cranial bone surface the site where the electronic component (CE) and the microphone (M) will be positioned

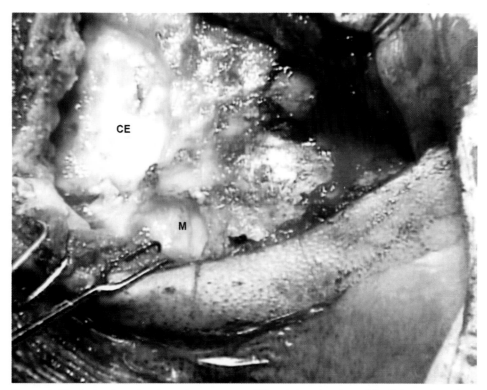

Figure 28 The beds where the electronic component (CE) and the microphone (M) will be positioned are prepared using a diamond burr

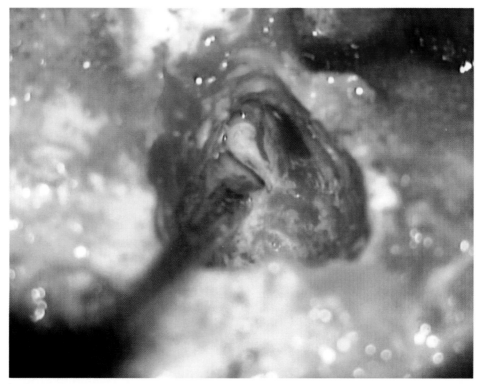

Figure 29 The middle ear is approached through a limited atticotomy until the body of the incus is visualized. Care must be taken not to damage the ossicular chain with the burr when accessing the atticus

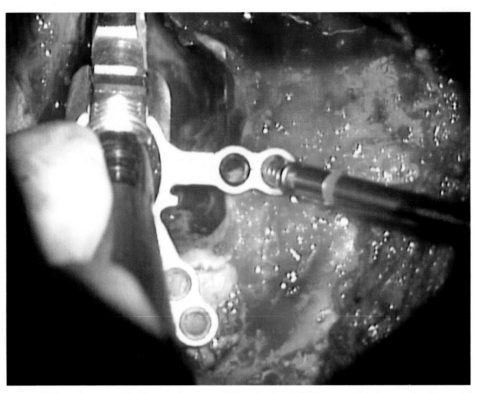

Figure 30 Next, the support for the transducer or ossicular stimulator MET is mounted and secured to the cranial bone with titanium screws. Every time a screw is placed it is important to check the right orientation of the support in relation to the ossicular chain

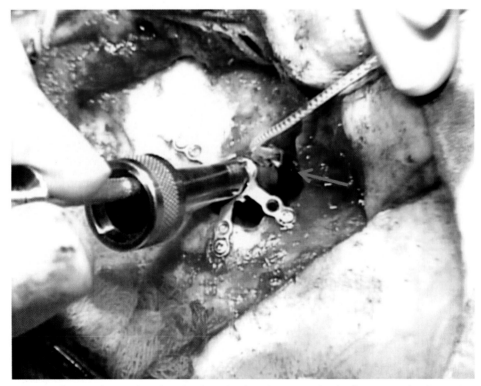

Figure 31 The ossicular stimulator (arrow) is then placed on the support that has been secured to the cranium facing the atticotomy cavity

5.4.4
Surgery of Totally Implantable Middle Ear Implant (Otologics)

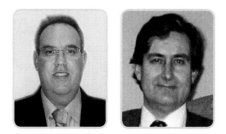

Angel Ramos Macias, Miguel Aristegui Ruiz

Carina® system (Otologics) is a fully implantable middle ear implant, using a digital multichannel acoustic signal processor and an electromagnetic stimulation (Figure 1). The system is attached to the ossicular chain supported by a support in the incus body.[1,2]

In the electromagnetic stimulation, the magnet is close to the ossicles or the inner ear (in the round window). A fluctuating magnetic field is generated when the coil is energized from a signal corresponding to an acoustic input initially collected by the microphone. This magnetic field causes vibration of the magnet, which is directly attached to the eardrum-ossicular chain and causes motion in the cochlear fluid (Figure 2).

The general indications are divided into two areas:[3-5]

1. *Sensorineural hearing loss:* Moderate to severe bilateral sensorineural hearing loss. Patient dissatisfied with hearing aids. Showing normal tympanometry and normal anatomy of the middle ear; speech understanding of 50% or better, in disyllabic words at 65 dB.

2. *Conductive or mixed hearing loss:* Secondary to radical cavities operated previously, disruption of the ossicular chain, atresia of external ear or middle ear malformations.

SURGICAL STEPS OF TOTALLY IMPLANTABLE MIDDLE EAR IMPLANT IN SENSORINEURAL HEARING LOSS
Incision

Normally it takes a retroauricular incision, about 1 cm posterior to the external ear. It is needed to make an extension upward

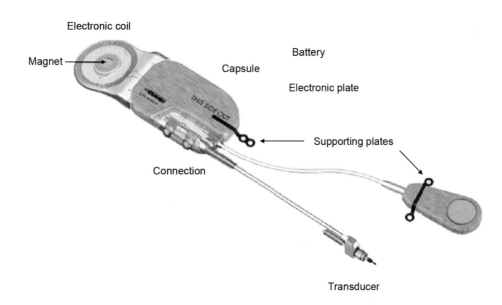

Figure 1 Schematic drawing of the totally implantable Carina® system (Otologics)

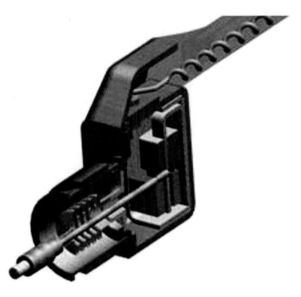

Figure 2 Electromagnetic transducer of the Otologics system

and backward at an angle of 45°, this incision should provide an adequate blood supply to skin flaps. Although there have been designed a lot of incisions, at present most surgeons use the retroauricular incision; with extension into the posterior temporal region, there is significant reduction in complications related to the incision (Figures 3A and B).

Cortical Bone

After incision we perform a flap by using a single cut through the layers that separate us from the cortical bone (skin, subcutaneous tissue, muscle and periosteum), we have direct access to the bone with a single flap, adequately expanded in order to fully expose the area of the receiver-stimulator and the area for mastoidectomy.

We dissect forward, in order to expose the spine of Henle and exposed the whole upper part of the external auditory canal (EAC). In this way, it is easy to drill further, atticotomy and especially at the time of placing the transducer correctly (positioning the transducer tip, upright microscope). At this point it is important to size position of the receiver-stimulator and microphone and make a pocket for its placement.

Atticotomy and Exposure of the Ossicular Chain

The upper limit is the temporalis line and the lower limit is at the top of the ear canal. So the atticotomy in total has about 20 mm long by 10–12 wide. Now drilling is required in order to

skeletonize the middle fossa dura and the EAC posterior wall. Occasionally, we may find the space between the dura and the EAC is too small for placement of the receiver transducer, so we are forced to drill at the level of the dura, creating an island of bone and push it up with a titanium plate fixation conveniently folded and fastened at the top of the temporal bone.

The drilling continues in order to expose the incus body. It is necessary to use a diamond burr and special care is taken not to touch or move the ossicular chain. Once you have exposed the incus body and the head of the malleous, sometimes you need to drill the area vertically above the atticotomy, about 5 mm in front of the incus body (Figures 4A and B).

Placing the Transducer Mount

Place to guide the transducer screw until the tip goes to the back of the incus body and it is placed about 2 mm. Subsequently, it is fixed with titanium screws support fins (Figures 5A and B).

Attaching the Microphone, Battery and Electronics

The goal at this time after small mastoidectomy, is to create a cavity housing the receiver-stimulator, so that it is stable, and far enough and away from the projection area or retroauricular region, to make place for the external processor behind the ear (BTE) correctly placed in this region (Figure 6).

Positioning the Transducer

The transducer is fastened with a joystick. We have to be especially careful in order to avoid falling into the cavity, because if this happens, the transducer may deteriorate. It is slowly tightening until the tip of the transducer is aligned to the incus body. At this time the thread is completely fixed so that the transducer remains stationary. With a small micromanipulator and driven by an external software that controls the advancement of the tip of the transducer, we gradually bring it to the incus body and put in contact with it. The software control is very important, because it allows the introduction of the transducer tip, but is not too tight and avoid the fixation of the chain. This system is called the "Load Wizard transducer" that provides real-time information to assist the surgeon in the placement and advancement of the transducer and provides an indication of the appropriate charge by measuring the electrical impedance of the transducer through a direct connection using a sterile adapter (Figures 7A and B).

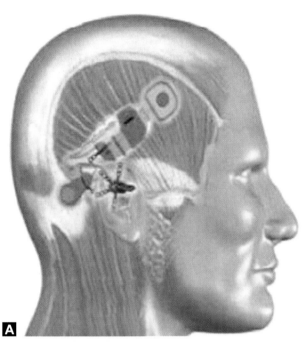
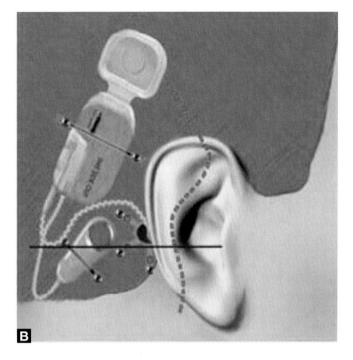

Figures 3A and B Incision in the totally implantable system

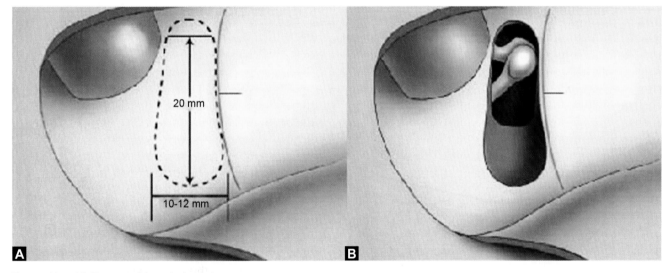

Figures 4A and B Exposure of the ossicular chain

Placement of the Receiver, Battery and Microphone

We introduce the implant into the pocket prepared above and anchored into the bone hole we had made. These were subsequently fixed with a screw to the bone. Place the microphone in the bone we had done and anchored with two screws that come prepared. The fixation of the implant in bone is important to avoid interference. The skin should not have more than

6 mm. Microphone placement in a pocket under the skin at the insertion of the sternocleidomastoid muscle is also used by many surgeons.

Suture

It is very convenient to suture in two planes. First suture the subcutaneous plane, ensuring that all the implant is covered. Be careful not to damage cables or the capsule with the suture

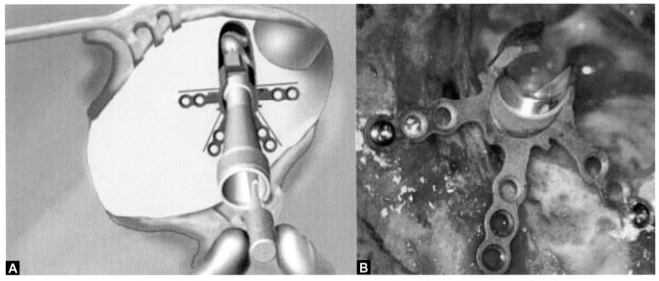

Figures 5A and B Placement of the support of the transducer

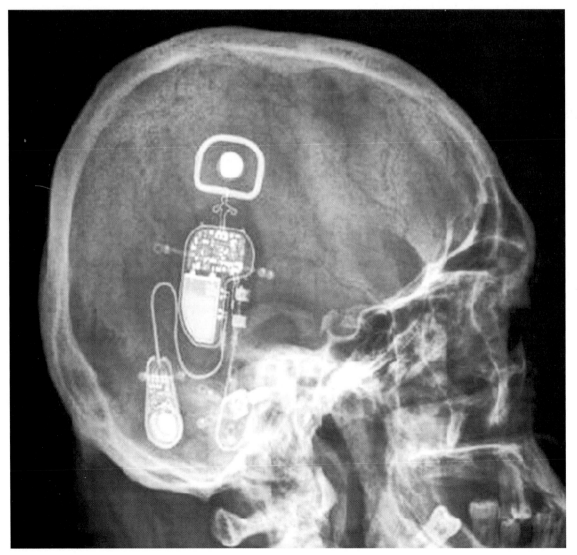

Figure 6 The totally implantable system in place

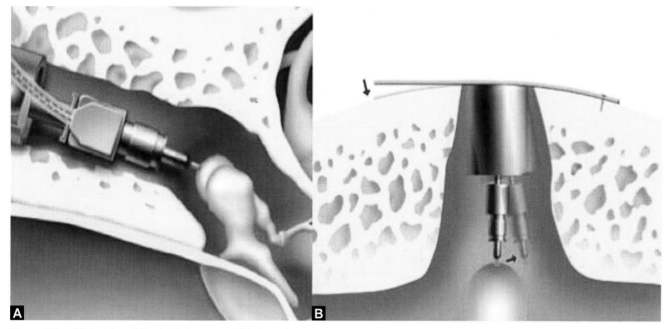

Figures 7A and B Location of the stimulating system of the transducer

needle. Once we locate the first subcutaneous plane to touch the status of the microphone, remove all the tissue that is left over it, because we have to try that there is no piece of muscle on the microphone, because when this happens the muscle contractions may produce undesirable noises to the patient.

TOTALLY IMPLANTABLE SYSTEM SURGERY IN CONDUCTIVE HEARING LOSS

Currently, the indication is given in ears with stable radical cavities and cases of atresia of external and middle ear, where the implant is connected directly.

Technical modifications have been made to adapt the system to different anatomical situations, such as adaptation of the transducer to the round window, oval window or stapes superstructure.[6,7]

In these situations, the stimulation through the round windows is the most frequently used. To fix the system, it is needed to prepare the bed of the round window so that the contact between the round window membrane is made through a middle ear prosthesis anchored to implant system for the stimulation. To complete these maneuvers, there should be placed an interface, primarily we used temporalis muscle fascia, thinning between the two surfaces and finally position the stimulation system, adapted to the anatomical situation (Figures 8 and 9).

Special Care and Complications

There are few complications that occur following surgery for the middle ear implant. The most common complications during the immediate postoperative period of surgery are those that occur at the level of the surgical wound and the flap, which in many ways are no different from skin complications in other surgical procedures. Most common are superficial infections and surgical wound seromas that resolved with local treatment, although sometimes it can lead to spread of infection to deeper tissues and are also a possible dehiscence of the wound.

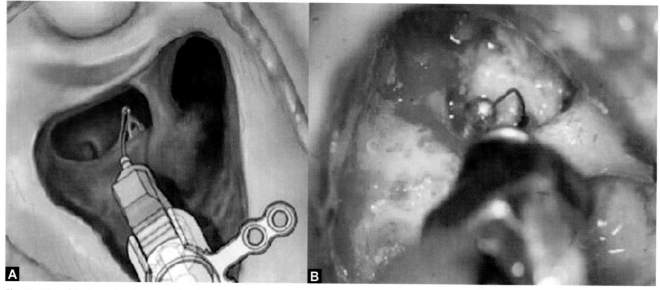

Figures 8A and B The system is anchored to the stapes

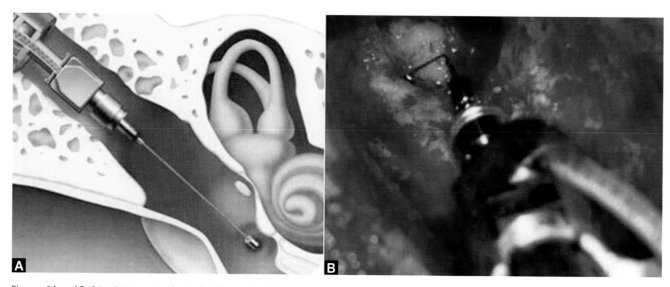

Figures 9A and B Stimulation system located in the round window

More important are flap necrosis with extrusion of the implant, which is unusual at present with the adequate incision and flap in order to maintain proper blood supply.

The risk of late implant infection is rare. It is important to use intravenous antibiotic treatment and occasionally reintervention for drainage, or removal of the contaminated device. This complication rate decreases when proceeding to close the cavity and sealing the ear, once the implant is placed.

Complications related to the facial nerve should be mentioned. For this reason, we recommend facial nerve monitoring during surgery. Even under these conditions the incidences reported by a number of communications are low and most of the time there was full recovery from paralysis after a few days.

REFERENCES

1. Kasic JF, Fredrickson JM. The Otologics MET ossicular stimulator. Otolaryngol Clin North A. 2001;34(2):501-13.
2. Fredrickson JM, Coticchia JM, Khosla S. Ongoing Investigations into an Electromagnetic Implantable Hearing Aid for Moderate to Severe Sensorineural Hearing Loss. Otolaryngol Clin N Am. 1995;28:107-20.
3. Jenkins HA, Pergola N, Kasic JF. Intraoperative ossicular loading with the Otologics Fully implantable hearing device. Oto-Laryngolgica Act. 2007;127:360-4.
4. HA Jenkins, Niparko JK, Slattery WH, et al. Otologics Middle Ear Transducer ossicular stimulator: Performance it is with varying degrees of sensorineural hearing loss. Acta Otolaryngol. 2004;124:391-4.
5. Baker RS, Wood MW, Hough JVD. The implantable hearing device for sensorineural hearing impairment: the Hough Ear Institute experience. Otolaryngol Clin N Am. 1995;28:147-53.
6. Siegert R, Mattheis S, Kasic JF. Fully Implantable Hearing Aids in Patients with Congenital Auricular Atresia. The Laryngoscope. 2007;117:1-5.
7. Tringali S, Pergola N, Ferber-Viart C, et al. Fully implantable hearing device as a new treatment of conductive hearing loss in Franceschetti syndrome. Int J of Pediatr Otorhinolaryngol. 2008;72(4):513-7. Epub 2008.

5.4.5A

General Concepts: Transcanal and Transmastoid Approach

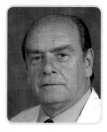

Marcos Goycoolea

The aim of the procedures discussed in this chapter is to re-establish safe continuity of the axons of the facial nerve that have been compromised by trauma or disease. This remains constant whether the procedure involves freeing, decompressing, or reanastomosing. A complete discussion of the indications for surgical exploration of facial nerve or any of its segments is outside the scope of this atlas; the comments here are intended only to contribute to a thorough understanding of specific procedures. Intratemporal facial nerve paralysis can be caused by different factors and can occur in different segments. Based on adequate preoperative assessment, the required procedure might involve a wide myringotomy, a transcanal or transmastoid approach, an exploration of the first nerve segment at the internal auditory canal, or a total facial nerve exploration.

MYRINGOTOMY

Facial paralysis may occur during an acute episode of otitis media. Performing a wide myringotomy for drainage of purulent effusion, obtaining a sample for culture, and placing a large-bore tube (along with adequate medical treatment) will suffice in the majority of cases. It is important to use a large tube. Small type I tubes tend to become plugged, requiring a second drainage procedure.

Transmastoid Approach

Surgical Steps

1. Those of a simple mastoidectomy
2. Those of a facial recess approach, if needed
3. Identifying the different segments of the facial nerve and skeletonizing the facial canal
4. Removing the bony covering
5. Opening the sheath of the nerve, if indicated.

Procedure

For practical surgical purposes, the facial nerve can be divided into three segments: (1) within the internal auditory canal and labyrinth; (2) the mastoid (vertical), and (3) the tympanic (horizontal middle ear).

The transmastoid approach provides access to the tympanic and mastoid segments of the nerve. Simple mastoidectomy and facial recess approaches have been described up to the point of clearly identifying the facial (fallopian) canal. The anatomy of the canal should now be reassessed (Figure 1A).

Mastoid segment: From the external genu, the nerve proceeds vertically to the stylomastoid foramen at the level of anterior edge of the digastric ridge (Figures 1A to C). The nerve usually is medial to the horizontal canal (a good landmark), but at times it may be lateral to it (congenitally or by inflammatory disease) or it may have a posterior projection at the genu, lending itself to potential damage. It is useful to visualize the nerve anterior to the digastric ridge, noting how lateral it becomes as it reaches the mastoid tip.

Tympanic segment: The nerve appears in the region of the cochleariform process at the geniculate ganglion, then runs posteriorly toward the oval window (not uncommonly, it is dehiscent at this point) to a point just inferior and generally medial (deeper) to the horizontal semicircular canal. Exposure of the tympanic segment is helped by enlarging the aditus ad antrum. This dissection, combined with enlargement of the facial recess approach, allows visualization anteriorly toward the cochleariform process. Drilling with a small burr is done under the incus without damaging or dislocating it; if this is not possible (which usually is the case), the incus can be removed with a joint knife (Figure 2A). If necessary, the tendon of the tensor tympani can be sectioned permitting elevation of the malleus;

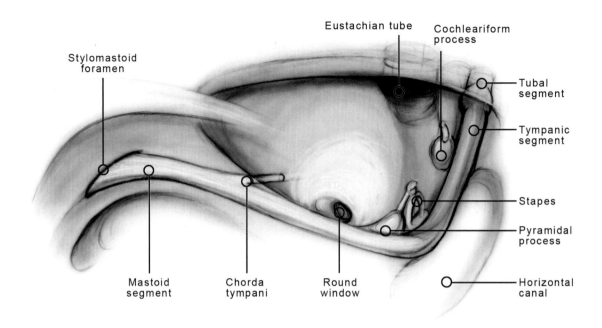

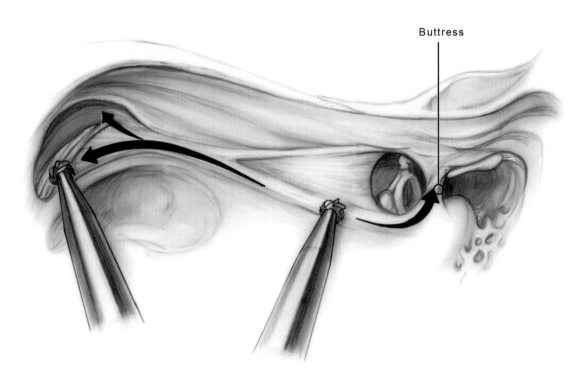

Figures 1A and B

Digastric muscle

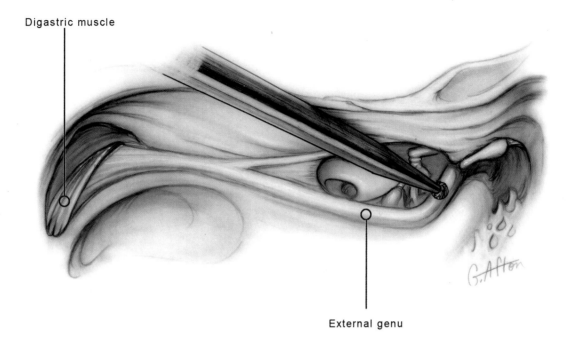

External genu

Figure 1C

Figures 1A to C Transmastoid approach. (A) Anatomy of the canal reassessed; (B and C) From the external genu, the nerve proceeds vertically to the stylomastoid foramen at the level of anterior edge of the digastric ridge

this will allow complete drilling toward the geniculate ganglion. If required for better exposure, an exploratory tympanotomy flap (previously described) can be elevated and additional transcanal exposure can be obtained. The mastoid segment can be dissected from the level of the fossa incudis or from the digastric ridge. From the ridge, it can be followed superiorly to the external genu; although this approach is perfectly acceptable, the authors tend to follow nerves peripherally rather than centrally and to start at the level of the fossa incudis. Drilling is done with parallel strokes in the direction of the nerve (superior to inferior or vice versa).

The entire facial canal should be thinned to eggshell consistency with a diamond or polishing burr. However, the facial nerve sheath should not be exposed with the burr. The thinned bone is fractured with a pick and the bone fragments are lifted gently with a Whirlybird, without using the facial nerve as a fulcrum (Figure 2B). The sheath is split open with a sharp sickle knife or a Beaver knife (Figure 2C). Special situations and handling of the nerve itself are described below. When closing, the incus is repositioned and held in place by several small pieces of Gelfoam®. Both articulations (with the stapes and the malleus) are carefully repositioned. Closure and packing are done as in a mastoid procedure. The exposed nerve

is then covered with gold foil (or a similar material) in order to avoid fibrosis and tissue ingrowth. Fascia should not be used directly over the nerve fibers.

Transcanal Approach

This approach allows access to the tympanic segment of the facial nerve and, if extended inferiorly, makes it possible to expose the mastoid segment down to the stylomastoid foramen. This can be used adequately in a sclerotic mastoid, but in a well-pneumatized mastoid it might result in a large cavity with an underlying exposed nerve. Risks of infection in these cases must be considered. This exposure can also be obtained by an endaural approach.

Procedure

A large tympanomeatal flap is created with vertical incisions at 2 and 6 o'clock, and the middle ear cavity is entered beneath the annulus. The posterior and superior walls are enlarged with burrs and curets to facilitate exposure. The incus is separated from the stapes with a joint knife. If necessary, the tendon of the tensor tympani is sectioned to allow elevation of the

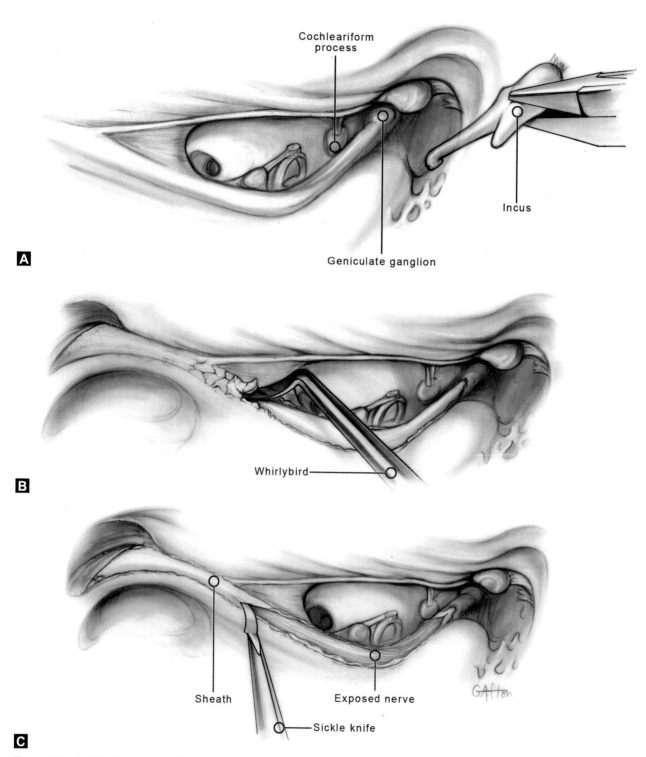

A Cochleariform process

Incus

Geniculate ganglion

B Whirlybird

C Sheath

Exposed nerve

Sickle knife

GAfton

Figures 2A to C (A) Drilling with a small burr is done under the incus or the incus removed with a joint knife; (B) Bone fragments lifted gently with a Whirlybird, without using the facial nerve as a fulcrum; (C) The sheath is split open with a sharp sickle knife or a Beaver knife

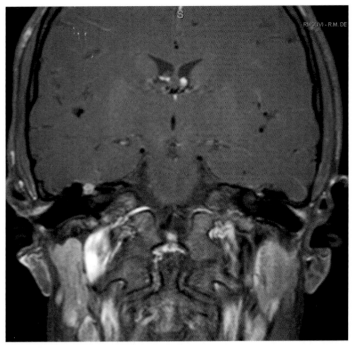

Figure 5 Right facial nerve schwannoma

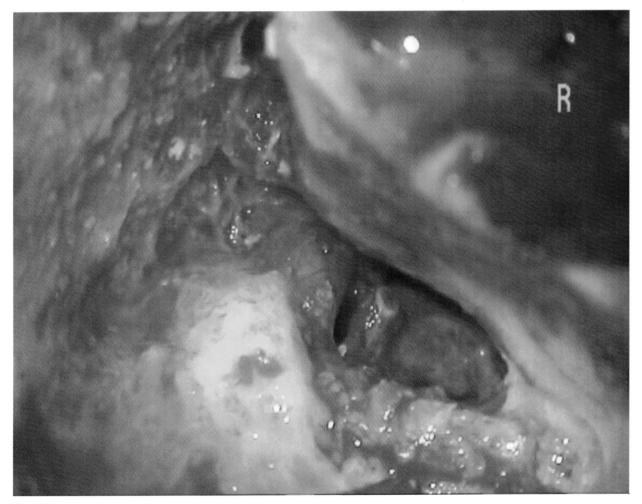

Figure 6 Intraoperative nerve schwannoma

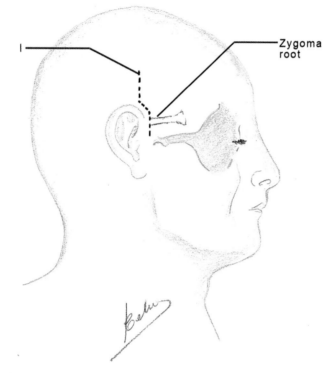

Figure 7 The Scheme: Invasive of access to middle fossa skeleton skulls

SURGICAL TECHNIQUES

1. Facial nerve decompression
   - Transmastoid/translabyrinthine
   - Middle fossa approach
2. End-to-end anastomosis of the facial nerve
3. Facial nerve grafting with sural nerve.

SURGICAL STEPS

Transmastoid/Translabyrinthine Approach

With the patient in dorsal position with lateral head rotation, a "C" postauricular incision is made 2 cm behind the postauricular crease and extended from mastoid tip to the squamous portion of temporal bone. The skin flap is dissected anteriorly to the cartilaginous external canal, and posteroinferiorly to expose the splenius capitis and sternocleidomastoid muscles. In the superior part of the incision, a large piece of temporal muscle fascia is taken to be used for closure. We make a muscular flap in "U" shape to mastoid defect closure. The lateral mastoid cortex is widely exposed.

A canal wall-up mastoidectomy is performed extending the posterior bony removal well posterior to the sigmoid venous sinus. With a large posterior tympanotomy, the descending and horizontal segments of the facial nerve are delineated. The bone decompression progresses until the stylomastoid foramen. The nerve sheath is opened all over the nerve extension from the horizontal to the descending segments until decompression of at least 180° of the nerve circumference.

For the translabyrinthine approach, a labyrinthectomy is undertaken and the internal acoustic meatus is opened. The labyrinthine and intrameatal segments of the facial nerve are also decompressed.

Middle Fossa Approach

With the middle fossa approach (MFA), the patient lies in the supine position with the head rotated to one side. The surgeon sits at the head of the bed. The skin incision is made from the edge of the zygoma root and extended superiorly for about 7 cm (Figures 7 to 9). After the temporal muscle flap is retracted (Figures 10 and 11), the craniotomy is made by opening a square bone flap of 4 x 3-cm size (Figures 12 to 15). A middle

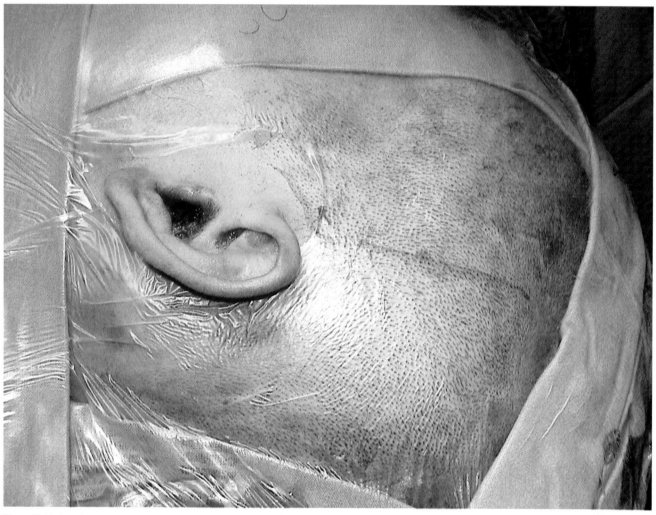

Figure 8 Marking intraoperative incision

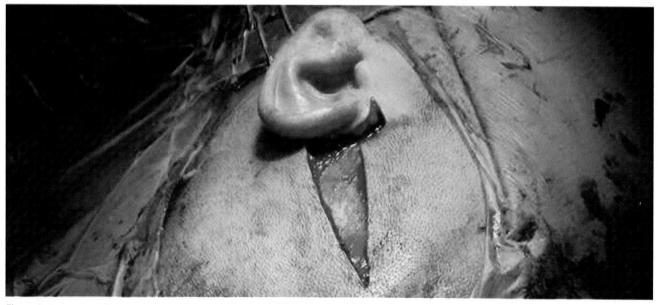

Figure 9 Fossa incision for access to media

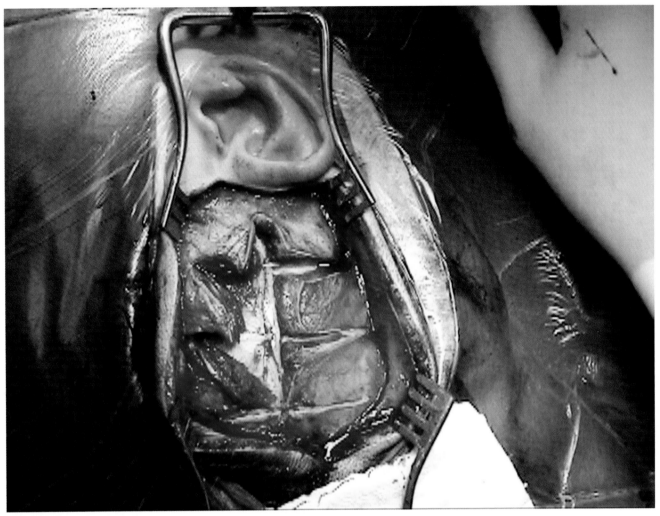

Figure 10 Longitudinal and transverse incision to remove the muscle

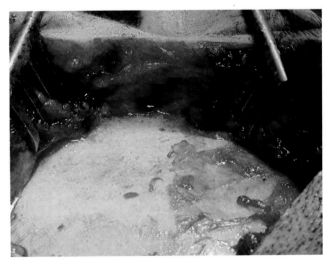

Figure 11 Exposure of cortical bone after freeing the muscle

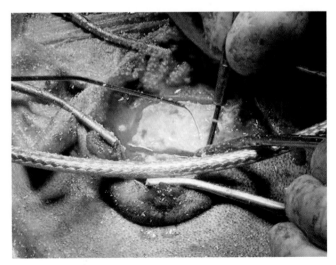

Figure 12 Top of craniotomy

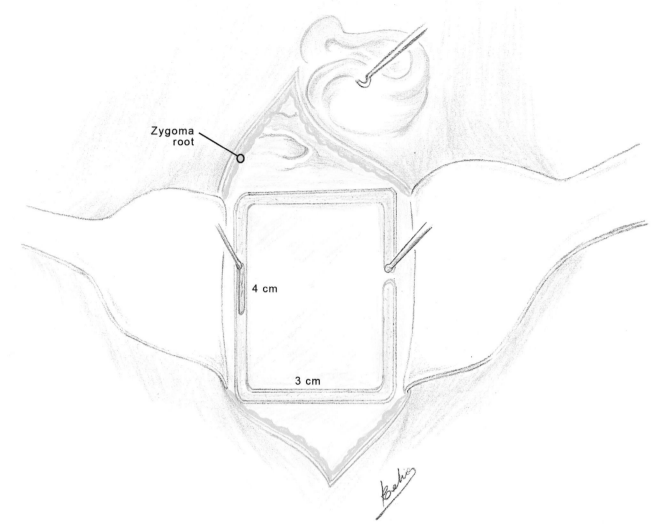

Zygoma root

4 cm

3 cm

Figure 13 Scheme of craniotomy of 4 x 3 cm

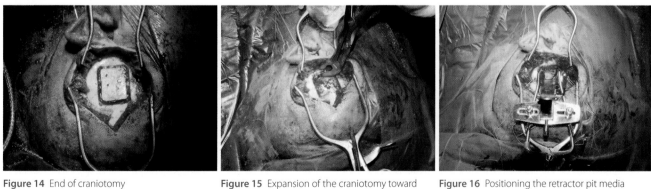

Figure 14 End of craniotomy

Figure 15 Expansion of the craniotomy toward the floor

Figure 16 Positioning the retractor pit media

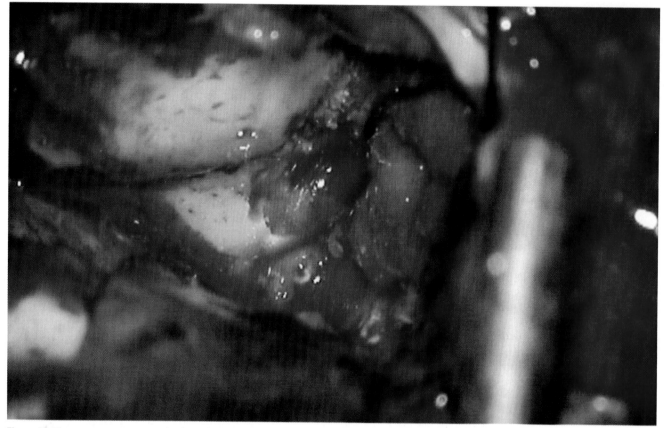

Figure 17 View arcuate eminence on the floor of the mouth

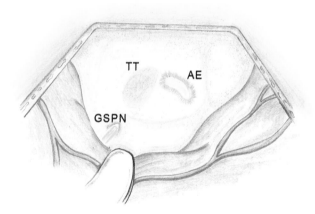

Figure 18 Outline of the floor of the middle fossa, with identification

Figure 19 Outline of the drilling of the tegmen tympani

ear retractor is positioned (Figure 16). The elevation of the dura must allow the visualization of the arcuate eminence and the superior semicircular canal (SSC), and the roof of the middle ear (Figure 17). The roof of the middle ear can be easily identified by its dark color (Figure 18). The surgeon opens a small hole with a diamond burr and identifies the cochleariform process,

and the adjacent segment of the facial nerve. The facial nerve is then followed until the geniculate ganglion is visualized (Figure 19). After the identification of the geniculated ganglion, the labyrinthine segment is easily exposed (Figure 20). In this point we begin the canal opening in proximal direction till the geniculate ganglion and labyrinthine portion of the facial nerve

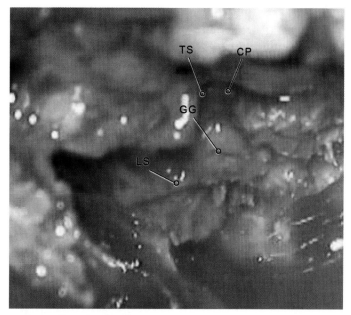

Figure 20 Geniculate ganglion

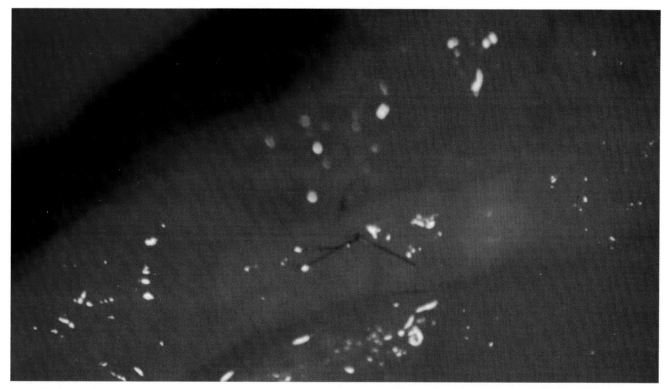

Figure 21 Epineural nerve suture

to its opening in the internal auditory meatus. The sheet of the nerve is opened and the entire portion is decompressed. The bone removed for the craniotomy is repositioned and fixed with nylon strips.

ANASTOMOSIS STABILIZATION TECHNIQUES

Epineural Suture

Traditionally, the most widely used nerve coaptation method. It is a suture of the nerve's external epineurium (Figures 21 and 22).

Advantages

- Short execution time
- Simplicity compared to the perineural suture
- Less necessity for magnification compared to the perineural suture
- The intraneural contents are not manipulated and therefore not iatrogenically hurt
- Minimum possibility of local foreign body reaction, since intraneural stitches are not done.

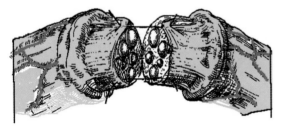

Figure 22 Scheme of epineural nerve suture

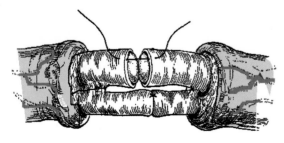

Figure 23 Scheme of fascicular nerve suture

Disadvantages

- Possibility of an incorrect fascicular alignment
- Necessity to put several stitches in order to prevent neuroma formation
- Requirement for 10-0 nylon.

Fascicular or Perineural Suture

The nerve fascicles are sutured (Figure 23). One should know the fascicular topography. This technique is more indicated in repairs of partial transections or in sites where the nerve has a good fascicular differentiation.

Advantages

Good fascicular coaptation, although it can be difficult to decide which distal fascicle corresponds to which proximal one.

Disadvantages

- Longer surgery time
- Greater technical difficulty
- Greater possibility of foreign body reaction and intraneural fibrosis because of intraneural manipulation
- Greater possibility of iatrogenic trauma
- Necessity for greater training in microsurgery technique.

Tubulization

A technique consisting of embracing the stumps with material to provide stabilization without the necessity of suture (Figure 24). Synthetic materials such as silicone tubes can be used, but are relatively contraindicated; otherwise homologous tissues or collagen can be used with biologic or synthetic glue.

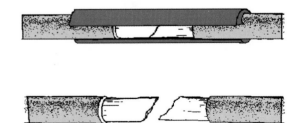

Figure 24 Tunneling scheme nerve

Advantages

- Short surgical time
- Technical facility
- Least possibility of intraneural foreign body reaction.

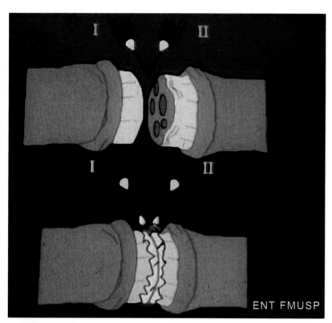

Figure 25 Schematic single fibrin anastomosis

Disadvantages

- Problems for stabilization of the anastomosis since there is no direct fixation
- Possibility of local foreign body reaction when homologous material is not used
- Problems for fascicular alignment.

Glueing with Fibrin Tissue Adhesive

The technique consists of approximating the stumps and stabilizing them with fibrin glue (Figures 25 and 26).

Advantages

- Least surgical time
- Greater technical facility
- Absence of local foreign body reaction
- Least iatrogenic trauma to the nerve.

Disadvantages

- Some difficulty for fascicular alignment.

When comparing the advantages and disadvantages of each method, we should bear in mind that the intratemporal facial

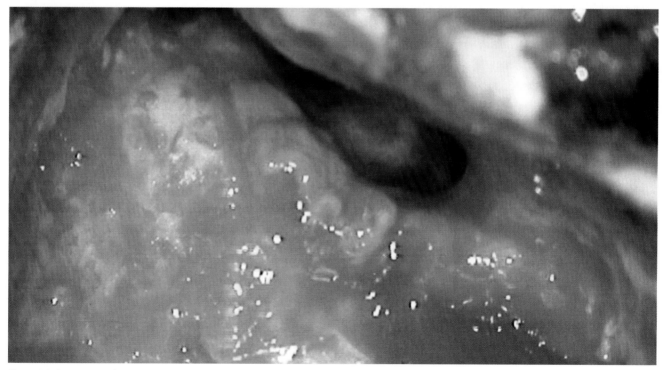

Figure 26 Appearance of intraoperative anastomosis queue

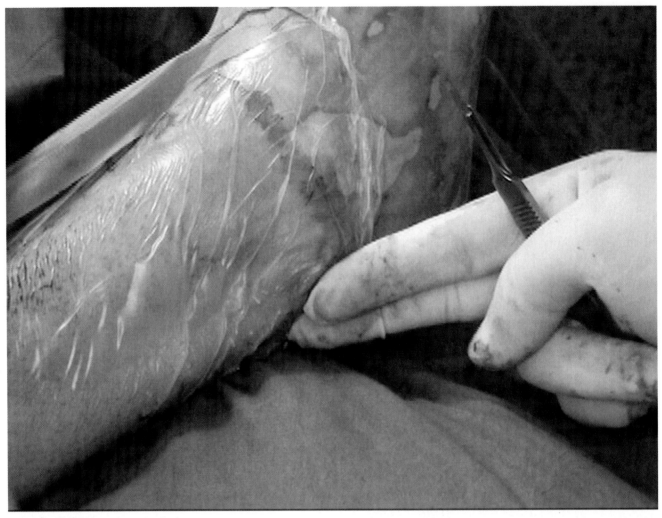

Figure 27 Identification of lateral malleolus-repair point

nerve does not have a very precise fascicular differentiation, especially the most proximal segment and that suturing in this location is technically very difficult due to the space limitations, the presence of important structures in the neighborhood, and in some cases the presence of cerebrospinal fluid. Based on our experience with the intratemporal facial nerve, we have developed the following order of preference for anastomosis in this location.

Facial nerve grafting with sural nerve

For grafts we prefer the sural nerve (Figures 27 to 32). The incision is made 2 cm above the lateral malleolus and extends superiorly 10 cm. The nerve is isolated from the parva saphena vein and incised according to the necessary extension of the graft. The anastomosis with the remaining facial nerve is made with fibrin glue.

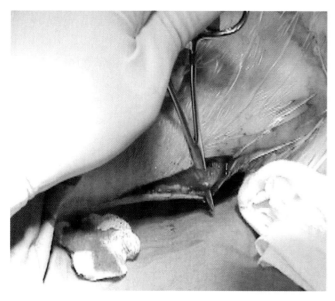

Figure 28 Neurovasculature identification

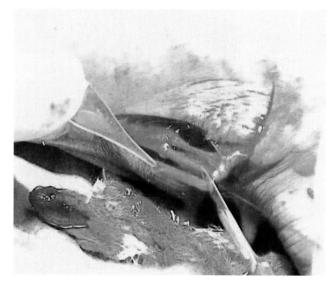

Figure 29 Identification of sural nerve and removal of graft

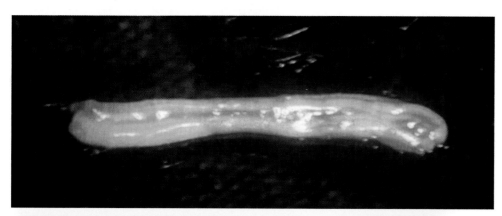

Figure 30 Sural nerve removed

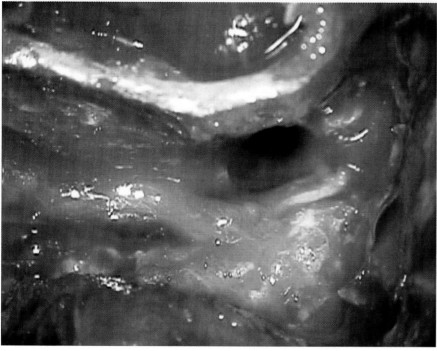

Figure 31 Sural nerve graft positioned with fibrin glue

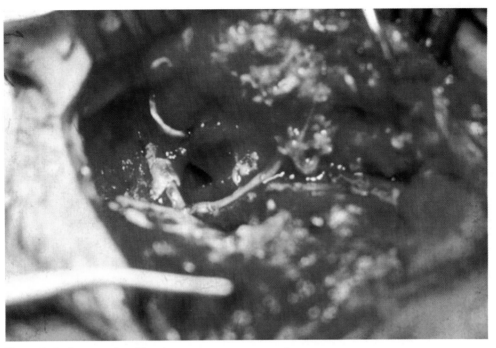

Figure 32 Sural nerve graft positioned

Potential Complications and How to Avoid Them

- *Iatrogenic injuries to the facial nerve:* An experience in ear surgery, careful dissection of the nerve and monitor use of the facial nerve.
- *Cerebrospinal fluid leaks in translabyrinthine approach with opening the internal auditory canal:* Filling with fat, temporal fascia and fibrin glue.

- *Epidural hematoma in the middle fossa approach:* Use of mannitol intraoperatively to facilitate retraction of the brain parenchyma.
- *Synkinesis:* Avoid electrical therapies.

POSTOPERATIVE MANAGEMENT

- Physiotherapy with facial exercises. Avoid electrical stimulation (galvanotherapy)
- Eyes care: lubrication
- Pertinent histopathology.

S